HEAVEN AND EARTH QIGONG

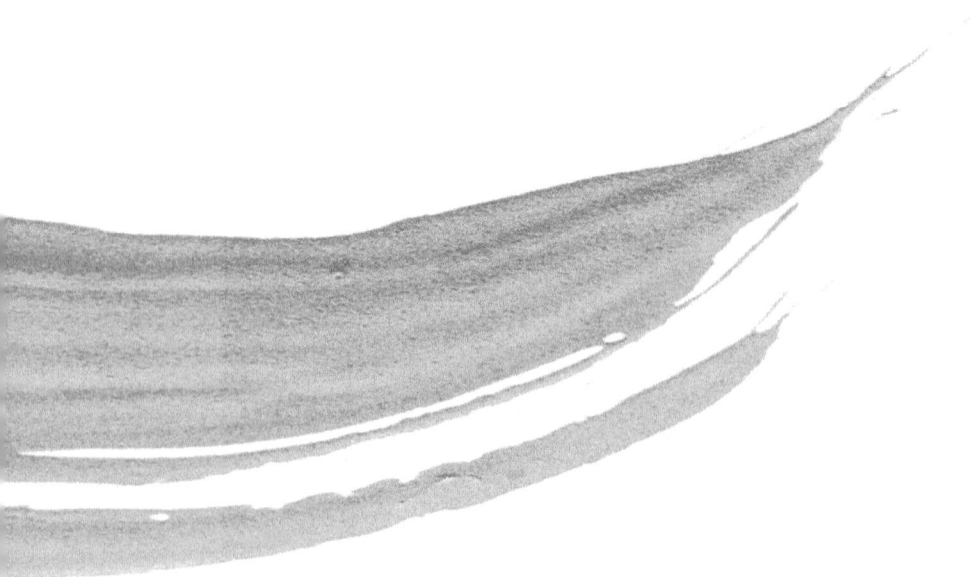

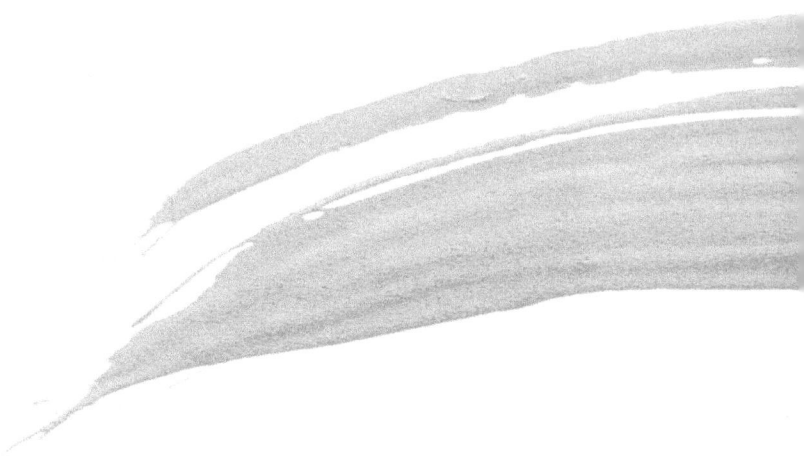

HEAVEN AND EARTH QIGONG

Heal Your Body and Awaken Your Qi

Bruce Frantzis and Paul Cavel

Energy Arts

Published by Energy Arts, Inc., P.O. Box 99, Fairfax, CA 94978, USA

The following trademarks are used under license by Energy Arts, Inc., from Bruce Frantzis: Frantzis Energy Arts™ system, Mastery Without Mystery®, Longevity Breathing® program, Opening the Energy Gates of Your Body™ Qigong, Marriage of Heaven and Earth™ Qigong, Bend the Bow™ Spinal Qigong, Spiraling Energy Body™ Qigong and Gods Playing in the Clouds™ Qigong.

Editing: H.L. Cavel
Cover design: Sarah Lim-Murray, Sarah Lim ART
Cover artwork: © Atichat/Adobe Stock
Interior design: Lisa Carta, Lisa Carta Design
Illustrations: Sophie Manham, London UK
Back cover photo of Bruce Frantzis: Richard Marks
Back cover photo of Paul Cavel: Ralph Heber

ISBN: 978-0-9982163-2-4
Printed in the United States of America

PLEASE NOTE: The practice of Taoist meditative and energy arts may carry risks. The information in this book is not in any way intended as a substitute for medical, mental or emotional counseling with a licensed physician or healthcare provider. The reader should consult a professional before undertaking any martial arts, movement, meditative arts, health or exercise program to reduce the chance of injury or any other harm that may result from pursuing or trying any technique discussed in this book. Any physical or other distress experienced during or after any exercise should not be ignored and should be brought to the attention of a healthcare professional. The creators and publishers of this book disclaim any liabilities for loss in connection with following any of the practices described in this book, and implementation is at the discretion, decision and risk of the reader.

DEDICATION

This book was made possible by Taoist Lineage Holder Liu Hung Chieh (1905-1986), who passed down the complete teachings of the Taoist Water tradition to Bruce Frantzis in the 1980s. It is Master Frantzis' wish that his senior students carry on the teachings for the benefit of future generations.

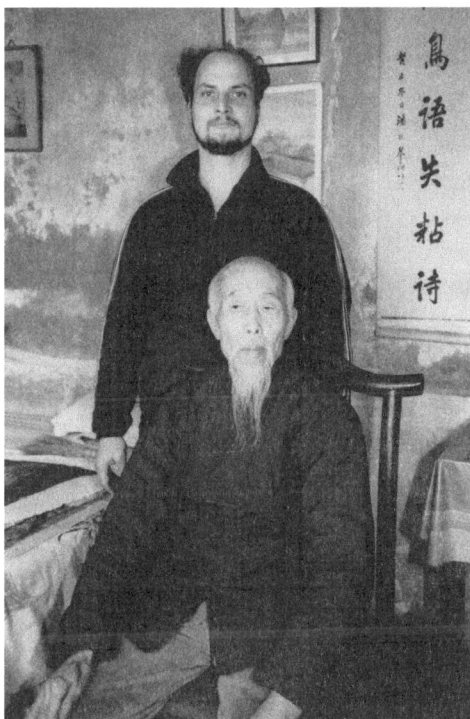

Taoist Lineage Holder Liu Hung Chieh with his disciple
Bruce Frantzis, Beijing, China, 1986

CONTENTS

ACKNOWLEDGMENTS

In addition to Taoist Lineage Holder Liu Hung Chieh, Master Frantzis would like to acknowledge two of his principal teachers who were instrumental in advancing his neigong studies: Huang Hsi I of Taiwan and Bai Hua, a fellow student of his teacher Liu.

Many people were a part of the creation of this text. My teacher Bruce and I would personally like to thank:

Heather Cavel for editing and project management. This book would still be in its infancy without her contributions, and would lack the cohesion and clarity essential to teaching neigong through the written word. Her skill is abundant and her tenacity is unsurpassed.

Mountain Livingston of Energy Arts, Inc. for project management and his unwavering support in bringing this project to fruition.

The invaluable readers: Energy Arts Senior Instructor Craig Barnes of New York for early comments, which particularly helped to develop the instruction sets; Caroline Frantzis for copyediting, ePub formatting assistance and helping to improve upon the overall presentation; Katy Rourke Wilson of Energy Arts, Inc. for proofreading; Energy Arts Senior Instructor Eric L. Peters of Massachusetts for providing feedback on the introductory chapters; and Energy Arts Instructor Dr. Alan Peatfield of Ireland for fact checking the Preface.

Lisa Carta of Lisa Carta Design for interior design and production, and especially for her persistent attention to detail in bringing together the many elements of this text for a seamless presentation.

Artist Sophie Manham of London for drawing more than 100 figures of models in Heaven and Earth postures, as well as most of the drawings throughout this text—a massive undertaking that is an integral aspect of conveying complex internal concepts in a clear and concise manner.

The talented Sarah Lim-Murray of Sarah Lim ART (www.sarahlimart.co.uk) for designing the cover artwork and modeling for the drawings.

Photographers: Sam Sapin for the photos in the pulsing section, Richard Marks for the meditation photo and headshot on the back cover of Master Frantzis; Ralph Heber of the Tai Chi Schule in Ulm for the back cover photo of Paul Cavel; Ian Shepherd (www.hawaiiphotography.net) for the photo of Craig Barnes; and Dan Winter, teacher at Toward Harmony Tai Chi and Qigong in Massachusetts, for the photo of Bill Ryan.

Energy Arts Instructor Jason Roberts of Sussex, England for being kind enough to take photos and demonstrate neigong techniques for photos amidst hectic days of training; and, most of all, for his invaluable teaching and supporting role in my courses, which enables me to focus on projects like this one.

Energy Arts Senior Instructor Jackie Smith of Scotland, my good friend, for his personal support and keeping my head straight.

Last, but certainly not least, I could not neglect to express my deepest gratitude for my teacher Bruce's many personal sacrifices sharing the Water tradition and teaching me the depths of Taoist neigong.

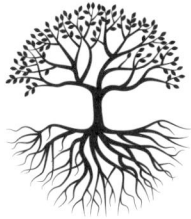

PREFACE

BY PAUL CAVEL

A Leaf in the Wind

The people of ancient China developed and, primarily through bloodlines, passed down health, healing and martial arts practices as a matter of their survival. The integrity of any lineage or tradition is a fragile matter though. If key individuals pass away before producing an heir or sharing their body of knowledge, the line is broken or downgraded. Throughout the ages, some lineages thrived and a few developed higher-level practices to do with spiritual pursuits, delving into realms that gave deeper meaning to life. Many more lineages went extinct. For example, during the Cultural Revolution when food was scarce, many Taoists and martial artists simply could not consume the raw energy required to study more rigorous techniques and achieve more advanced stages of practice. The emperor, and later the Communist Party, targeted lineages that threatened their power, a legacy which unfortunately continues on in Tibet as this text goes to print. These power structures and belief systems have contributed to the demise and dramatically reduced the number of surviving authentic lineages today.

Of course examples of the extermination of lineages can be observed all around the globe, on both small and large scales, and sometimes not even with the intent to do so. In Feudal Japan, swordsman Miyamoto Musashi single-handedly took out the Yoshioka lineage by prevailing in three matches against the brothers of that famous clan. In Medieval Europe, the Catholic Church embarked upon a rampage to rid the planet of "heathens," almost completely annihilating Gnosticism and paganism. We are left with only fragments of their very sophisticated and once well-documented teachings.

Perhaps the fiercest threat of all now looms at our doorstep—the instant-gratification, push-button, big-data age spurred on by market capitalism. Many people do not even consider that they are losing pieces of their humanity through ever-growing expectations and by chasing after material objects. Many ancient teachings, including Taoist ones from China, cautioned people against unabated expectations.

In the 13th century in Western Europe, the Cathars had great influence over the society in which they lived. Living frugally and following a spiritual path was held in high esteem, while being overly concerned with material objects, including money—especially loaning money for profit—was frowned upon. Eight-hundred years later we have the direct opposite scenario with banking at the top of the hierarchy, dictating world affairs, while following a true spiritual path is fodder for big-budget films, primarily regarded as intangible or irrelevant to modern living.

Lao Tzu's Water Tradition

The most well-known Taoist text is the *Tao Te Ching* (also transliterated as *Daodejing*) authored by the Sage Lao Tzu (also known as Laozi) twenty-five hundred years ago, which is among the most translated books in the world. Its wide distribution validates assertions that the teachings are as relevant today as they were in ancient times. What is not widely known, however, is that Lao Tzu was an adept of the Water tradition, Old Taoism, and he was encapsulating deeply developed Taoist concepts previously only shared by oral tradition in that terse, instructive manuscript.

Taoist philosophy is quite unique in its approach to life in that it does not impose arbitrary rules or codes of conduct that can be limiting to some individuals or negate other religious belief systems. Instead, the purpose of the teachings is to guide practitioners through a process of looking inside themselves and discovering their personal truths. Finding your path in life is a way of discovering your essence, according to Taoist philosophy. Rather than telling you how to live your life, the Water method leads you into yourself. Since you are here on this planet in physical form, Taoists reason that all practices should start with the physical body and beginning methods are, therefore, extremely pragmatic. You first seek to clear out your stagnancies, then progressively move through healing old injuries, strengthening your body and life-force energy, balancing your emotions and calming your mind. From a Taoist perspective, physical-qi practice is precisely what enables a spiritual path to become a reality since most people would not otherwise have the strength, stamina and focus required for the journey.

There is no expectation for any practitioner to go beyond the mundane levels of qi practice, which is basically to do with keeping the body and mind healthy, and is within the realms of qigong and foundational meditation practices. It is considered a personal matter whether any individual chooses to continue on to deeper neigong and genuine Taoist meditation to cultivate their body, mind and spirit. Indeed, many students find that qigong practice relieves their aches and pains, gives them more energy, smoothes out their emotions and helps them to think more clearly. Just this level of practice alone goes a long way toward creating satisfaction and contentment in their lives.

For others, becoming healthy and creating stability in their lives are merely stepping stones, the necessary prerequisites for delving deeper into their being, discovering what is there and systematically beginning to release everything that holds them back from reaching their human potential. For these Water method practitioners, they simply adjust and refocus the practices they have already embodied, allowing them to seamlessly transition into deeper studies.

The Time for Secrets Has Passed

Many schools and lineages have pieces of the Taoist neigong system, on which the Water tradition is based, but it is extremely rare to find the entire 16 neigong present within a single lineage—both inside and outside of China. Over the millennia, especially since the more superficial, New-Age, fusion-style approach to health and spirituality has blossomed, aspects of the neigong system have been passed on and mixed in with pieces of other systems that may or may not integrate well with one another. All of the information presented in this book comes from Lao Tzu's Taoist Water tradition as passed down by lineage holders, grandmasters to masters, for four millennia, since the time of the Yellow Emperor, Huangdi—completely intact and in the purest form possible.

Even after thorough investigation by many scholars, Bruce Kumar Frantzis is the only known lineage master publicly teaching the Taoist Water tradition in the West today. Frantzis, who was a disciple of the late Grandmaster Liu Hung Chieh of China (1905-1986), was officially recognized as a master by his teacher in the 1980s. In previous publications Frantzis shied away from using the title of "master" and has actually discouraged his students from addressing him as such. The reason is due to the advice he received from Grandmaster Liu when he received his endowments. "Even though you have the skill, insight, understanding and perception of a master, in China it is customary to be accepted as a true master only at age 70." Frantzis turned 70 this past spring and now accepts his rightful title of master in this and all following publications. This was not the only advice given to him by his late teacher. Liu also encouraged him to to openly share the once closely guarded inner tradition, declaring, "The time for secrets has passed." For this reason, Master Frantzis openly teaches the authentic internal technology of the Taoist arts in-depth. He offers the opportunity to study the inner teachings without the restrictions to which practitioners throughout ages have been bound and which many schools or teachers in the East and the West do not offer to the masses. This fact, along with his ability and willingness to directly transmit, mind to mind, the critical qi techniques to his students, enables them to experience deeper levels of practice and states of consciousness.

This does not mean that his students do not have to devote considerable time and energy to reaching more advanced stages of training, that other schools are not based on internal neigong technology or that teachers outside of his school do not teach genuine spiritual traditions. However, for one tradition to contain the *entirety* of the health, healing, martial and spiritual aspects of the fully integrated 16 Taoist neigong system is increasingly rare.

A Form of Indra's Necklace

In the 3rd century AD, the Mahayana Buddhists popularized the concept of Indra's necklace. Composed of many threads, with each one containing many jewels and each jewel offering a reflection of all others, the necklace represents the interconnectedness of all things in the universe. The clasp represents the integration point at which all threads link together and become unified into one whole.

The neigong system is itself an Indra's necklace with each of the 16 components containing many pearls of wisdom that shed light on and help to develop the deeper aspects of an individual's body, mind and qi. The Marriage of Heaven and Earth Qigong is a microcosm of the metaphor. This 3,000-year-old self-healing practice has never been put into print and shared publicly, with its deeper aspects of neigong traditionally being reserved only for disciples. Its many threads of neigong are activated and integrated in a way that gives practitioners a taste of what is possible from ongoing study of Taoist arts—without the complex choreography associated with other qigong sets. Heaven and Earth Qigong bridges the beginning to advanced levels of neigong, yielding much more than a powerful form of exercise for health, healing and relaxation. It is a journey into the systems, substructures and layers of your body, energy and mind. Practice is an exploration of what you are made of and the potential you hold deep inside yourself—that which most human beings never put in the effort to discover.

From a much broader view, practice of ancient arts—such as those within the Taoist Water tradition, which have a rich history and a living representative with whom to study the inner teachings—serves as an antidote to the trends toward materialism and the obliteration of ancient knowledge. Through practice of Heaven and Earth Qigong, you not only help to keep the Water tradition alive for future generations, but honor the many personal sacrifices that have been made by some very wise and generous folks over millennia to help us realize who we really are.

—Paul Cavel, Andalusia, Spain (January 2019)

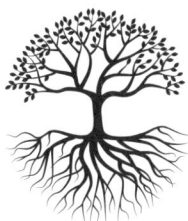

INTRODUCTION

The purpose of learning Taoist qigong is not necessarily to move your body better, but rather to move and balance your qi according to the principles of Chinese medicine. In this sense, the primary function of qigong practice is to exercise your body and mind in ways that allow you to relax and build your qi for health, physical healing, overall wellbeing and possibly spiritual pursuits—if you so choose.

HEAVEN AND EARTH QIGONG

The terms qigong (also chi gung) and neigong (also nei gung) are often used interchangeably; however, *qigong* is a blanket term that generally means "energy exercise"; whereas *neigong* refers to the original 16 broad-ranging and in-depth internal techniques of the qi cultivation arts (itemized in Appendix A) with each taking many years of dedicated study to fully embody.

At the most fundamental level, the Marriage of Heaven and Earth is a Taoist neigong system based on circular movement, both physically and energetically.

WOOD ELEMENT NEIGONG

According to Taoism (also Daoism), the Five Elements—Water, Fire, Wood, Metal and Earth—are the five energies which comprise the energy matrix of the material universe. That is to say, the Five Elements give rise to the realm of manifestation and serve as templates for understanding reality as we experience it. In Chinese medicine, each of the five dynamic energies are associated with and govern the internal organs of the human body, which are themselves associated with and govern specific body systems, emotions and personality traits. In this model, the vital organs support positive attributes and emotions when they are healthy and balanced, and unbalanced attributes and negative emotions when compromised.

Heaven and Earth Qigong is categorized as a Wood Element practice. In China it is quite common to find many different forms called the same or very similar names because it is the underlying methodology that provides the basis for the name—not a set of movements *per se*. However, the opposite is also true: just because you practice a specific set of movements, it does not mean you necessarily embody the energies of that level of practice.

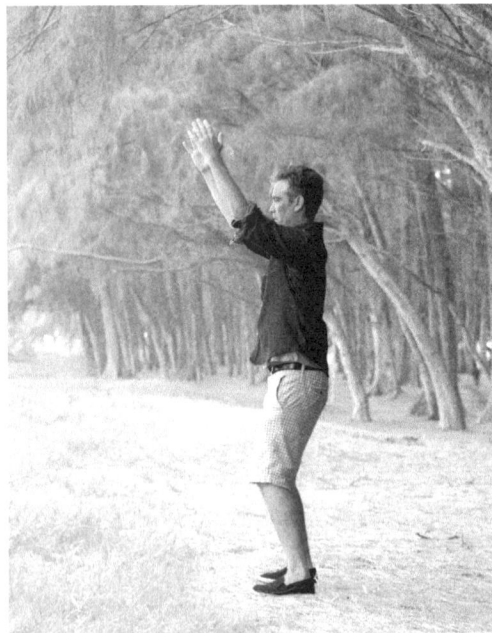

PHOTO BY IAN SHEPHERD

Craig Barnes, Senior Student of Master Frantzis,
connecting to the energy of Heaven

In the case of the Wood Element's methodology, there are many qigong forms with names that point to the joining or marrying of Heaven and Earth energies since, when the seed of a tree is planted, the roots grow downward, deep into the earth, while the branches reach upward, high into the sky. In so doing, the tree connects and joins the energies of Heaven and Earth and serves as the living representation of the directive of all Taoist Wood Element qigong, where Heaven and Earth energies become balanced and unified into one whole inside the practitioner's body.

THE MACROCOSMIC AND MICROCOSMIC ORBITS OF ENERGY

The first of the two-part Heaven and Earth exercise is meant to activate the macrocosmic orbit of energy, as will be discussed in-depth in Section Four. Ultimately, the aim is for an adept practitioner to:

1. Extend their qi deep into the ground.
2. Bring it up, through their body and into the sky.
3. Bring it back down, through their body and into the ground once again.

During the macrocosmic orbit, as the practitioner cultivates their sensitivity to qi, they can gain the ability to link with the energies of Earth and Heaven, and then circulate those energies throughout their entire body.

The second part circulates qi through the microcosmic orbit—the torso, neck and head (also covered in Section Four)—whatever energies the practitioner has contacted and mobilized. The few seconds of letting go to neutral at the end allows them to absorb the circulated energies. Over many repetitions they hook into, run through their body, and bank the abundance of natural energy available in the Earth and heavens. This generates a resonance that attunes the individual to the natural world in which they live.

Even though this is the aim of Wood Element practice, Taoist philosophy dictates that first you must focus on your physical body or else you can too easily become disconnected, space out and simply visualize or fantasize about what could be happening, rather than actually and tangibly achieving the goals of training. For this reason, all the instructions in this book cover the first level of Heaven and Earth Qigong training and remain within the physical body. Once a practitioner embodies what is presented in this volume, they will be ready for the next level of practice: that is to direct their qi outside of their physical body, yet remain anchored and grounded within it. By slowly increasing the depth and range of motion of your qi—that is how far you can extend and project your qi into the earth below and sky above, and how deeply you can penetrate your body toward its core—you can progressively and systematically grow and develop your health, vitality and mind.

INTEGRATING LAYERS OF NEIGONG

With most qigong systems, the aim is to develop an aspect, layer or neigong thread in one move and then focus on different and/or deeper content in the next move. In this way, the qi generated in the preceding move is passed up to the next (if and only if executed correctly). Many internal exercises are designed to amplify qi circulation through a series of coordinated movements that together form a set. Most of the other qigong sets in the Energy Arts System (all except Bend the Bow), tai chi (also taiji) and bagua intrinsically operate in this way to generate qi and cultivate resiliency and vitality—albeit with caveats specific to their unique composition and primary *modus operandi*.

Heaven and Earth Qigong is different.

With only one continuous motion, the emphasis is on building layer upon layer of internal qi content through many repetitions instead of varying movement sequences. As you develop depth, content and quality of motion at each stage, energy cultivation naturally follows.

Energetically Efficient

The secret behind exponential energy growth lies in Heaven and Earth's specialized technology, which is designed to engage everything in the human body and its energy, from the skin to the internal organs, and the etheric field to the central channel—including all the layers in between.

The *etheric field* is the layer of energy that exists directly outside the physical body and is sometimes referred to as the "aura" (see Figure A-1). Starting from the skin and projecting outward in all directions, the etheric field can be very shallow (e.g. several inches from the surface of the skin) in an unhealthy person to several feet from the surface of the skin in a vibrant individual. The size, density and quality of the etheric energy is strongly correlated with immune function as the etheric field is connected to and born out of wei qi.

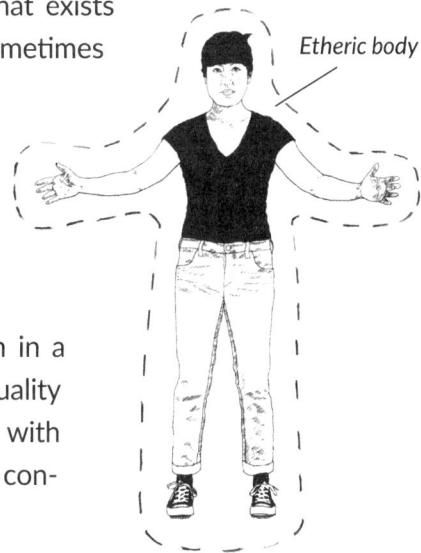

Etheric body

Figure A-1

Wei qi is the layer of energy between the skin and the muscles, which flows at the level of the fascia and protects the body from disease and the external environment.

Fascia is primarily composed of a structural protein (collagen), which runs head-to-toe, inside-to-out and forms an all-encompassing and interwoven system of fibrous connective tissue throughout the body. It supports and protects individual muscles, internal organs and the entire body as a unit.

In terms of the learning progression, Heaven and Earth is the first Water tradition neigong system to work at this depth, developing the bulk of physical content found in tai chi, hsing-i and bagua, as well as developing the foundational material necessary for advanced qigong systems, such as Bend the Bow Spinal Qigong and Gods Playing in the Clouds Qigong.

Take a look at Heaven and Earth's wide range of internal-energetic layers—with each containing incredible potential depth:

- Biomechanical alignments
- Bending and stretching the body
- Taoist breathing
- Twisting the soft tissues
- Opening-and-closing techniques (a.k.a. "pulsing")
- Activating the spinal column as one integrated whole
- Lengthening (yin-yang energy flows)
- Wrapping the soft tissues (collateral qi flows)
- Feeling, moving and transforming internal energies
- Techniques for working with the etheric field
- Activating the macrocosmic and microcosmic orbits of energy
- Outer Dissolving
- Techniques for working with the left and right channels of energy
- Techniques for working with the central channel of energy
- Techniques for working with the internal organs
- Techniques for working with the lower tantien

The real effort is in developing your ability to integrate all of the above exceptionally well. When you do, you can practice Heaven and Earth to support healing, increase physical or mental performance, develop martial power and more.

THE FIVE PRIMARY QI FLOWS

For new students, learning Heaven and Earth will help you begin to use many letters of the neigong alphabet. However, whether you are building your form for the first time or you are a long-term practitioner, you will systematically and progressively deconstruct and weave into your form

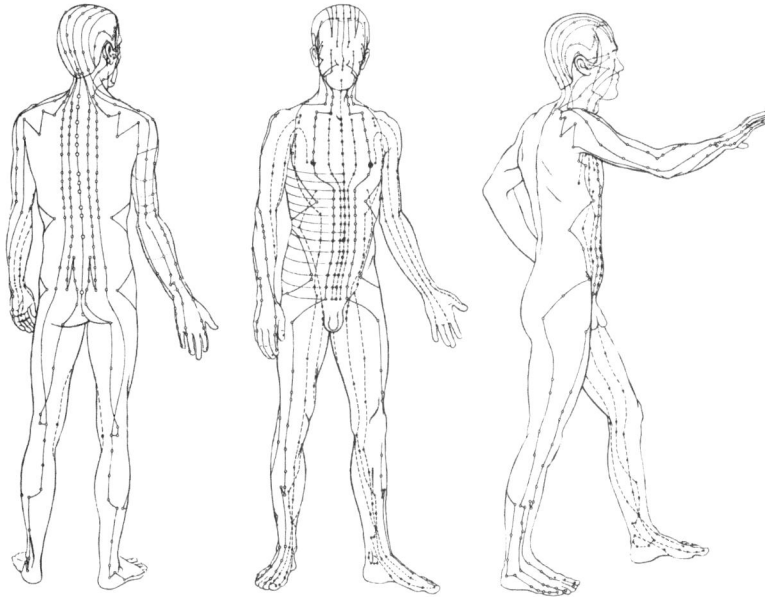

Figure A-2:
Acupuncture Meridians

*Wei qi flows through the ascending, descending and collateral meridians
located at the level of the fascia*

the five primary qi flows. This is the process that allows you to fine-tune and upgrade your practice.

The five primary qi flows, which will be covered in-depth throughout this text, are:

- Opening and closing the skeletal frame.
- Activating and developing the ascending and descending qi flows (acupuncture meridians). See Figure A-2.
- Activating and developing the body's collateral qi flows.
- Cleansing the tissues inside the brain.
- Joining the above qi flows to generate and boost the great and small heavenly orbits of energy, more commonly known as the macrocosmic and microcosmic orbits.

FOUR ESSENTIAL COMPONENT PRACTICES

Four component practices will allow you to develop skill working with the five primary qi flows. Progressive, step-by-step instructions are provided in the chapters that follow to teach you how to:

- Shift your weight along the centerline of each foot, which encourages qi to move up and down your body through the ascending and descending energy channels, as well as your spine.

- Bow and straighten your spine to open up the back (posterior) and front (anterior) aspects of your vertebrae, an exceptionally important exercise that is almost non-existent in other exercise systems.

- Lengthen your body's fascia in order to gain access to, release and stretch your muscles, nerves, ligaments and blood vessels.

- Energetically penetrate your legs from your spine, through your tailbone and down to your feet.

These essential foundational practices will help you differentiate between physical and energetic exercise, then fuse them within the two-part Heaven and Earth form. With these, your Heaven and Earth practice will become a physical framework through which qi circulates throughout your body with minimal resistance.

WHY LEARN HEAVEN AND EARTH QIGONG?

The Wood Element governs the liver and the liver enables the power to get things done. When positively charged, the liver gives the ability to achieve personal goals and express compassion. When negatively charged, there is a tendency toward irritation, anger and rage, which can lead to exhaustion and downgraded bodily functions. Simply put, anger shatters qi.

As a Wood Element qigong, Heaven and Earth is particularly valuable for helping to heal a variety of physical and emotional imbalances associated with the liver as well as the body's soft tissues (fascia, muscles, ligaments and tendons), which are governed by the liver. What follows is not the complete list, but covers many of the common ailments for which Heaven and Earth has been prescribed by Chinese doctors in-the-know for three millennia.

PHYSICAL HEALING

Benefits of Soft-Tissue Techniques

The physical motions of the Heaven and Earth form, along with foundational soft-tissue techniques, such as bending-and-stretching and twisting (to be covered in Sections One and Two), can:

- Relieve tension in the body, mind and qi.
- Dredge up and release blockages from old injuries.
- Increase flexibility and range of motion.
- Improve circulation and digestion.
- Reduce high blood pressure and improve venous return.
- Reduce back, neck and shoulder restrictions, and pain.
- Strengthen the arms, neck, legs, spine and internal organs.
- Seal inguinal hernias.

Benefits of Pulsing Techniques

When opening-and-closing (pulsing) techniques (to be covered in Section Three) come online and are woven into the fabric of the Heaven and Earth form, all of the previous positive effects are amplified, and deeper blockages and restrictions can drop away.

Additional benefits of pulsing:

- Relieves constipation by inducing peristalsis—movement within the large intestine.

- Repairs joint and soft-tissue damage from repetitive-strain injuries and blunt-force traumas, and relieves pain from both.

- Profoundly releases the nerves.

- Takes pressure away from the heart by directly pulsing the blood vessels, which tones them and increases circulation.

- Reduces stress and soothes the nerves by strengthening the synapses and regulating smoother and more regular signals in the central nervous system.

Benefits of Adding Deeper Energetic Techniques

When the specific energetic and Wood Element techniques are woven in (as covered in Section Four), another boost in the efficiency and effectiveness of all the previous benefits takes place.

Additional benefits of weaving in deeper energetic techniques:

- Mitigates the effects of alcohol, including reducing hangovers and long-term damage to the liver from alcoholism.

- Circulates blood and relieves energetic congestion in the brain, which has the knock-on effect of improving sleep and rest cycles.

- Improves digestion by balancing the liver and gallbladder.

- Tonifies and improves liver and gallbladder function as a whole, which has the potential to relieve more serious ailments, such as hepatitis, over time.

EMOTIONAL BENEFITS AND QUALITIES

The body, mind and emotions are influenced by qi. When qi becomes inhibited, clogged up or stagnant, there is a tendency not only for physical problems to emerge, but also irregular and raw emotions. If left unaddressed for too long, an individual can become volatile—potentially explosive, depressive or swing between the two.

Getting the liver qi moving well can smooth out the emotions and, with long-term practice of Heaven and Earth, a practitioner can reach a more stable baseline and healthier outlook. In terms of stress, because anger is stored in the liver, Heaven and Earth practice can strengthen the body's qi to dispel the physical-energetic components of anger, including excessive heat, rising yang energy and erratic breathing.

In general, a balanced and healthy liver with strong qi flow supports the ability to bond and emotionally engage. This enables you to persevere and remain committed to overcoming obstacles, which at the most fundamental level, can dramatically reduce stress.

IMPROVED INTELLECTUAL PERFORMANCE

Intellectual work can literally cause the brain to "eat" the body, as the Chinese say. Mental overload requires more blood and qi, so the brain starts pulling from the internal organs to keep going. Then, after the stressful event is over, blood and qi often stagnate or become trapped in the brain. In a healthy, relaxed person, blood naturally drains out of the brain and returns to the torso to become re-oxygenated in the lungs, where it can be re-circulated by the heart to both the body and the brain.

The movements of Heaven and Earth are designed to cleanse the brain (as will be covered in-depth in Chapter 21), balance qi flow in the macrocosmic and microcosmic orbits (explained in Chapter 22), and amplify alternating opening-and-closing rhythms in the body. All of these techniques are unique, classic Water tradition practices that support your ability to maintain healthy blood and qi circulation in your brain. Over time you can increase your intellectual capacity, and become more awake, present and aware. This ability allows you to see things clearly and, from that place, decide what warrants your focus and attention to further your knowledge and continue down your true path.

VALUE FOR MEDITATORS AND HEALING

Opening and closing is also key to Taoist meditation. Internally pulsing specific points within your body and mind gives you the ability to target places inside where you feel blocked energy. Pulsing these areas with regularity and focus very often makes accessible the energy of the emotional, mental and psychic states that can be bottled up, repressed and trapped inside. When they become accessible, they can be released through deeper meditation techniques. Heaven and Earth is a very simple movement form that can enable you to access inner spiritual blockages, which is a rare and invaluable tool for meditation.

Qigong can also serve as a warm-up before other therapeutic practices to gain access to and more effectively address psychological issues.

Heaven and Earth Qigong has the potential to contain an incredible quantity of internal techniques that can address a wide range of health issues. It is like a high-quality multi-tool that has many applications. The one constant in life is change and, as you age and your requirements and goals change, so can the focus of your practice. In this way, Heaven and Earth has the capacity to aid you in growing and evolving, regardless of where your personal path might lead you.

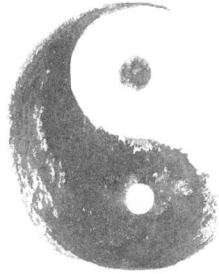

BUILDING THE HEAVEN AND EARTH FORM

Components covered in this section:

- The neutral standing posture
- Arm movements
- The weight shift
- The kwa squat
- The C-curve.

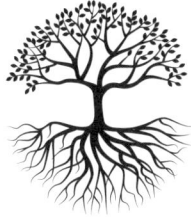

CHAPTER 1:

SETTING THE STAGE FOR MOVEMENT

OVERVIEW OF HEAVEN AND EARTH QIGONG

The Marriage of Heaven and Earth Qigong is a two-part movement with six phases that can be divided into 14 steps (see Table 1).

TWO-PART MOVEMENT	SIX PHASES	14 STEPS
1. MACROCOSMIC ORBIT	First-Phase Stretch	1, 2, 3
	Second-Phase Bend	4, 5, 6, 7
	Third-Phase Stretch	8
2. MICROCOSMIC ORBIT	Fourth-Phase Bend	9, 10, 11
	Fifth-Phase Stretch	12, 13
NEUTRAL	Sixth-Phase Release	14

Table 1: Heaven and Earth Qigong

The two parts are the macrocosmic and microcosmic orbits.

- The macrocosmic orbit is made up of three phases (steps 1-8).
- The microcosmic orbit is made up of two phases (steps 9-13).
- The final, sixth phase (step 14) is simply a release or let go, so your body returns to the neutral standing posture before the beginning of the next repetition.

Initially the six phases are referred to as "stretch-bend-stretch-bend-stretch-release" and later, as you will see, they become "open-close-open-close-open-release." Opening-and-closing techniques are the deeper objective and become the primary *modus operandi* of Heaven and Earth Qigong. That said, more likely the exercise will be confined to activating layers of your soft tissues (skin, fascia, muscles, ligaments and tendons) until you develop your ability to connect to and feel inside yourself.

For this reason, in the early stages of the instructions that follow, the authors will use the terms "bend" and "stretch." Once you develop a good degree of skill deeply penetrating your body with your mind and you can directly activate your joints and the synovial fluid inside them at will, the terms "open" and "close" are more appropriate. In Section Three, where pulsing is covered in detail, the authors will describe how to generate the pulse, but do not confuse knowing the information with having developed the skill. Reading a menu is not the same experience as eating the food. Remember the deeper neigong within Heaven and Earth has traditionally been reserved for disciples, who would have already fulfilled prerequisite training to do with opening their bodies and releasing the bulk of the tension that resided there.

If a group of practitioners at various levels of skill practice Heaven and Earth together, such as in a class, beginners might be activating their soft tissues, intermediate students their joints and fluids, while more advanced students are directly activating their qi—all with the same basic external form. If you have a trained eye, you will be able to pick up on the distinct differences that morph the quality of their movements, but generally you cannot judge a book by its cover.

When learning any qigong form, including Heaven and Earth, the ideal method is to first practice the basic choreography and then systematically and progressively add internal neigong techniques to imbue that form with qi. In the beginning, the most important aspect to grasp is what causes a stretching or bending action in your whole body. This is because bending-and-stretching techniques both initially connect the body into one whole and prepare the body for deeper neigong. Opening-and-closing techniques literally sit inside of bending-and-stretching techniques, yet can only become fused within the Heaven and Earth form once the practitioner has sufficiently opened and released their body's soft tissues. Therefore, while learning and practicing the instructions in Sections One and Two, focus only on where to stretch or bend, so that later you can activate other deeper internal processes in the correct sequence and at their specific, relevant points.

TAOIST PRINCIPLE OF SEPARATE AND COMBINE

The Taoist Principle of Separate and Combine is an ancient guideline for training, which states that once a basic movement, set or form has been learned, the individual components that comprise it must be teased out, deconstructed and trained independently of all others until it is upgraded (to some degree) in its own right. Then that component or thread is recombined and practiced along with other components. The continual cycle of separate-combine, deconstruction-reconstruction is precisely what allows any practitioner to find what is not working well in their form and diminishing overall results, so they can tune into and fix any parts that are not functioning optimally. This process is necessary because what typically prevents someone from progressing is not entirely apparent to them and may even be hidden within their subconscious mind.

TWO STREAMS OF INTEGRATION

The efficiency of your qigong practice depends upon two streams of integration. The first stream concerns your body parts, such as your arms, legs, spine, torso, internal organs, neck and head. The second stream has to do with the 16 neigong components, such as alignments, breathing, twisting, pulsing, lengthening and energy flows. All qigong forms set the body into motion to achieve a specific weave of internal neigong content or qi, which yields a particular flavor or quality of movement.

First you must understand how each body part moves in each exercise. Once you have some idea about the choreography, you can focus on the ways in which neigong components function individually, in pairs, in small groups and, finally, when everything is combined, as one exercise. The multilayered nature of qigong systems is what makes them complex and warrants the deconstruction-reconstruction process in order to achieve the full depth and range of potential benefits.

Many students, including those who train daily for years, find their development stunted even though they are dedicated to their practice by all accounts. The lack of appreciation for the Principle of Separate and Combine is often at the heart of the issue. Human nature and Western culture drive students to focus on their favorite or the perceived more advanced aspects of practice. But chains break at their weakest links, so all threads must be developed and honed in their own right, or overall results from practice are diminished.

Traditional Taoist training dictates that you learn each new technique, piece by piece, then refine and integrate it through many training cycles. No matter how long you practice a qigong set, tai chi style or bagua palm, this process prevails. Each time you stabilize some degree of flow in your art, you once again take it apart and explore the increasingly fine layers that give rise to the flow. The aim is to improve that which is present before adding to the depth and complexity, or setting about the next deconstruction-reconstruction cycle to advance your practice.

The application of the Principle of Separate and Combine to achieve high-performance results can be observed outside the context of Taoism, such as in Formula One racing. Engineers observe how their car performs on the track, then they strip it down, make changes to upgrade particular components, rebuild the machine and then once again take it for a test run. Lap times reducing by tenths of a second are considered a real success and, over time, significant gains can be made. The car's essential components always remain the same—an engine, a gearbox, suspension, etc.—but each part is constantly being monitored individually and in terms of how it functions in relation to all others. This process yields seamless integration and incredibly high-performance vehicles.

FIVE CORE GUIDELINES FOR MOVING IN QIGONG

Whenever learning a form of qigong, five core guidelines allow you to accurately, efficiently and safely learn form movements. Without incorporating these essential principles, practice lacks the fundamental internal connections that define internal energy arts training.

1. KEEP THE BODY ALIGNED

The Neutral Standing Posture

In qigong, movement is usually preceded by a standing practice. The neutral standing posture sets up the body for correct and accurate practice to achieve the goals of the form (Figure 1-1 on the next page).

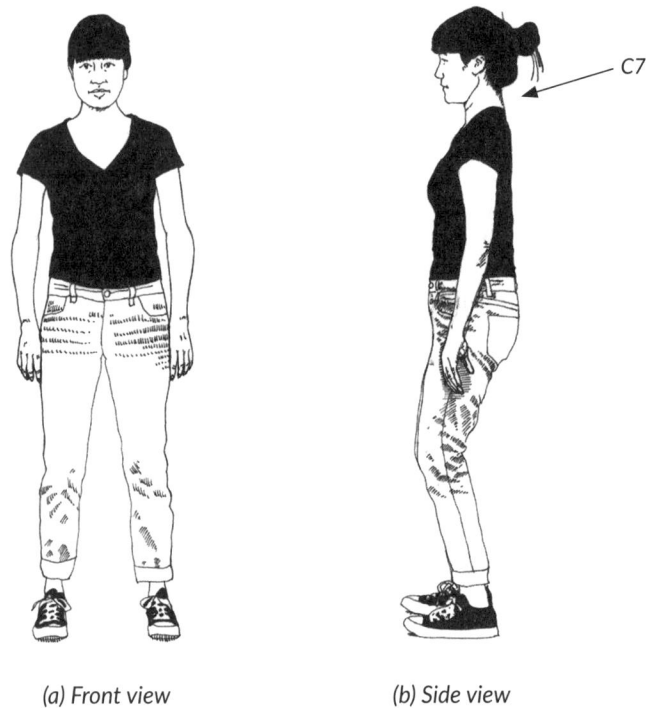

(a) Front view   (b) Side view

Figure 1-1:
Neutral Standing Posture

The key points of the neutral standing posture follow.

- Feet are parallel and shoulder width apart. Your weight is evenly distributed between both feet and runs through the center of your arches. You want an even pressure on the balls, heels and outside edges of your feet.

- Knees are slightly bent: first lock your knees, then bend them just enough to unlock them and engage your thighs, making sure your kneecaps do not project forward of your toes, collapse in or splay out.

- Gently drop down the back of your pelvis, sacrum and tailbone in order to open up your lower (lumbar) spine and sink your weight into your feet—without bending your knees any farther.

- Slightly raise C7 (the seventh cervical vertebra)—without distorting your lower spine or locking your knees.

- Relax your neck and gently raise your occiput to open up your neck—without losing any of the previous alignments.

- Release your shoulders, arms, chest and belly, and let them all hang down off your spine (from C7)—without collapsing your torso, neck or head.

- Rest your thumbs and index fingers against the outside of your thighs, and relax your arm and hand muscles.

The importance of the standing posture cannot be overemphasized since the outcome of your practice session is directly linked to how well you begin. Always spend a few minutes focusing on and making micro-adjustments to your standing posture and settling in before you start moving. Then, during any motion, attempt to maintain all of your alignments, especially those associated with your spine, to prevent over exuberant arm movements that create distortions.

See the Bibliography for Master Frantzis' book, *Opening the Energy Gates of Your Body*, which covers standing alignments in more depth.

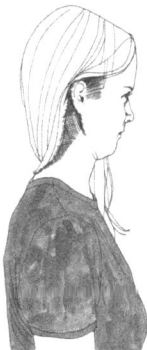

Figure 1-2

Look Forward and Slightly Downward

During standing and qigong practice, look forward and slightly downward, while keeping your gaze soft (see Figure 1-2). These two points will allow you to keep the occipital area open, and give you a sense of whether you are tipping or leaning during any motion. They also help you tune into *feeling* your body rather than thinking about or visualizing yourself doing something that does not match reality.

The Left and Right Channels of Energy

The left and right channels are located deep inside the body (Figure 1-3). They run through the arms, legs, torso and head. These channels extend on each side of the torso from:

- The shoulder's nest—the soft space between the pectoral/upper chest muscles and deltoid/upper arm muscles.
- The hip fold (or "inguinal groove," covered in Chapter 4) at the front of the pelvis/thigh.

By moving your arms along these lines, you can affect the qi running through your left and right channels.

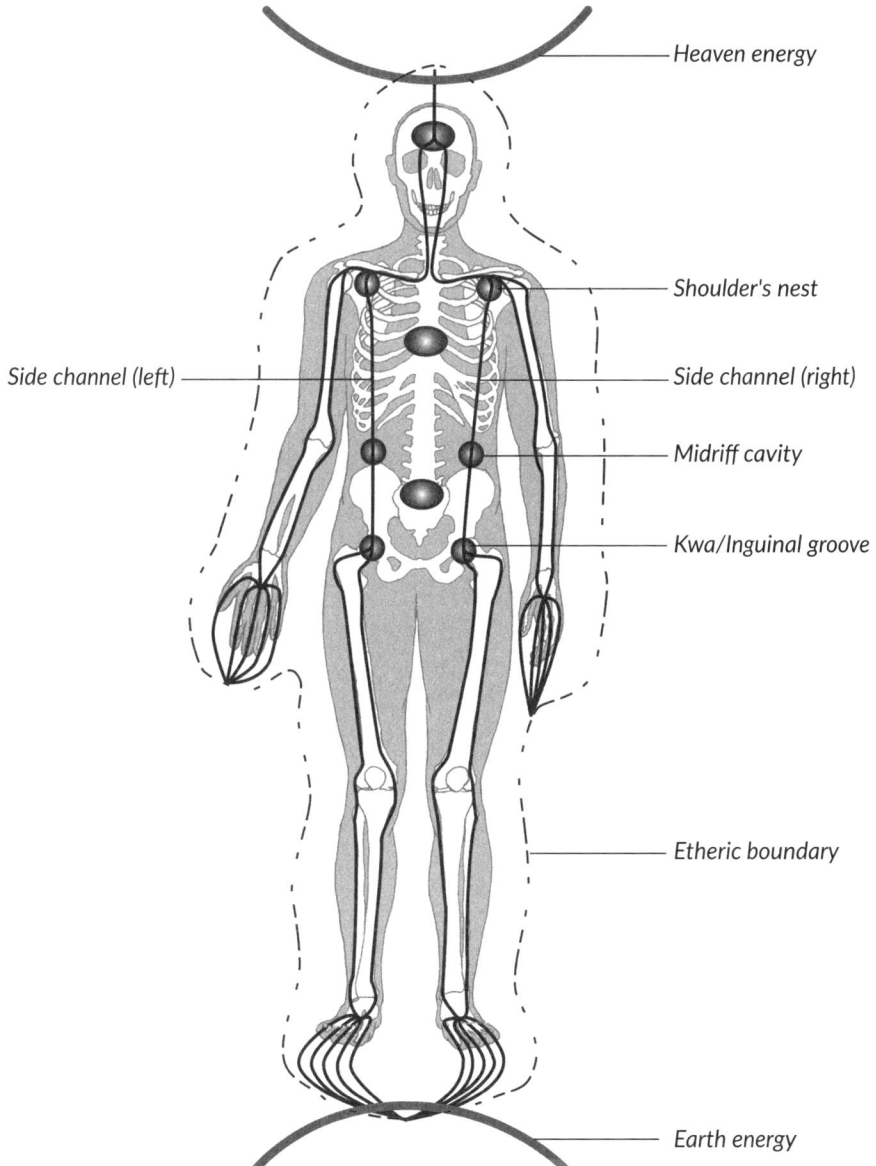

Figure 1-3:
Energy Anatomy

The left and right channels, which guide Heaven and Earth
form movements, run deep inside the body

2. KEEP A BEND IN THE LIMBS

When bending or stretching an arm or a leg—the primary method of moving in qigong—never completely bend or straighten your limb (Figure 1-4). Doing either causes disconnection and, thereby, reduces qi flow and downgrades internal motions to external ones. That is to say, forms are empty without the fundamental internal connections that enable qi to flow uninhibited. Freely flowing qi is precisely what is responsible for the health and healing benefits associated with internal arts training, such as tai chi and qigong.

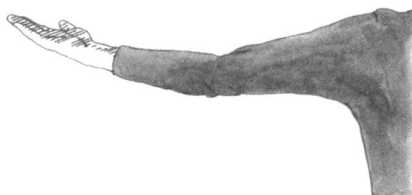

(a) Incorrect: Too Straight

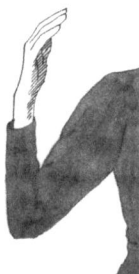

(b) Incorrect: Too Much Bending

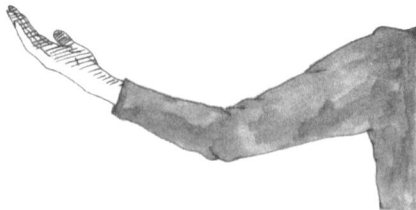

(c) Correct: Stretch

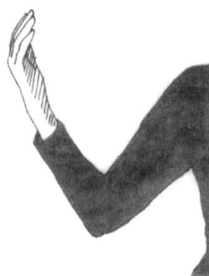

(d) Correct: Bend

Figure 1-4:
Maintain a Slight Bend in the Arms at All Times

Always maintain a slight bend in the limbs

3. KEEP THE HANDS SOFT

When bending and stretching the hands or forming a fist, as in the second part of the movement, do so in a soft, smooth way. When a fist is completely formed, the ideal is to maintain a space in the middle about the size of the width of your index finger. This allows blood and qi to circulate freely, the name of the game in qigong. To find the sweet spot, gently wrap the fingers of one hand around the index finger of your other hand. Then pull out your finger, leaving your fist with space in the middle and a soft quality (Figure 1-5).

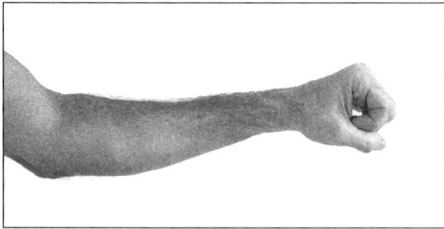

(a) Correct: Soft fist   *(b) Incorrect: Tensed fist*

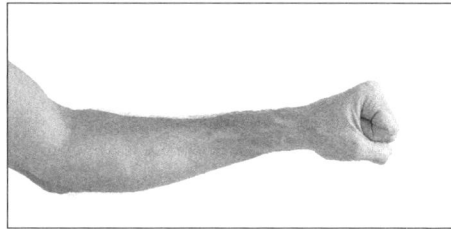

Figure 1-5:
Maintain a Soft Fist

4. KEEP SPACE IN THE ARMPITS

In neigong, maintain a space in your armpits to help connect your arms to your spine, and aid blood and qi flow to and from your hands and torso (Figure 1-6). That space can increase and decrease in size, but never completely closes down. If you maintain a distance of one fist width between your upper arms and your chest, as well as between your hands and your torso/thighs, you will never shut down your armpits while moving.

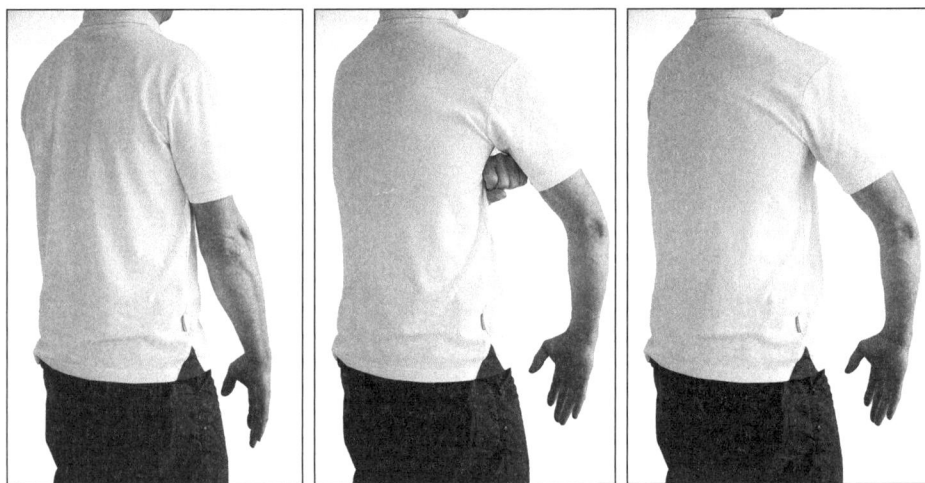

(a) Incorrect: Armpit closed   (b) Correct: Armpit open—
one fist width   (c) Correct: Armpit open

**Figure 1-6:
Maintaining Space in the Armpits Supports Qi Flow**

5. KEEP A RELAXED INTENT

Stress and tension inhibit blood and qi circulation, so the first goal of qigong is relaxation to stimulate blood and qi flow. For this reason, you never push your body, mind or qi beyond its upper limits during practice. Once you exceed your comfortable capacity, resistance is naturally generated. This resistance creates stress, whereby the nerves tighten and contract the muscles, which diminishes qi flow. Conversely, staying within your comfort zone, allows the nerves to let go, so that blood and qi can be mobilized and more powerfully circulated around the body.

The 70-Percent Rule

The 70-Percent Rule is fundamental to Water method training protocols and states that healthy individuals should use about two-thirds of their full effort and energy while always leaving about one-third in reserve. This principle of moderation is applied to:

- The length of time they practice or engage in any activity.
- The intensity of their practice or the degree to which they engage in any activity, such as how far their arms bend/flex and stretch/extend.
- The depth of their practice, such as moving the tissues on the surface of the torso versus the internal organs underneath.

If you are compromised or operating below normal capacity for any reason, e.g. a muscle strain or due to a serious cold or flu, flip the equation and use only 30 percent (or even less) of your effort and energy while leaving at least 70 percent in reserve.

The 70-Percent Rule prevents injury and damage to your body, exhaustion of your energy, as well as mental strain and internal resistance, which allows you to train regularly. By keeping at least one-third in reserve, you will always be left feeling you could do more and, therefore, can continue long-term training.

SAFETY TIPS

Heaven and Earth Qigong, like all Taoist arts, is designed to take you deeper into your body, mind and qi in progressive stages while always adhering to the 70-Percent Rule. If at any point you experience serious discomfort or pain, stop practicing immediately and rest. Return to the basic component exercises and rebuild the form while using less effort and reducing your range of motion with a focus on relaxation.

FOCUS ON THE RELEASE

Qigong is a healing art in large part because it is practiced softly. At the end of each open and at the end of every repetition, soften and release in order to let go of any tension created from excess effort or hyper focus. Otherwise tension compounds and, over time, practice can cause or exacerbate body-mind-qi imbalances rather than ease them.

WEAK LINKS REQUIRE CARE

There are several body parts that are more vulnerable to injury than others and require more attention and care (Figure 1-7). They are:

- The knees.
- The lower back (lumbar spine).
- The occipital region, where the head meets the neck.

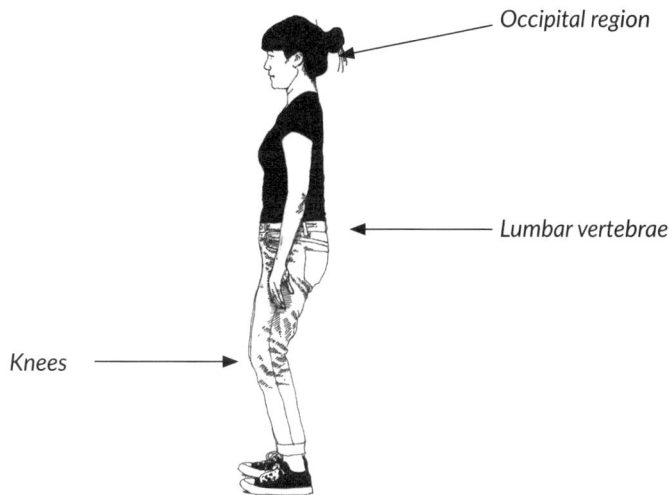

Figure 1-7:
Weak Links Require Care

Pay special attention not to strain these areas by following all instructions carefully. If you find you cannot practice without igniting strain or tension, STOP! Seek out live instruction from a qualified instructor who can help you make the adjustments you might not recognize that you require.

FOR WOMEN

Whenever doing any form of exercise, do not allow your arms to rub against your breasts as it can be detrimental to your health. When practicing qigong, always keep your arms and hands a minimum of one fist width distance from your breasts. This may require you to adjust form movements as women have done in China for millennia.

MORE EXPERIENCED HEAVEN AND EARTH QIGONG PRACTITIONERS

The form that is presented in this book might vary slightly or significantly from the form you have previously learned. This is the *definitive beginning method* of initiating practice of Heaven and Earth Qigong since it aims to open up the whole skeletal frame, activate the pulse and create a sense of growing and expanding—the primary *modus operandi* of Wood Element neigong.

Wise students repeatedly return to fundamental neigong in order to strengthen their foundation, refine their skill set and prepare for deeper qi development, allowing more advanced stages of practice to flourish. Once you have gained full control over all of the material presented in this volume while simultaneously being able to fully bring alive the pulse throughout all the joints of your body, at will, form movements begin to morph. This allows more advanced neigong to take root—without losing any of the internal techniques presented herein. Take this opportunity and spend the next year or so deepening your skills at this level of practice. The time and energy required will be well worth the effort.

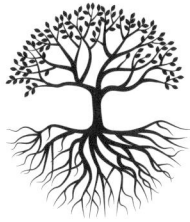

CHAPTER 2:

ARM MOVEMENTS

BENDING AND STRETCHING THE HANDS

Right from the start you can begin moving your hands in synchronization with a stretching or a bending action.

- During a stretch, lightly extend your fingertips, initially from your elbows and eventually your shoulder blades—without locking the joints in your elbows, hands or fingers.
- During a bend, release and relax your wrists, hands, fingers and arm muscles, while lightly "cupping" your hands.

HOW TO FIND THE CORRECT HAND POSITIONS

Stand in the neutral posture (Figure 2-1) and:

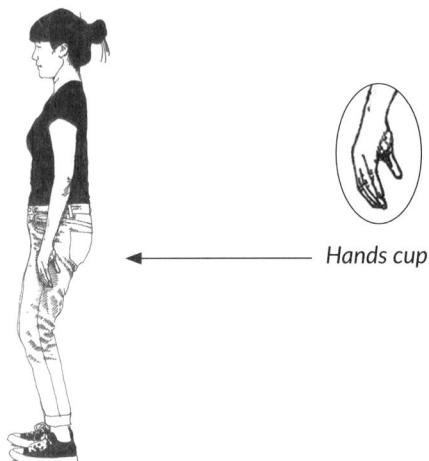

Hands cup

Figure 2-1:

Hands Relax and Lightly Cup

1. Relax your arms and hands at the sides of your body, and notice how your hands naturally assume a curved form. This is the neutral hand position (Figure 2-2).

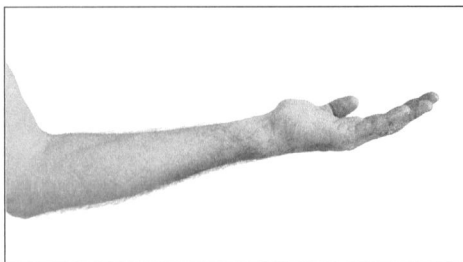

Figure 2-2:
Neutral Hand Position

2. Next slowly stretch and expand your hands and notice how they become less curved (Figure 2-3a). Do not stretch them so much that they go flat or to the point of locking the joints (Figure 2-3b).

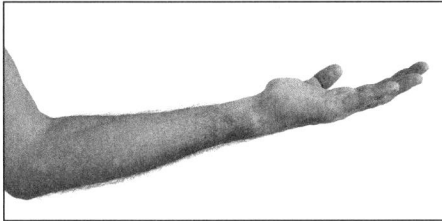

(a) Correct: Stretch   *(b) Incorrect: Too stretched*

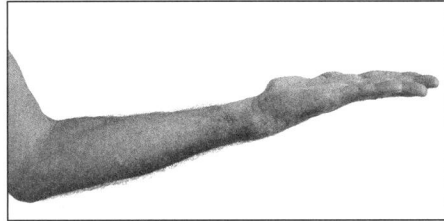

Figure 2-3: Stretched Hand Position

3. After the extension, release your hands back to neutral and then continue curving them. Notice how they come to form a shallow cup with your fingers lightly touching each other (Figure 2-4a)—yet they are not overly curved either (Figure 2-4b).

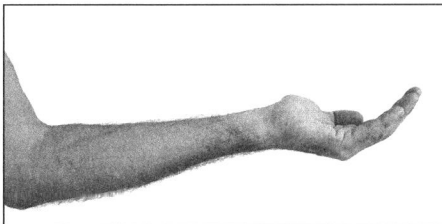

(a) Correct: Bend/Cup   *(b) Incorrect: Too much bending/cupping*

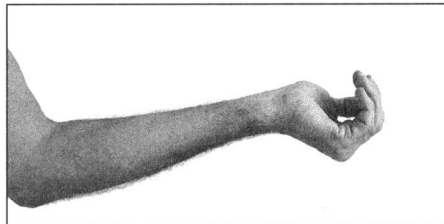

**Figure 2-4:
Cupped Hand Position**

HOW TO MOVE THE ARMS

Figure 2-5: How to Move the Arms—Snapshot

MACROCOSMIC ORBIT

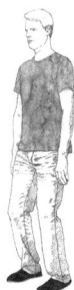 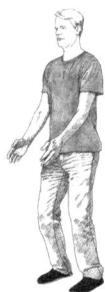 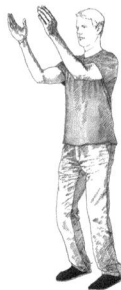 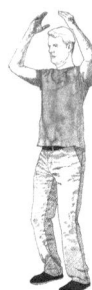 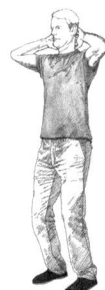

(a) Neutral posture   *(b) Step 1*   *(c) Step 2*   *(d) Step 3: Midpoint*   *(e) Step 3: Endpoint*

Stretch ⟶

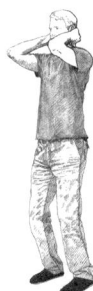 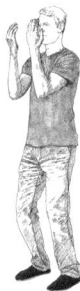 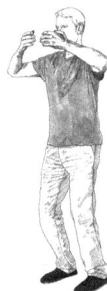 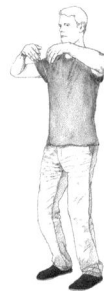

(f) Step 4   *(g) Step 5*   *(h) Step 6*   *(i) Step 7*

Bend ⟶

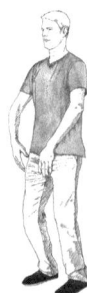

(j) Step 8

Stretch ⟶

MICROCOSMIC ORBIT

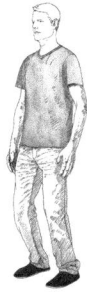 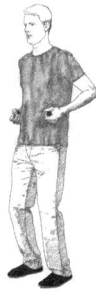 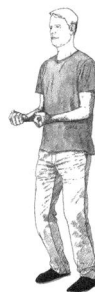

(k) Step 9   (l) Step 10   (m) Step 11

Bend ⟶

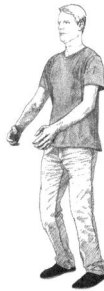 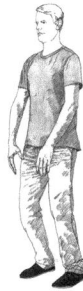

(n) Step 12   (o) Step 13

Stretch ⟶

NEUTRAL

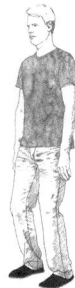

(p) Step 14

Release ⟶

NEUTRAL STANDING POSTURE

Start in the neutral standing posture with your arms relaxed and your hands resting on your outer thighs (Figure 2-6) as covered in Chapter 1.

MACROCOSMIC ORBIT

First-Phase Stretch

Pay special attention not to raise your chest or arch your back during all three steps of the first phase.

Step 1 - Bring your hands forward while rolling under your elbows such that your elbow tips turn to point to the ground, while your forearms turn until they become parallel with each other (Figure 2-7).

- Your arms are shoulder width apart and your palms come to face each other.

- The rolling under of your elbows prevents your shoulders from rising or bunching up.

- During this and all stages of the first phase, slowly and lightly stretch open your hands.

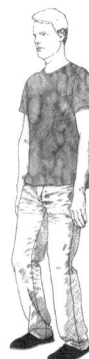

**Figure 2-6:
Neutral Position**

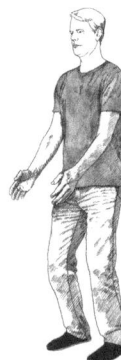

**Figure 2-7:
Step 1**

Step 2 - Once your arms are parallel and about shoulder width apart, lead from your hands to raise your arms, sink your elbows and drop your shoulders (Figure 2-8)—without:

- Letting your arms drift sideways.
- Bending your elbows more than when you started the movement.
- Hardening or tensing your muscles.
- Raising or bunching up your shoulders.

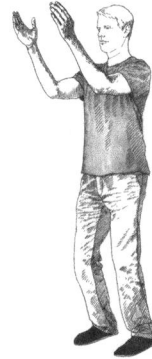

Figure 2-8:
Step 2

Continue until you reach the natural barrier where you cannot raise your arms any farther—without generating one or more of the distortions referenced above.

Step 3 - When you hit that barrier, which is caused by the restrictions in your body, do not push through it.

- Relax and spread your elbows to the sides while drawing your palms over the crown of your head and extending your fingertips toward each other (Figure 2-9).
- Continue to extend your fingertips until they come to touch your occiput (Figure 2-10).
- The tips of your middle fingers will also touch each other if your hands and wrists are fully open and not scrunched up.

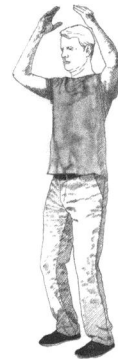

Figure 2-9:
Step 3—Midpoint

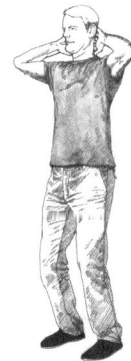

Figure 2-10:
Step 3—Endpoint

Second-Phase Bend

Pay special attention to keeping your spine still in space, not allowing your head to jut forward or crunching up your neck to scrunch up during all steps of the second phase.

Step 4 - While keeping your middle fingers touching at your occiput, bend your wrists and bring your elbows forward, ideally until your forearms become parallel to each other (Figure 2-11).

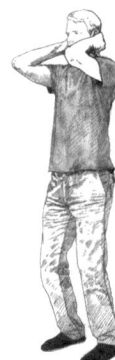

Figure 2-11: Step 4

- Be sure not to squash your ears. If you find you make a strong contact with your ears, then you know you did not sufficiently bend your wrists. A light contact is normal, but you do not want a heavy contact.

- During this and the following three steps of the second-phase bend, your hands continuously soften and lightly cup.

Step 5 - Release your fingers at your occiput and bring your hands over the crown of your head (not shown) by dropping your elbows down in front of you (Figure 2-12). Do NOT allow your hands to separate and come forward by moving around the sides of your head and past your ears.

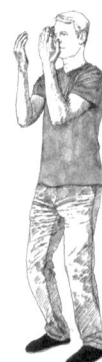

Figure 2-12: Step 5

- Continue until your forearms are parallel and more or less perpendicular to the ground. Your palms will come to in front of your face.

- Do not close your armpits or allow your arms to touch your chest.

- Your hands and arms will be one to two fist(s) width from your face and your torso.

Step 6 - Rotate on the center of your palms and raise your elbows to the sides in such a way that your hands do not descend and your elbows come up to roughly shoulder height. Keep your shoulders sunk during this and all other steps to ensure that they do not rise. See Figure 2-13.

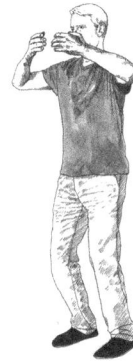

**Figure 2-13:
Step 6**

Step 7 - Drop your fingers downward by softening your hands and wrists. Your palms remain facing your body and your arms do not move upward, downward, forward or backward. Your hands finish fully cupped. See Figure 2-14.

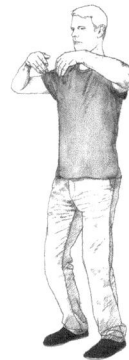

**Figure 2-14:
Step 7**

Third-Phase Stretch

Throughout the third-phase stretch, keep C7 lifted and stable.

Step 8 - Sink your hands down toward the ground, while your palms face and trace the left and right channels of energy within your torso, until your hands arrive in front of your thighs fully stretched open (Figure 2-15).

Keep your elbows slightly bent as your hands finish dropping, so your elbows do not lock, your hands remain one to two fist(s) width from your body and you do not close down your armpits (as covered in Chapter 1).

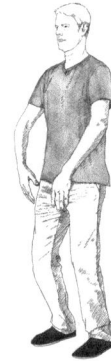

Figure 2-15: Step 8

MICROCOSMIC ORBIT

Fourth-Phase Bend

Through all three steps of the fourth-phase bend, you will inscribe a half circle with your hands—using a backward-upward-forward motion—from beginning to end.

Step 9 - Relax your arms and hands, and allow them to naturally draw away from one another toward the outside of your thighs, while your hands release from the stretched position and begin to form fists. Your palms come to face your outer thighs. See Figure 2-16.

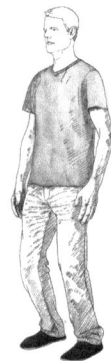

Figure 2-16: Step 9

Step 10 - As your hands reach the outside of your thighs, begin bending your elbows and continue forming fists with your hands as they rise and turn to face up. Continue up to the height of your midriff, where your forming fists also make contact with your midriff (Figure 2-17).

If for any reason you encounter tension in your body when trying to achieve the contact between your forming fists and your midriff, relax and use less effort while trying to maintain the circular motion. Over time your body will open up and allow you to achieve the ideal.

During steps 10 and 11, be sure not to bend or twist your wrists, keeping each hand, as it forms a fist, in a straight line with the elbow.

Step 11 - From the height of your midriff, continue forming fists and turning your palms to face up, as your hands circle slightly upward and forward in such a way that your forearms gently rub against your lowest ribs. Continue to bring your hands forward until your elbows come just forward of your lowest ribs while your fists come to completion (with the hole in the middle as covered in Chapter 1). See Figure 2-18.

During the microcosmic orbit, allow your armpits to close, but not completely shut down. Women must also take care not to rub their breasts, which takes precedence over the forearms rubbing against the lower ribs. For this reason, women might have to experiment with the fourth-phase bend to calibrate their arm movements.

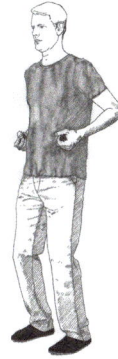

Figure 2-17: Step 10

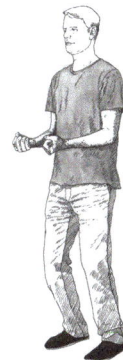

Figure 2-18: Step 11

At the end of the fourth-phase bend, your forearms are horizontal and parallel to the ground, and your palms face up in a fisted position. Your fists are forward of your torso in line with your left and right channels of energy. Your fisted hands are soft and free from any tension or strength whatsoever (as covered in Chapter 1).

Fifth-Phase Stretch

Throughout both steps of the fifth-phase stretch, you will inscribe a half circle with a forward-downward-backward motion.

Step 12 - Your elbows move forward as your fists begin to open and your hands begin to drop downward. Your palms turn to face each other. See Figure 2-19.

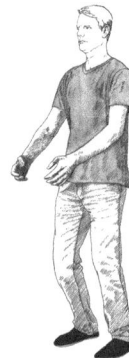

Figure 2-19: Step 12

Step 13 - Your hands continue to turn, drop and open, and your palms naturally circle backward to face toward your body—more or less finishing in the same position as the end of the third-phase stretch of the macrocosmic orbit (Figure 2-20).

Keep one to two fist(s) width between your hands and the front of your thighs, and keep your armpits open.

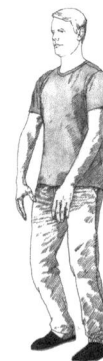

Figure 2-20: Step 13

NEUTRAL

Sixth-Phase Release

Step 14 - The neutral position is achieved by slowly and progressively releasing all the effort out of your arms and your upper body, and allowing your hands to come to and rest against the outside of your thighs (Figure 2-21).

- Release all your soft tissues, all your joints and your nerves before repeating the six phases anew.

- The neutral position is both the finishing position of the previous movement and the beginning position of the next, so take your time and let everything in your system settle.

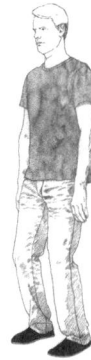

Figure 2-21:
Step 14

LINKING THE ARMS DEEPER INTO THE BODY

The following instructions allow arm movements to link deeper into the body by engaging the shoulders and upper body tissues to a further extent. This training loosens and releases the shoulders, neck and upper body tissues more so than in the introductory method for moving the arms, and can greatly diminish tension held in the upper body. It also prepares the body for deeper neigong threads that will be woven into the Heaven and Earth form, such as opening-and-closing and lengthening techniques.

GENTLY LIFT FROM C7

Find a stable stance with your feet placed firmly on the ground and maintain it. Do not let your arm motions pull you off your root or diminish your balance. At this stage, you want an even pressure on all parts of the soles of your feet with your weight centered over both arches throughout the whole motion.

When standing in the neutral posture (Figure 2-22) and throughout the entire movement, lift your torso up from the seventh cervical vertebra (C7). This action is what holds the body stable and prevents distortion in the spine from the arms attempting to take over the motion. It is also what creates the foundation for the neck and head to lift yet remain soft.

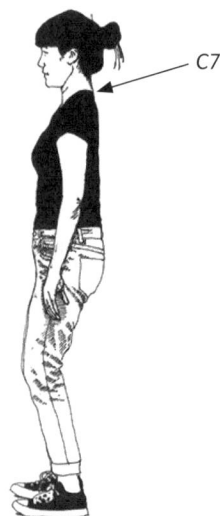

Figure 2-22

OPEN THE SOFT TISSUES AND NERVES

When you move your arms correctly, you will stretch the soft tissues in your upper body in a number of ways. The aim is to progressively open up the tissues over many repetitions, not suddenly in only one or two rounds. When practiced correctly, the tissues will open while the nerves let go, which allows stretches to more deeply penetrate the body. Conversely, pushing too hard binds the nerves, and restricts blood and qi flow. When returning to neutral at the end of each round, spend a few seconds completely releasing your nerves before starting the next repetition. If the nerves release, the soft tissues can release, which increases blood and qi flow, and enables deeper stretching on the next round.

TWO VECTOR FORCES IN THE STRETCHING PHASES

There are always two vectors or forces in the arms during the stretching phases, which prevent you from locking your elbows and enable access to your insides (Figure 2-23).

- The first vector affects how the elbows extend away from the spine.
- The second affects how the fingertips extend away from the elbows.
- During these two integrated components of a stretch, always keep a bend in your elbow joint.

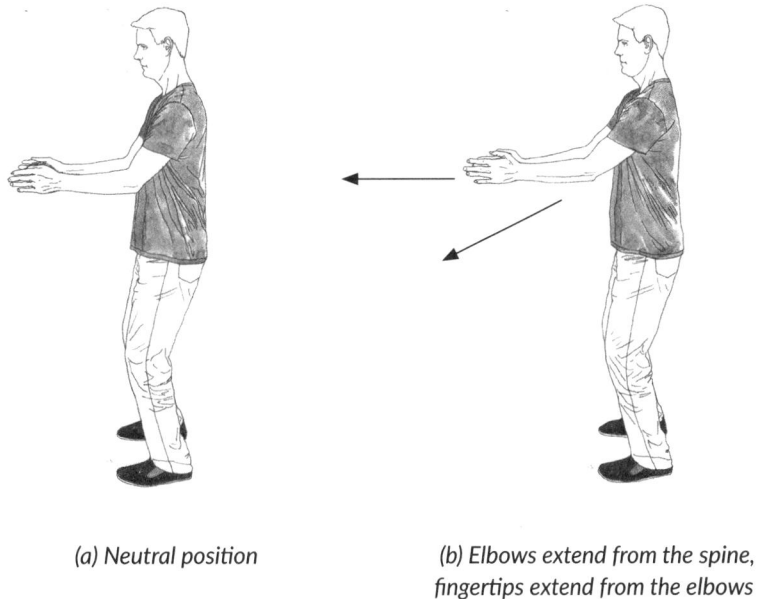

(a) Neutral position

(b) Elbows extend from the spine, fingertips extend from the elbows

Figure 2-23: Two Vectors of the Arms

With these vectors in mind and as a doorway into neigong practice:

1. Bring your arms parallel at about the height of your diaphragm/ solar plexus. The position is found about halfway through the first-phase stretch, step 2 (Figure 2-23a).

2. Sink your elbows slightly forward and downward (first vector) and project your fingertips directly forward (second vector)—without extending your elbows (Figure 2-23b). This movement is small and opens up the tissues of the shoulders, neck and upper back while connecting the arms to the spine, but only if the spine remains stable by keeping C7 lifted and anchored in place.

FOCUS ON THE RETURN IN THE BENDING PHASES

In the bending phases, the main focus is on the return, specifically how stretched tissues return to neutral. If, for example, during a stretching phase you manage to elongate the soft tissues of your arms, hands and fingers, then during the following bending phase, the release of those tissues should be slow, smooth and continuous (and not sudden). Think of slowly stretching an elastic band, then slowly guiding the release back to the neutral state as opposed to just letting go at the most stretched point and allowing it to snap back to neutral.

MOVE FROM THE ELBOWS

The movement of the elbows is a key focus in early Heaven and Earth practice as they allow you to link with and connect the soft tissues of your upper body. If your elbows move, your hands will move, and you will stretch or release the soft tissues from your elbows to your spine. Conversely, if you move from your hands, you will very likely overly straighten or bend your elbows, which fails to engage the soft tissues between your elbows and your spine. Along with these foundational bending-and-stretching techniques, twisting and opening-and-closing neigong can open your body and aid the release of both superficial and deeper, accumulated tensions in your body.

Macrocosmic Orbit

First-Phase Stretch

Steps 1-2 - Your elbows drop and extend forward out of your spine and your fingertips extend out of your elbows. Keep C7 still, lifted and anchored, and do not straighten or lock your elbows.

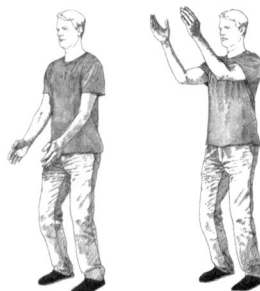

Step 3 - When your fingers reach their maximum 70-percent height, spread your elbows away from each other and extend your fingers toward each other in continuum as your hands pass over your head. Continue until your fingers touch your occiput at the back of your head. This generates a stretch throughout the arms, shoulders, back and chest, which is why, even though the elbows are physically bending, this motion is considered a stretch.

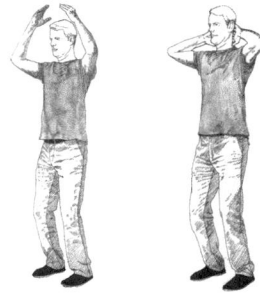

By projecting your elbows out to the sides while stretching your fingers in toward your centerline, you increase the stretch in the soft tissues of your arms. Be sure to maintain an even stretch across both your chest and your back:

- If your elbows are too far forward, you will only achieve a stretch across your back.
- If your elbows are too far back, you will only stretch the tissues across your chest.
- When you find the sweet spot, the stretch is equal across both your back and your chest, and it continues all the way to your fingertips.
- Let your chest relax downward instead of puffing forward. When the chest puffs up, qi flow becomes distorted.

Second-Phase Bend

During the second phase, even though this is a bending action, certain tissues will stretch open, especially those between your shoulder blades.

Step 4 - Your elbows project forward as they come around to the front of your body, ideally until your arms become parallel with each other. Keep your fingers on your occiput and C7 anchored in place as you draw out your shoulder blades with your elbows and relax your hands and wrists. This action stretches open the tissues in the back, especially behind the heart.

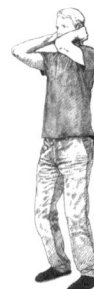

Steps 5-7 - Keep your elbows extended forward, softening your wrists and cupping your hands, as:

- Your hands come over the crown of your head (not shown) and in front of your face.
- Your elbows rise and you rotate on the center of your palms.
- Your fingers drop down.

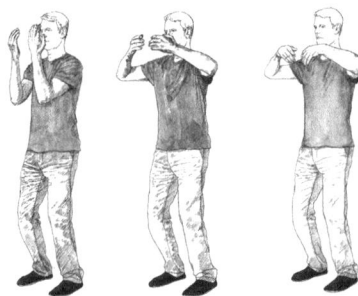

Third-Phase Stretch

Step 8 - As your hands descend, extend your elbows slightly forward and to the sides.

- Your hands remain the same distance apart throughout the entirety of the motion.
- Keep a minimum of one fist width between your torso and your arms, as well as your thighs and your hands.

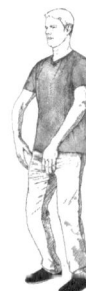

- By keeping the elbows bent and C7 raised while extending the fingers away from the elbows, all the soft tissues of the arms, shoulders, neck and upper torso open up quite profoundly.

Microcosmic Orbit

Fourth-Phase Bend and Fifth-Phase Stretch

During the fourth and fifth phases, if you were to watch your hands from the side, they trace a complete circle:

Steps 9-11 - On the bending phase, the hands travel backward, upward and then forward.

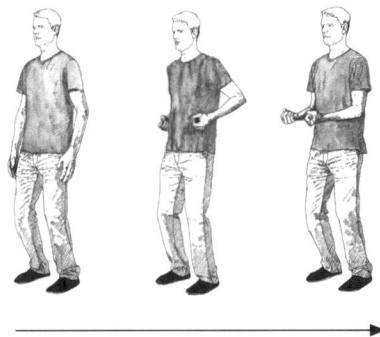

Steps 12-13 - On the stretching phase, the hands travel forward, downward and then backward.

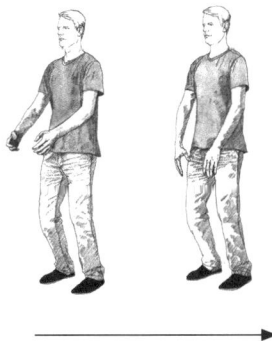

This circle is one of three aspects that must be seamlessly blended together in order to perform these two phases of the form well. The three aspects are:

- The circle (as just described).
- Turning the arms—palms facing upward, then palms facing backward.
- Closing and opening your fists.

The hands do not move in space without turning and either opening or closing the fist, so all three aspects begin and finish together.

As you bend, circle your hands to the top of the circle while your palms turn up and your fists close. Continue until your elbows come to just forward of the sides of your lower ribs with your forearms horizontal, where all three change to the opposite:

- Your elbows and hands travel forward, downward and then backward.
- Your forearms rotate, so that your palms first come to face each other, and then they face the front of your thighs.
- Your fists gradually open while your fingertips stretch out from your elbows.

All three aspects finish when your hands are one fist width from the front of your thighs. The same distance is maintained between your upper arms and your chest. Be sure not to close down your armpits.

INTERMEDIATE PRACTITIONERS AND THE NATURALLY FLEXIBLE

The images and explanations in the previous section approach Heaven and Earth Qigong from a beginner's perspective. However, the goal of the form is to open up the body considerably more than what is possible from external forms of exercise. It is not that the parameters shift over time, but rather that you gain access to and can open your body and nervous system progressively more with ongoing training. Therefore, if you have been practicing qigong for some years and you have become more flexible—or happen to be naturally flexible from the start—what you are trying to achieve from practice (while always adhering to the 70-Perecent Rule) changes or is different, respectively.

Over time your range of motion increases throughout the movement, so your tissues elongate farther during the stretching phases—without use of excessive force. As a result, the return to neutral takes longer. The real difference is in the first stretch.

Macrocosmic Orbit
First-Phase Stretch

Step 1 - Bring your arms parallel by rotating your elbows under and slightly sinking your elbows and hands down. This will create a deeper connection through the soft tissues of your back, neck and spine.

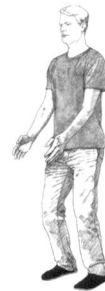

Step 2 - Keeping the connection from step 1 by continuously allowing your elbows to remain heavy throughout the motion, raise your arms high while your spine remains straight and your shoulders sink down.

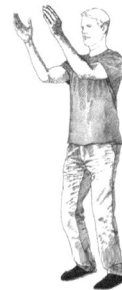

- The arms remain parallel and the distance between them remains the same throughout this step.
- Ideally, you are looking for your arms and hands to point directly up toward the sky—without raising your shoulders whatsoever (Figure 2-24); however, this is difficult to achieve without losing at least one of the previously covered parameters—even for the

naturally flexible. There is no need to do a super stretch in the beginning to get your arms vertically above your head. Initially, your fingertips might only comfortably reach as high as the top of your forehead, which is sufficient. However, as your body's soft tissues release and elongate in progressive stages—in both a single practice session and from ongoing practice over time—you might find that your fingertips can comfortably reach higher and higher until they are vertically above the crown of your head.

- Always adhere to the 70-Percent Rule and do not push, force or rush the process. Allow your body to open at its own pace, which may take longer than you project.

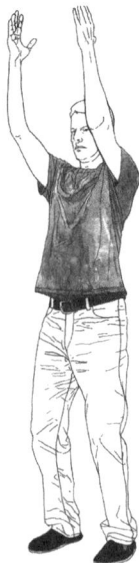

Figure 2-24:
First-Phase Stretch—End of Step 2
(Intermediate Practitioners)

Once the body has opened to a significant degree from regular and long-term training, ideally the arms and hands point directly up toward the sky without raising the shoulders or igniting any tension

Step 3 - From the apex of this much higher position, simply bend and separate your elbows to the sides and draw your hands straight down until your fingertips contact your occiput.

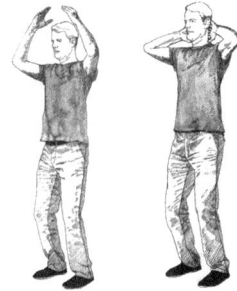

Second-Phase Bend

Steps 4-7 - Your elbows continue to draw forward smoothly and come around to your left and right channels. After your hands have come over your head, your elbows spread and rise to the sides slightly higher than your shoulders.

Be sure not to raise your shoulders at any point throughout the four steps of this bending phase.

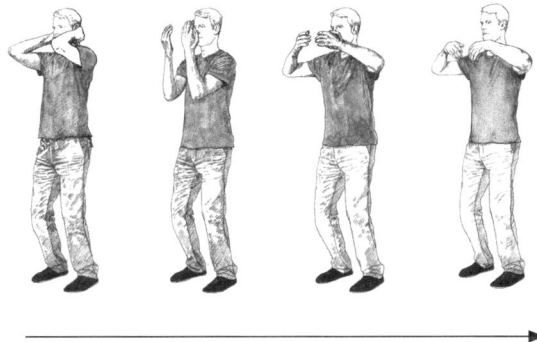

Third-Phase Stretch

Step 8 - The third-phase stretch is the same as the beginning method from the perspective of choreography. The difference is that the extension through the fibers of your hands, arms, shoulders, neck and upper torso will be greater than in the beginning method.

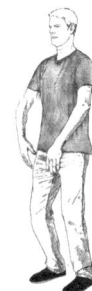

Be mindful not to devolve into pushing and forcing your arms to extend farther, which would cause you to disconnect or generate tension.

Microcosmic Orbit
Fourth-Phase Bend and Fifth-Phase Stretch

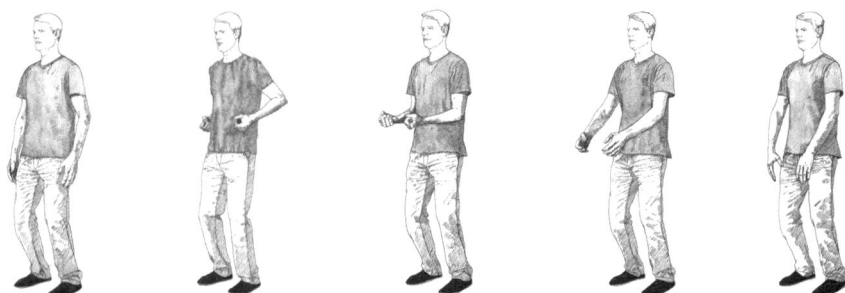

Steps 9-13 - In the fourth-phase bend (steps 9-11) and the fifth-phase stretch (steps 12-13), the size of your circle will noticeably increase, especially in step 12, where your elbows drive forward as your hands descend to open your shoulder blades and the soft tissues behind your heart—before you release the tissues between your shoulder blades during step 13.

- Even though your circle increases in size, your hands never rise above the height of your elbows and your forearms remain horizontal at the top of the circle.

- Be sure your hands do not travel behind your torso during the bending phase (steps 9-11).

- If you apply too much force, your nerves will shut down to protect your body from potential injury. Practice slowly and diligently and be gentle with yourself.

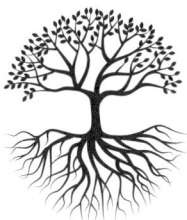

CHAPTER 3:

THE WEIGHT SHIFT

A primary technique for mobilizing the ascending and descending energy in the body is shifting weight back and forth along the center of the feet. When practiced correctly, other neigong threads come to assist in boosting and supercharging these specific qi flows, as will be covered in the following sections.

SETTING THE STAGE FOR MOVEMENT

Start in the neutral standing posture, but this time drop the back of your pelvis to the best of your ability—without forcing your body or squatting down.

- Simply stand, release your lower back muscles and drop your buttocks (gluteal muscles), sacrum and tailbone to open up your lower (lumbar) spine and increase the pressure in your feet. Keep this "extra" pressure in your feet at all times during the exercise.

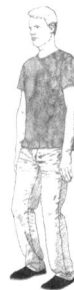

- If you stand correctly, your weight should be centered over the arches of both feet, creating an even pressure in the heels, balls and outside edges of your feet.

You will learn the weight shift in three layers. First you will learn how to do a correct weight shift, next you will learn the specific weight-shift pattern for Heaven and Earth Qigong, and then you will join the weight shift with the arm movements of the form.

THE WEIGHT SHIFT

PRELIMINARY EXERCISE: BASIC WEIGHT SHIFT

From the newly modified standing posture, draw your mind to your tailbone at the base of your spine and pelvis, and let it rest there for a minute or two.

1. When your mind has fully contacted your tailbone and pelvis, move them forward half an inch to an inch, until more of your weight is on the balls of your feet than is on your heels. Your heels remain firmly on the ground at all times.

2. Next move your tailbone and pelvis back to your arches again with your weight evenly distributed between both feet, as in the beginning position.

3. Continue to use the backward motion of your tailbone and pelvis to draw your body back half an inch or so, until more of your weight is on your heels than is on the balls of your feet. Do not allow your toes to lift involuntarily. If this happens, you know you have gone back too far as lifting the toes indicates you are losing your balance.

4. Once again, shift your tailbone and pelvis forward, so your weight returns to the arches of your feet.

5. Repeat steps 1-4 a dozen times or so, until you have tuned into this fundamental and essential neigong technique.

Important Points

You can increase qi flow and, thereby, health and healing benefits of this basic weight shift by adhering to the following points:

- All weight shifts originate from the tailbone while the tailbone remains connected to the pelvis and the spine. Therefore, if the tailbone moves one inch, the pelvis, whole spine, torso and head move one inch, as does the sternum and the chin. There is no leaning or swaying to influence the weight to shift to specific points on the feet.

- Weight shifts should be done slowly, smoothly and continuously— not suddenly, sharply or in staccato fashion.

- The sacrum and gluteal muscles always remain relaxed and sunk with the full weight of the body completely over the feet. There is no arching of the back, rising of the chest, or distortion of any kind in the torso, head or neck.

- The knees remain slightly bent (as in the neutral posture) and they do not project forward beyond the front of the toes. There is no rising or descending as in the kwa squat (to be covered in Chapter 4).

Intermediate practitioners: You will learn how to energetically penetrate your legs with your tailbone during the weight shift in Chapter 7.

THE SIX-PHASE, WEIGHT-SHIFT PATTERN FOR HEAVEN AND EARTH QIGONG

In the Marriage of Heaven and Earth, the idea is to bring your qi up and down your body at specific points throughout the exercise. Putting weight onto the balls of the feet naturally brings energy up the body, whereas putting weight onto the heels encourages energy to go down the body. When the body's weight is equally distributed between the two, on the arches, the upward and the downward flows become balanced and the collateral (horizontal) qi flows around the body are supported.

The following weight-shift pattern generates the correct qi flows for the six-phase Heaven and Earth exercise. The motion is subtle and therefore should be practiced separately until it becomes second nature to you. Later your mind must be free to focus on other techniques without losing this essential component.

The correct pattern begins with your weight on the arches of your feet and your mind in your tailbone and pelvis (Figure 3-1a), then:

- **First Phase** - Shift your weight forward onto the balls of your feet (Figure 3-1b).

- **Second Phase** - Shift your weight backward onto the arches of your feet (Figure 3-1c).

- **Third Phase** - Continue shifting backward onto the heels of your feet (Figure 3-1d)

- **Fourth Phase** - Shift your weight forward onto the balls of your feet once again—without stopping as your weight transfers through your arches (Figure 3-1e).

- **Fifth Phase** - Shift your weight backward onto your heels once again—without stopping as your weight transfers through your arches (Figure 3-1f).

- **Sixth Phase** - Shift your weight forward onto your arches (Figure 3-1g).

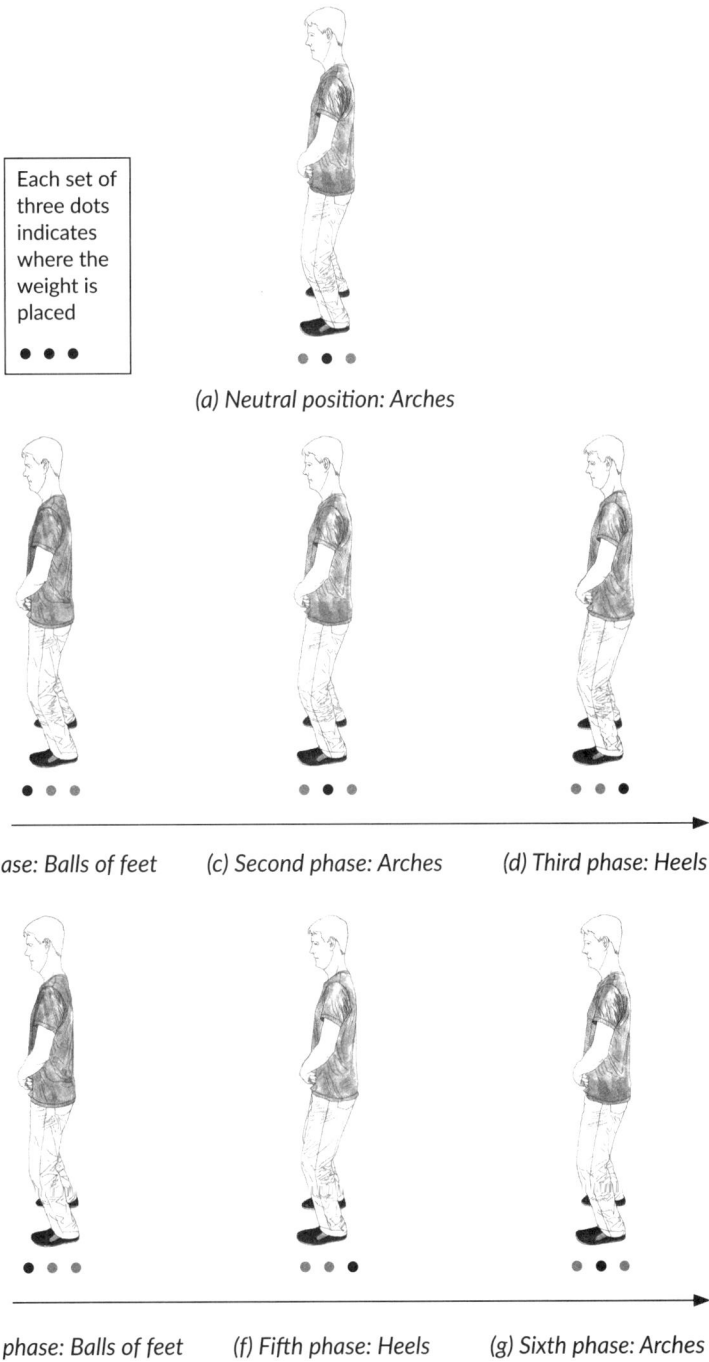

Each set of three dots indicates where the weight is placed

● ● ●

(a) Neutral position: Arches

(b) First phase: Balls of feet   *(c) Second phase: Arches*   *(d) Third phase: Heels*

(e) Fourth phase: Balls of feet   *(f) Fifth phase: Heels*   *(g) Sixth phase: Arches*

Figure 3-1: Six-Phase Weight-Shift Pattern

When practicing this sequence—shifting your weight from the arches, to the balls, to the arches, to the heels, to the balls, to the heels and back to the arches of your feet—move smoothly and slowly. At each point, rest for a few seconds, so your nerves and mind can register whether or not you arrived at the correct destination. Note the quality of your connection to your feet at each point. If you rush the process, you will jumble your nerves and confuse your mind. Moving slowly and taking your time will cultivate the correct quality of motion, allowing the technique to become second nature to you.

Practice this weight-shift pattern until you can move smoothly and continuously. Be sure you can recognize the upward and downward flows of energy, and easily activate them as directed before moving on to the next exercise. This essential component practice will be woven into form movements time and time again, and thereby serves as a means by which you can amplify and cultivate your qi.

JOINING THE WEIGHT SHIFT WITH THE ARM MOVEMENTS

The next stage in building the Heaven and Earth form is combining the weight-shift pattern with the arm movements from Chapter 2. Practicing just these two components will help you join the physical motion with the beginning method of bringing qi up and down the body before adding in many more layers and details that comprise this simple-looking yet complex qigong form.

Eventually the aim is for the weight shift to move the arms. The legs, spine and kwa always move and power the arms in neigong, so you want to put the right signal in your body from the outset to prevent your arms from taking over control. Since the weight shift ever so slightly leads the movement, it will be just ahead of any arm movement. You will start with the weight shift and allow your arms to follow. In the beginning, there is no requirement for the shift to last for the entire movement of the arms, so shift forward or backward according to the instructions, and remain there until your arms have completed that phase of the exercise.

Macrocosmic Orbit

As always practiced in qigong, begin in the neutral standing posture with your weight evenly distributed and centered over the arches of both feet (Figure 3-2a).

First Phase - Shift forward while simultaneously raising your arms up toward your crown. Once your weight is on the balls of your feet, wherever your arms may be at that moment, stay on the balls of your feet until your fingers meet at your occiput (Figure 3-2).

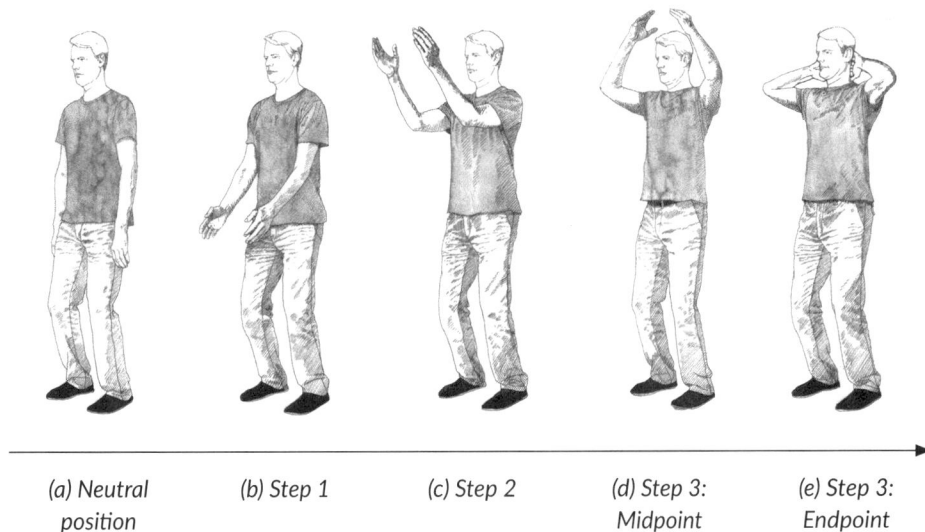

| (a) Neutral position | (b) Step 1 | (c) Step 2 | (d) Step 3: Midpoint | (e) Step 3: Endpoint |

Figure 3-2:
Combing the Weight Shift and the Arm Movements—First Phase

Shift forward onto the balls of your feet and remain there

Second Phase - Shift backward to the arches of your feet during the second-phase bend:

- Maintain the contact between your fingertips and your occiput and move your elbows around to the front of your body.
- Bring your hands over your head.
- Your palms pivot and your elbows rise.
- Then your hands and fingers sink down.

Once your weight is on the arches of your feet, stay there until your elbows are high and wide and your fingers point down toward the ground at the end of step 7 (Figure 3-3).

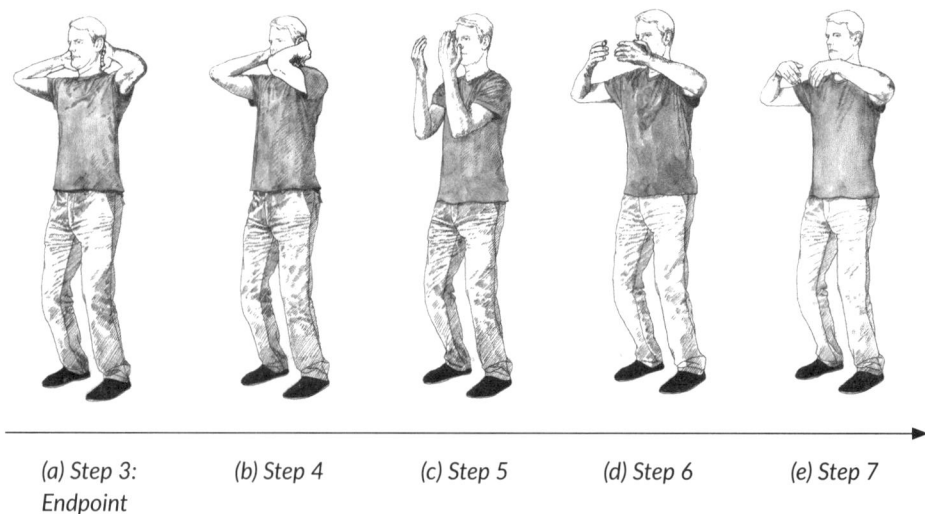

(a) Step 3: Endpoint (b) Step 4 (c) Step 5 (d) Step 6 (e) Step 7

Figure 3-3:
Combing the Weight Shift and the Arm Movements—Second Phase

Shift backward onto the arches and remain there

Third Phase - Continue shifting backward onto your heels and sink your hands down toward the ground. Once your weight arrives on your heels, remain there until your hands are at their lowest position in front of your thighs (Figure 3-4). Keep your armpits open.

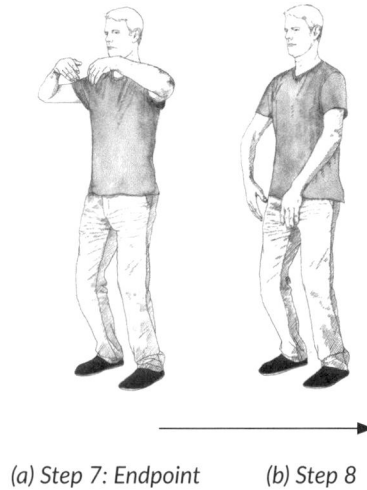

(a) Step 7: Endpoint   (b) Step 8

Figure 3-4:
Combing the Weight Shift and the Arm Movements—Third Phase

Continue shifting backward onto the heels and remain there

Microcosmic Orbit

Fourth Phase - Shift forward onto the balls of your feet as you circle your hands backward, then upward and forward. Once your weight arrives on the balls of your feet, remain there until your elbows are just in front of your lower ribs (Figure 3-5).

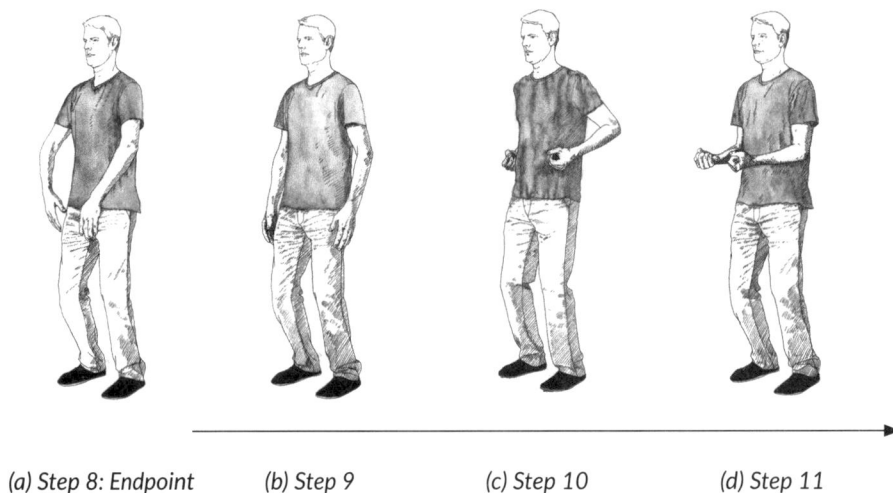

(a) Step 8: Endpoint   (b) Step 9   (c) Step 10   (d) Step 11

Figure 3-5:
Combing the Weight Shift and the Arm Movements—Fourth Phase

Shift forward onto the balls of your feet and remain there

Fifth Phase - Shift back toward your heels as your opening fists circle forward, downward and backward. Once your weight arrives on your heels, remain there until your hands have reached their destination (Figure 3-6).

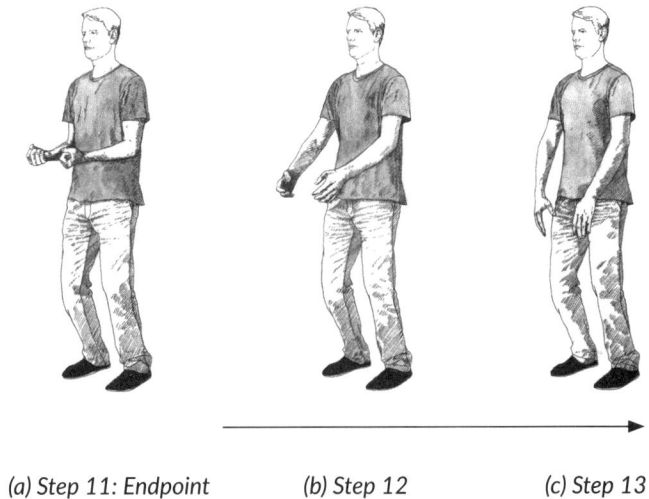

(a) Step 11: Endpoint   (b) Step 12   (c) Step 13

Figure 3-6:
Combing the Weight Shift and the Arm Movements—Fifth Phase

Shift backward onto the heels and remain there

Neutral

Sixth Phase - Shift forward onto your arches, and soften and release any tension in your arms until they come to rest on your outer thighs (Figure 3-7).

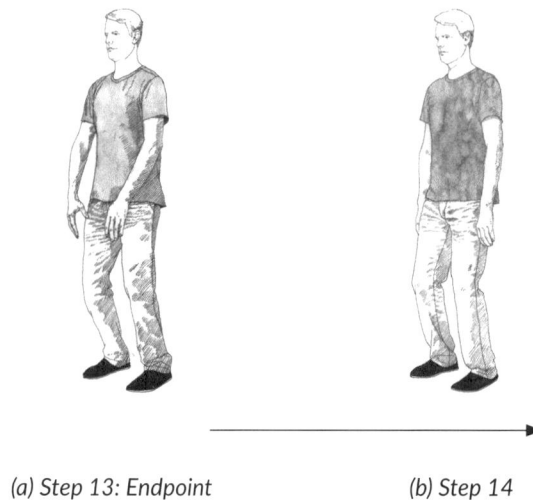

(a) Step 13: Endpoint   (b) Step 14

Figure 3-7:
Combing the Weight Shift and the Arm Movements—Sixth Phase

Shift forward onto both arches as the arms release and come to rest on the outer thighs

Important Points

Together the two components of the weight shift and the arm movements increase qi flow, which help to move your physical body. It works like this:

- **First and Fourth Phases** - As you shift your weight forward onto the balls of your feet, your *arms and qi rise* in the first-phase stretch and the fourth-phase bend.

- **Third and Fifth Phases** - As you shift backward onto your heels, your *arms and qi descend* in the third-phase and fifth-phase stretches.

- **Second Phase** - As you shift backward onto your arches, the *upward and downward qi flows become balanced* in the second-phase bend as your hands begin at your occiput and finish in front of your face/throat. There is no significant rise or fall of the hands or qi.

- **Sixth Phase** - As you shift forward on your arches, allow the mobilized qi to gather and bank at your lower tantien as you *release* to neutral—again without any significant rise or fall of your hands.

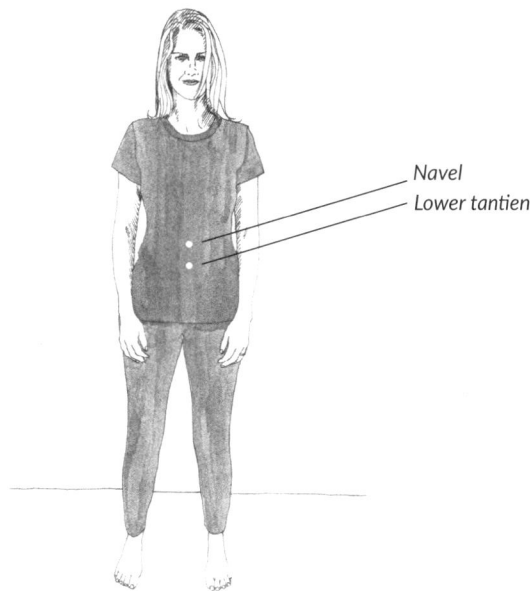

Navel
Lower tantien

Figure 3-8

The *lower tantien* is located an inch or two below the navel in the center of the body and is the central energy gate, which governs the entire physicality and subtle energy anatomy of the body (Figure 3-8).

The arm movements and qi techniques reinforce one another. In the beginning, the process of clearing out the channels is initiated by moving the arms and shifting weight. Later the movement of energy up and down the body assists in raising and sinking the arms. As qi techniques come online, the arms require less effort to move and so generate a deeper sense of relaxation, which mobilizes more qi. Over time the effort required by the arms becomes absolutely minimal and the flow of qi becomes far stronger.

Intermediate Practitioners

All of the beginning instructions apply except, once you become familiar with the beginning method, each weight shift should last for the entirety of the corresponding arm movement. The shifting motion remains constant and never becomes static. In this way, you will arrive at the designated weight-shift points in the exact moment your arms complete each phase of motion, and both the weight shift and your arms will change at the same moment in time.

REVIEW

So far you have learned the basic Heaven and Earth exercise with some internal content. Continue practicing these component exercises while learning the next few in order to:

- Become familiar with the material and begin the process of embodying each individual technique in its own right.
- Easily, correctly and seamlessly layer in additional techniques set out in this section—without errors or distortions.

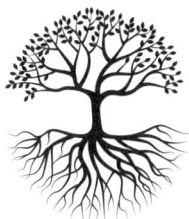

CHAPTER 4:

THE KWA SQUAT
AND THE C-CURVE

THE KWA

The *kwa* is a Chinese energetic concept that does not have a specific physical equivalent in Western anatomy and physiology. It encompasses the area on each side of the body extending from the hip fold, through the inside of the pelvis to the top of the hip bones (iliac crest) and back to the lower spine (Figure 4-1). One of the primary functions of the kwa is to connect the legs to the spine via the pelvis; at the center of this area is where the psoas muscles are situated. These muscles enable you to sit upright in a chair and walk around. There are many other muscles engaged in these actions, but all of these are subordinate to the psoas. The psoas muscles directly connect the thigh bones (femur) to the lower back (lumbar vertebrae) and, in so doing, run deeply through the pelvis. These are the muscles you will attempt to activate and engage when doing a kwa squat.

Psoas muscle

Lumbar spine

Iliac crest

Sacrum

Pelvis

Tailbone

Hip joint

Adductor
muscles

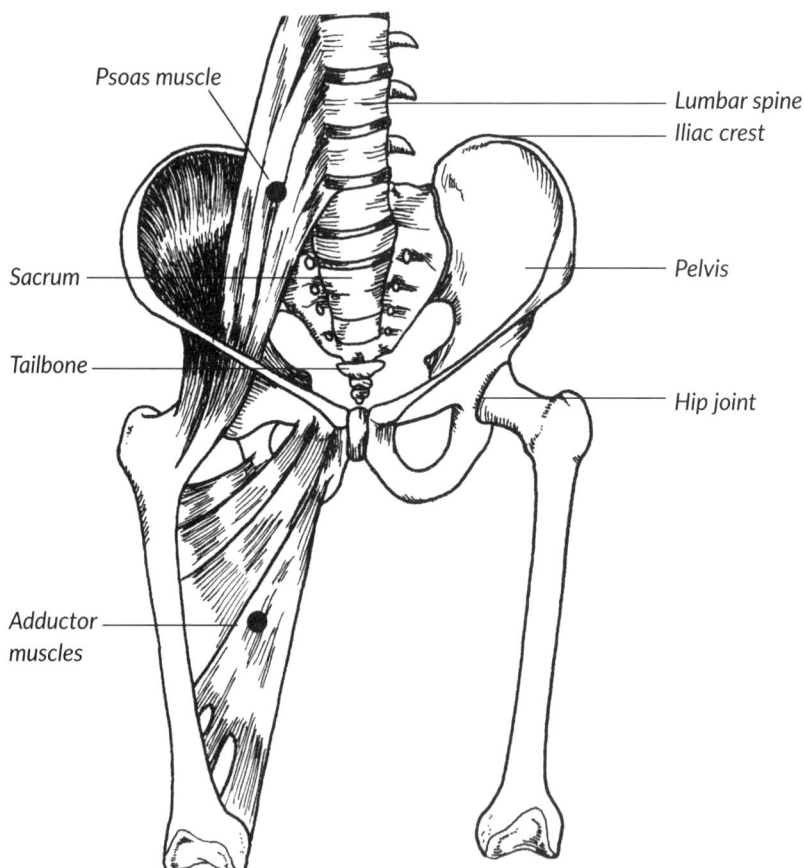

Figure 4-1:
The Kwa

THE KWA SQUAT

The kwa squat is both a preliminary exercise for correctly activating the kwa and psoas muscles, and the technique that leads, drives and powers physical motion in Heaven and Earth Qigong. The importance of developing refined control over and skill with engaging your kwa cannot be overstated. There are many levels and layers to activating the kwa with various ways each can be applied. In this section, you will learn the guidelines for engaging and activating your kwa with more in-depth considerations presented in stages and sprinkled throughout this text.

PRELIMINARY EXERCISE: SIT IN A CHAIR

To get an idea of the basic motion:

1. Sit on a dining-room-style chair and place your feet directly under your knees.
2. Stand up and sit down a few times without moving your knees.

In this exercise, you will actually squat much more than when integrated in both the kwa squat and the Heaven and Earth form, but it helps to get the basic rhythm.

PRELIMINARY EXERCISE: FIND THE INGUINAL GROOVES

Notice how when you sit down, you fold at the hips and when you rise, they unfold. The places where the hips fold are called the "inguinal grooves," which you can locate by simply standing on one leg and raising your other knee. The place where the hip naturally folds and a woman's bikini line cuts diagonally across the leg is the inguinal groove (Figure 4-2).

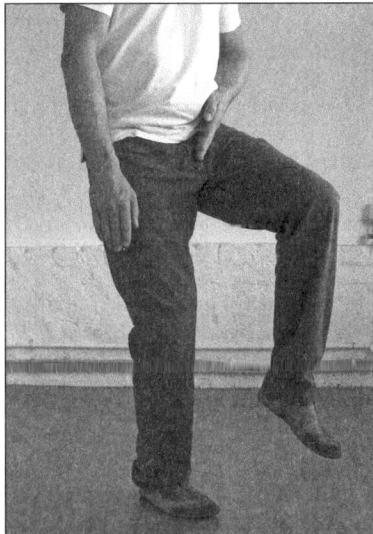

Figure 4-2: Find the Inguinal Groove

Place your hands in your inguinal grooves for feedback and:

- Squat down a little by folding in your inguinal grooves (Figure 4-3a).
- Then slowly come up and return to the neutral position.

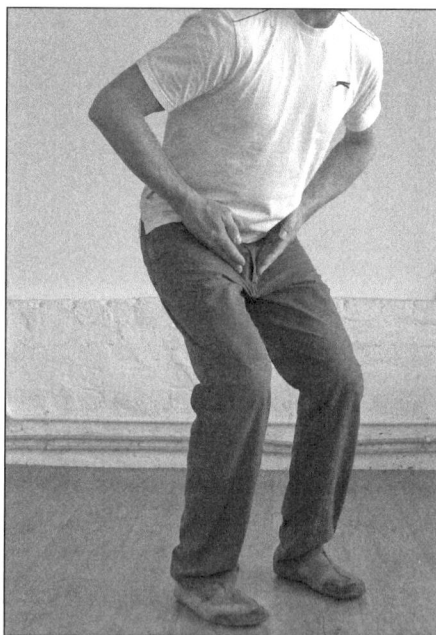

(a) Fold at the hips

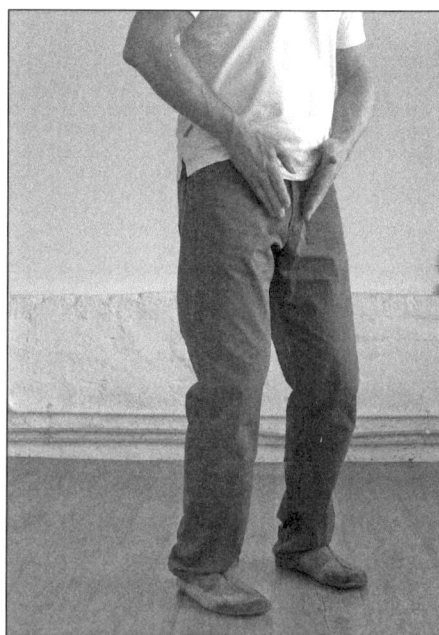

(b) Neutral position

Figure 4-3: Fold in the Inguinal Grooves

BASIC KWA SQUAT

Begin in the neutral standing posture with your hands on your lower belly and relax (Figure 4-4a). Nothing significant happens in qigong without softness and relaxation.

1. Slowly lower your buttocks (gluteal muscles) as if you were going to sit in a chair, but only go down a few inches (Figure 4-4b).

2. Slowly come back up to return to the neutral position (Figure 4-4c).

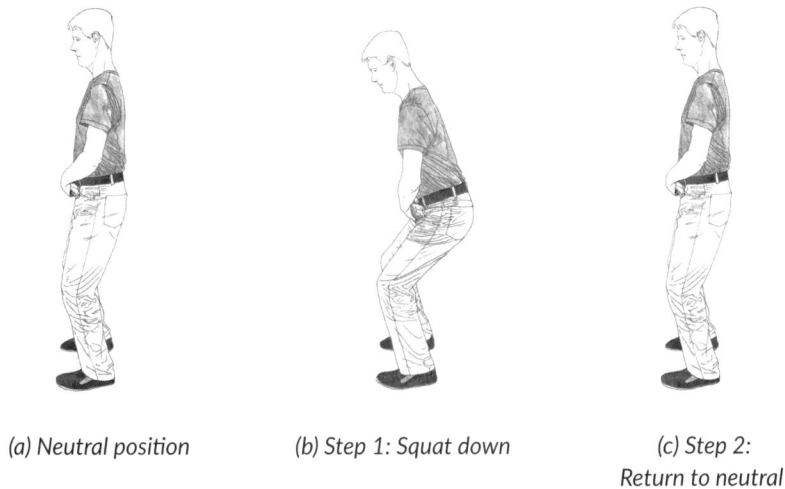

(a) Neutral position   (b) Step 1: Squat down   (c) Step 2:
                                                           Return to neutral

Figure 4-4:
Basic Kwa Squat

Important Points

Practice this exercise a few times and feel your body through all aspects of both the downward and upward motions with the following parameters in mind:

- Your knees stay absolutely still in space—without any forward, backward or sideways movement as you sink down and rise up.

- Keep your spine straight through both steps and do not arch your back, stick out your buttocks, raise your chest or collapse your neck.

- Fold in your inguinal grooves on the descent and unfold on the ascent.

BENDING AND STRETCHING THE KWA

Begin in the neutral standing posture and take a few moments to relax (Figure 4-5a).

1. To descend, drop the back of your pelvis, sacrum and tailbone, fold in your inguinal grooves and allow the weight of your body to naturally shift backward onto your heels (Figure 4-5b).

2. To rise up, stretch your kwa open as you lift and drive your tailbone forward onto the balls of your feet (Figure 4-5c).

3. Release into the neutral position as you relax back onto the arches of your feet (Figure 4-5d).

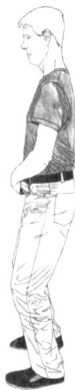

(a) Neutral position   (b) Step 1:
Squat down   (c) Step 2:
Stretch open onto
the balls of the feet   (d) Step 3:
Return to neutral

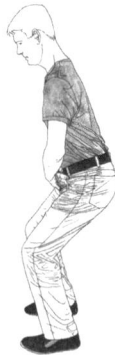

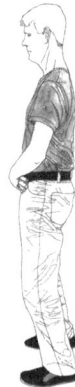

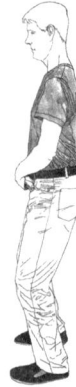

Figure 4-5:
Bending and Stretching the Kwa

Important Points

- As you descend and ascend, your knees act as hinges: they do not project forward beyond your toes on the descent; and they do not move backward as you rise up. This action is responsible for bending and stretching the psoas and the kwa.

- Fold in the inguinal grooves to bend your kwa on the descent and slightly stretch your kwa upward on the ascent.

- As you descend, do not push your buttocks backward; as you rise, do not lift your chest or arch your back.

- Your spine remains relatively straight throughout the whole process, but you can lean forward a little as you descend—as long as your shoulders do not project forward beyond your knees. As you rise up, bring your spine to the vertical position once again.

BOWING AND STRAIGHTENING THE SPINE

The next step in building the Heaven and Earth form is learning how to correctly bow and straighten your spine. The spine is central to all neigong, especially high-level practice, since it connects the arms to the legs and supports the internal organs. Without this fundamental connection, the arms and legs move independently of each other, which is never practiced in neigong training.

The Tai Chi Classics, a collection of articles that cover all the once closely guarded and secret internal principles of tai chi (see Bibliography), states, "When one part moves, all parts move; when one part stops, all parts stop," which has two primary levels of meaning:

- If any body part is moving, such as an elbow, hand, knee, foot, spine or joint, then every other body part is also moving.

- If one neigong thread is active, then all other neigong threads are active and integrated within the form. This is the goal and definitely not the starting point.

This principle also applies to unifying the entire spinal column to move as one seamless, integrated unit, instead of only moving parts of the spine while others remain dormant or out of sync. This is why the first port of call for spinal techniques within the Wood Element is to unify and integrate the entire spinal column, pelvis and skull. After some weeks or months of focused practice, the spine can be efficiently and effectively integrated into the Heaven and Earth form to create further unity.

THE ORIGIN OF MOVEMENT IN THE SPINE

In order to fully integrate spinal motions, start by focusing on feeling the back and front of your spine as you move from each at different points in the form.

- When bowing your spine, move from the back of your spine.
- When straightening your spine, move from the front of your spine.

These markers allow you to open up the back and front of your spine independently of one another, enabling more profound access to your spine, so you can contact and release progressively deeper tensions over time.

This independent control and movement of the spine does not break the Taoist Principle of "one part moves, all parts move" because the whole spine moves. You cannot move and stretch open the back of your spine without the front being affected and the opposite is also true. It is only the point of focus and origin of the motion that changes—either the back or the front.

THREE DISTINCT MOTIONS OF THE SPINE

Heaven and Earth Qigong uses three distinct motions in the spine, which are:

- Hooking the neck
- Rolling the lower (lumbar) spine/pelvis
- Drawing back the middle of the spine

You will learn how to move each part independently before combining the three motions to form one complete C-curve.

1. Hook the Neck

The hooking-the-neck component practice is for the upper spine. The aim is to stretch open the back of your neck/spine as you bend/bow, and the front of your spine as you straighten/stretch up. At the end of each bowing-and-straightening cycle, spend a few seconds relaxing and releasing your spine, neck and nerves before repeating the exercise. Failing to relax and release can lead to excessive force being put through the neck and occipital region on the next repetition, which could cause a soft-tissue strain. As covered in Chapter 1, the occipital area is one of the most vulnerable places in the body, so practice extra carefully and softly in the beginning, until you have a good sense of how the exercise affects you and you can accurately gauge the right amount of effort required.

Safety Tip: Practice with a chair or sofa behind you, so that if you experience any dizziness or become disorientated, you can easily sit down and rest. Do not force your body. The stretching process is slow and progressive in terms of the number of repetitions you can do in a single practice session and over the weeks, months and years of regular training. All comes to those who practice with patience.

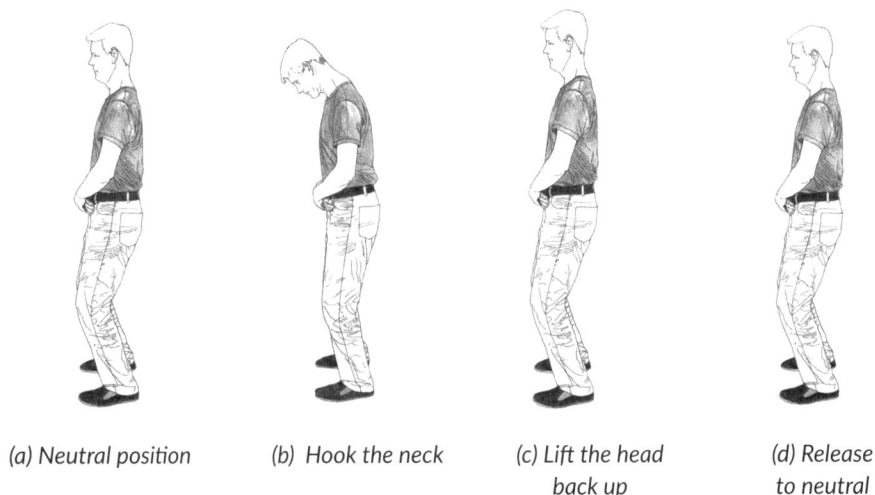

(a) Neutral position   (b) Hook the neck   (c) Lift the head back up   (d) Release to neutral

Figure 4-6: Hook the Neck

*Hooking the neck opens the back of the spine
while lifting the head backward and upward opens the front of the spine.*

Always take the time to set up the correct standing posture (Figure 4-6a).

1. First, to understand what NOT to do:

   (a) Place your fingertips in your throat notch—the space between the two collar bones (clavicles), where they join with the top of the breast bone (sternum)—to give you a point of reference and feedback (Figure 4-7).

   (b) Just allow your chin to drop down and make contact with your fingers.

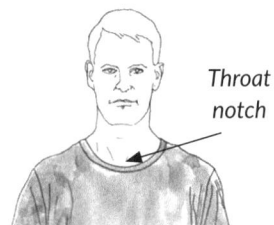

Throat notch

Figure 4-7

   Notice how the space between your chin and the top of your sternum diminishes dramatically. This is a disconnected motion, lacking the connectivity through the neck that enables the hooking action to open up the top part of the spine.

2. Then, to hook the neck correctly, keep your fingers on your throat notch and realign your head, so it is vertical and not tilting backward or to either side.

   (a) Put your mind in your occipital area, where your fingers would touch at the end of the first phase (step 3) of the macrocosmic orbit.

   (b) From this place, lift your occiput slightly and bend your neck forward; the crown of your head moves up toward the sky ever so slightly, then forward and finally downward in a continuous arc (Figure 4-6b). When done correctly, the space between your chin and the top of your sternum hardly reduces at all *and* you obtain a good stretch in the back of your neck. In the newly acquired position, you should be able to place your fist between your chin and your sternum.

3. Bring your head back up to the neutral position, albeit a little higher than before (Figure 4-6c). You do not simply move your head back, which would cause the stretch to dissipate in the back of the neck and would close down the occiput. Instead, bring your head upright by your mind contacting the front of your spine (behind your throat) and lifting your head backward and upward from that place. When done correctly, some of the space you have previously created in the back of your spine will be maintained, you will open up the front of your spine and you will keep your occipital area open. The center of your eyes should be on a horizontal line with the center of your ear and your skull sits on top of your spine without jutting forward.

4. At the end of the move, relax and release everything in your head, neck, jaw, eyes and mind, and let your neck shrink slightly to return to neutral. This step is essential to prevent any tension from building, and for developing a healthy neck and spine (Figure 4-6d).

5. Repeat steps 1-4 several times while monitoring how this action affects your system.

2. Roll the Lumbar Spine/Pelvis

This rolling-the-pelvis component practice is for the lower spine.

From the neutral standing position, put one hand on your lower belly and the other hand on your sacrum/tailbone to give you feedback as you perform this intricate motion (Figure 4-8a). The aim is to roll your pelvis so that your back hand drops and your front hand rises, which requires the center of your pelvis to pivot.

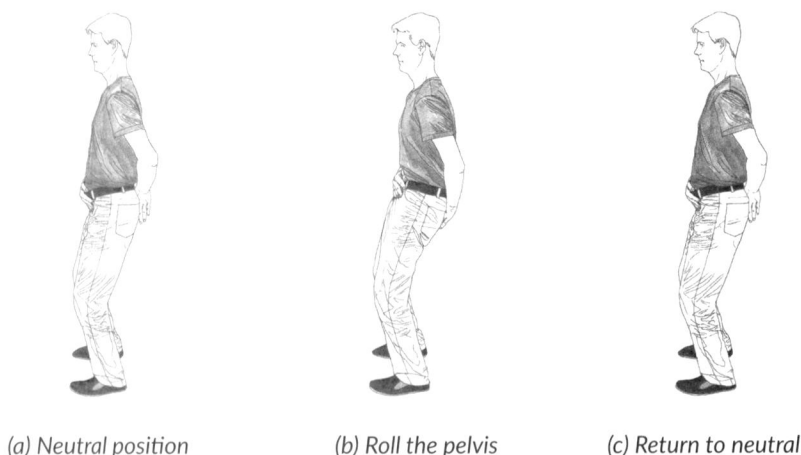

(a) Neutral position   (b) Roll the pelvis   (c) Return to neutral

Figure 4-8: Roll the Pelvis

In the isolated pelvic roll, the inguinal grooves go flat

1. Your tailbone drops and gently tucks under, stretching open the lower back (lumbar vertebrae). See Figure 4-8b.

    (a) The height of your body/head does not descend and you will not lean backward.

    (b) The area of the inguinal grooves becomes flat, which is acceptable for an isolated component practice, but not for the standing position, the kwa squat or moving in Heaven and Earth Qigong.

2. From the tucked under position, roll your pelvis backward to the original standing position.

(a) Make sure you do not roll backward too far, which will cause your back to arch.

(b) When you have completed the return, you should be in the neutral standing posture.

Practice a few repetitions to get the hang of it.

3. Repeat one more roll of your pelvis to tuck under your tailbone. Then, from the tucked position, this time put your mind in your tailbone (at the very bottom of your spine) and, as you engage the return of your pelvis, feel for the sense of smoothly and gently driving your tailbone down toward your feet (Figure 4-8c). Feel your tailbone and do not exert any excess physical force during the process—this is a soft, internal motion.

    (a) There is no need to focus on the backward motion of the pelvis as this will happen naturally *if* the tailbone goes down. If you focus on the backward motion, you will not get the downward motion and instead will more likely find yourself pushing your buttocks backward and arching your back, which disconnect the upper and lower parts of your spine.

    (b) When you get the downward motion of the tailbone, the pressure in your feet will increase slightly and you will naturally open up the front of your lower spine, which is the purpose of this part of the exercise.

    (c) Relax and release to neutral.

4. Repeat step 3 several times gently encouraging your spine to open up. The lumbar spine is a vulnerable area, so do not force your body. Also, make sure the downward pressure goes through the back of your knees onto your feet, and never allow the pressure to go into the knee joints themselves.

Important: The knee is a weight-transferring joint, not a weight-bearing joint (as will be covered in detail in Chapter 17). The space at the back of the knee is designed to transfer the body's load to the foot. If you experience any excess pressure or pain in your lower back or knees, it is a sign that you are misaligned or using too much force. Stop, rest and revisit this exercise after a break.

Many back problems originate in the lower spine and are caused by the front spinal vertebrae being too closed or tense. When done correctly, the tucking process opens up the back of the lumbar spine, while the downward motion of the tailbone on the return maintains some of that space and opens up more space on the front of the spine. The increased pressure in your feet may raise your torso slightly, which is a sign that you are on the right track—as long as you do not extend your knees.

3. Draw Back the Middle of the Spine

So far you have learned how the top part of the spine curves over and the bottom part curves under. These two forces alone can stretch a large part of the back of your spine. Now you will learn how to activate the middle part of your spine, the area behind your solar plexus/diaphragm (Figure 4-9).

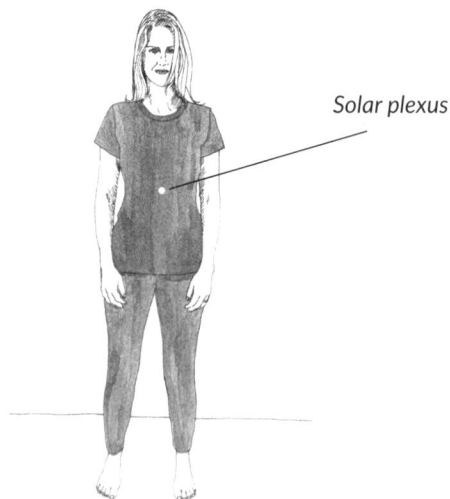

Solar plexus

Figure 4-9:
Solar Plexus

The solar plexus is just below the breast bone (sternum)

If done correctly, the middle part of your spine drawing directly backward will stretch open the back of your mid spine. When done in unison with the first two exercises, the whole spine becomes connected in a single flex. However, for now, stay focused on activating only the mid spine itself.

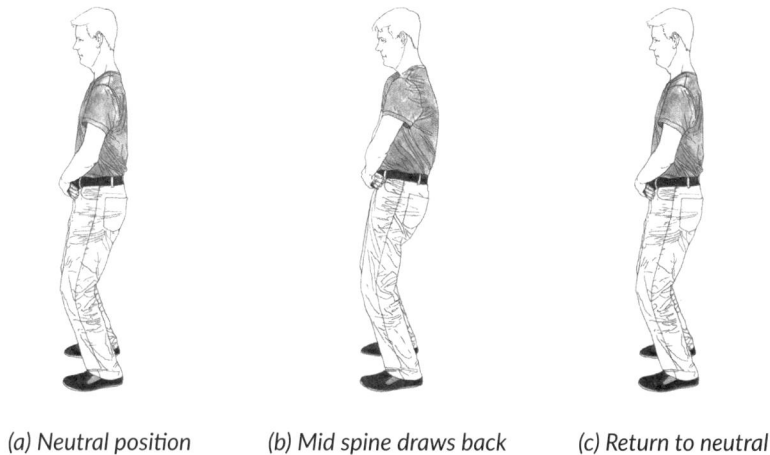

(a) Neutral position   (b) Mid spine draws back   (c) Return to neutral

Figure 4-10:
Draw Back the Mid Spine

From the neutral posture, bring your mind to the back of your spine and into the space opposite to your solar plexus (Figure 4-10a). You can ask a training partner to touch and maintain contact with that area of your spine, so your mind can more easily connect to the exact space you wish to feel for the duration of the following exercise.

1. Keeping your pelvis, shoulders and head still in space, slowly draw back your mid spine a few inches. Move as smoothly as possible, without any sudden or jerky motions (Figure 4-10b).

2. When you have drawn back your mid spine as far as you can without excess force, slowly allow your spine to naturally return to the neutral posture once again (Figure 4-10c). As before, the feeling is like slowly guiding the release of a rubber band back to the neutral state as opposed to just letting go at the most stretched point and allowing it to snap back to neutral.

3. Repeat steps 1-2 several times while attempting to gain control over moving from your mid spine and stretching open the back of your mid spine.

Important: If you draw back your mid spine and allow your pelvis, shoulders and/or head to come with it, you simply displace your bodyweight and unplug from your feet. For this reason, you must anchor in place these body parts. The backward motion of the mid spine is meant to stretch the tissues in and around the middle of your spine and torso.

The action of drawing back the mid spine creates a lot of space for the chest to sink into the belly, an important aspect of neigong training. If you try to force your chest downward without first creating the internal space for it to travel inward through your torso, you will simply put unwanted tension and pressure into your heart and other internal organs. Conversely, if you retract your mid spine, your internal organs will come along for the ride and your chest can naturally sink into the newly created space. Practice drawing back your mid spine several times, while gently dropping your chest as you do so.

THE C-CURVE:
BENDING AND STRETCHING THE SPINE

Once you are familiar with the three component exercises for creating a spinal curve, and you have gained some understanding and skill from practicing each of them individually, you can join them together into one exercise.

The C-curve exercise has three parts:

*   Bend to create the "C" form.
*   Release back to the neutral position.
*   Stretch to open the spine.

When working with the spine as a standalone exercise, you will begin by moving from the mid spine. This initiation point changes when you put the spinal C-curve into Heaven and Earth, which will be covered in the following section.

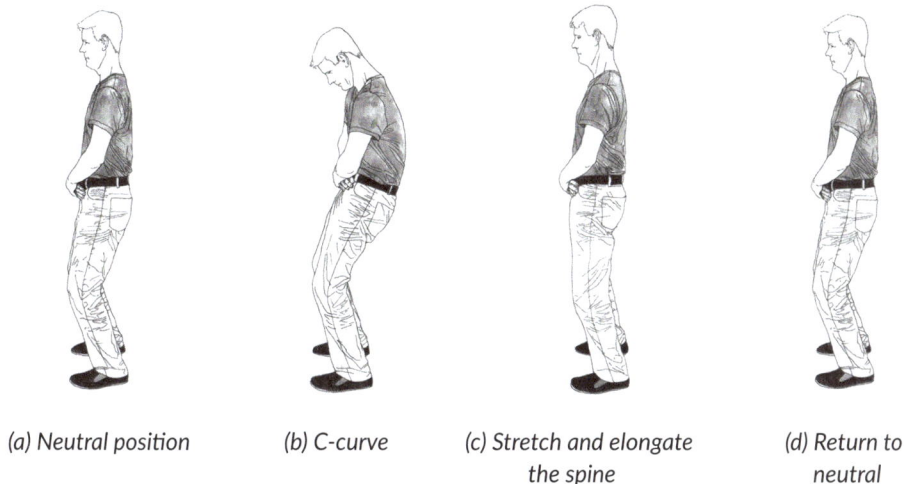

(a) Neutral position   (b) C-curve   (c) Stretch and elongate the spine   (d) Return to neutral

Figure 4-11: Spinal C-curve

First, begin in the neutral standing posture and take a minute to relax and contact your spine with your mind (Figure 4-11a).

1. Bend - From your mid spine, start to draw back and, as soon as you do, simultaneously begin hooking your neck and rolling your pelvis under. All three motions should be coordinated in tandem yet are initiated from the mid spine (Figure 4-11b).

2. Stretch - From the C-curve, you will once again initiate the next motion from your mid spine by moving forward (Figure 4-11c). Immediately your tailbone starts to drive down and your neck stretches up until you reach the original position—albeit a bit more open than when you started from your tailbone and neck having extended in opposite directions.

3. Neutral - The last action is to slowly release and soften your whole spine—without collapsing—and return to the neutral position (Figure 4-11d).

4. Repeat steps 1-3 half a dozen times, then rest and feel what this deep, spinal exercise does to your system before training any further.

Important: Once moving, ensure all three areas of the spine are active—the mid spine draws back, and the skull and tailbone move forward. Ideally, all three movements finish at the exact same moment in time to ensure an even stretch throughout the back (posterior) of the spine and to create more internal space into which your chest can sink. When you have reached the final position, from the side your spine will look like the letter "C," at least to some degree, hence the name "C-curve."

BENEFITS OF THE C-CURVE

The benefits of this component exercise go far beyond creating flexibility in and control over your spine. Many people have stiff, inactive, dormant, closed or even partially fused vertebrae. The four exercises covered in this section that target the three parts of the spine as well as the complete C-curve give you a means for recognizing, locating, accessing and opening up the various parts of your spine, especially those needing attention. Once you begin to open up your spine, the nerve roots—the exit points for the nerve pathways from the spinal cord—and the spinal cord itself become freer and, thereby, allow all the signals travelling along this information superhighway to flow unobstructed, or at least less obstructed. Since the spinal cord plugs directly into the brain, the junction through which every signal between the brain and the body travels, the occipital region, where the spinal cord connects to the brain, requires the utmost care and attention.

When the complete exercise is done correctly, the whole ribcage also flexes and loosens, which releases tensions that can otherwise trap the internal organs within the thoracic cavity, thereby literally giving those organs more space to breathe. The combination of the thoracic spine flexing and opening up is the mechanism by which tension is released from both the spine itself and the ribcage to take pressure off the upper internal organs, especially the heart. The same release of tension also occurs in the lower organs and the diaphragm via the lumbar vertebrae, all of which are attached to the spine through a series of ligaments and which stretch and release along with the abdominal muscles. All of this goes toward releasing deeply bound tension both externally and internally, in and around the belly, so your internal organs can function properly. Your organs are responsible for your health as they pump blood, digest food, regulate immune functions and oxygenate your body. All deep, internal exercise physically and energetically targets the organs—since they determine your state of health and wellbeing—which the C-curve brings alive.

JOINING THE KWA SQUAT AND THE C-CURVE

Both the kwa squat and the C-curve activate the lower (lumbar) spine, so this area where the two link is of particular importance.

Another area of interest is that of the inguinal grooves (hip folds). In the C-curve, as a standalone exercise, it is permissible (and even encouraged to get the full range of motion in the lumbar spine) to allow the inguinal grooves to disappear from sight, that is to go flat. However, in the kwa squat, you will disconnect from your psoas muscles and deactivate your kwa if you allow your inguinal grooves to go flat. Therefore, to integrate the two, you must adhere to the following instructions carefully.

PREPARATORY EXERCISE: BASIC KWA SQUAT

From the neutral standing posture, practice the basic kwa squat from the beginning of this chapter (Figure 4-4) a few times with your palms contacting your inguinal grooves to provide feedback.

1. To bend - fold in your inguinal grooves as you squat down and release your gluteal muscles, sacrum and tailbone, sinking them down toward your feet as your weight goes into your heels.
2. To stretch - drive your tailbone forward, bringing your weight onto the balls of your feet as you lift up your torso and stretch open your kwa.

COMBINE THE KWA SQUAT AND THE PELVIC ROLL

Now we will combine the kwa squat and the pelvic roll, the second part of the spinal curve (Figure 4-12). All you need to do is join these two pieces together correctly as follows.

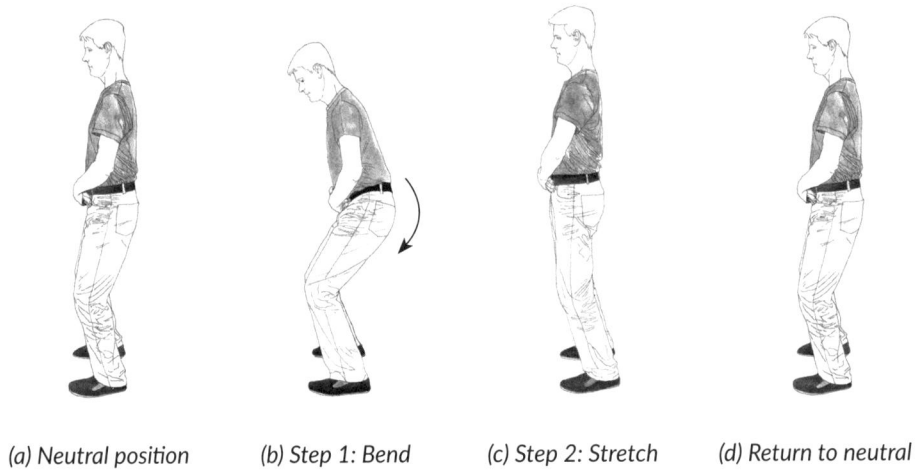

(a) Neutral position   (b) Step 1: Bend   (c) Step 2: Stretch   (d) Return to neutral

Figure 4-12:
Combine the Kwa Squat and the Pelvic Roll

Beginning-level students:
Place the edge of your hands in your inguinal grooves to give you
more feedback as you practice this intricate motion

Bending/Curving

Start in the neutral standing posture and place the edge of your hands on your inguinal grooves or your lower belly to provide feedback (Figure 4-12a).

1. Begin by dropping the back of your pelvis (gluteal muscles, sacrum and tailbone) and folding in your inguinal grooves. As soon as your hands register that the inguinal grooves are folding, begin to roll the back of your pelvis by tucking your tailbone under and forward as it descends. See Figure 4-12b.

(a) Do not overdo it by applying too much force.

(b) Keep your tailbone descending all the time you roll under the back of your pelvis and always maintain a crease in your inguinal grooves.

(c) If done correctly, your weight will shift backward onto your heels and your knees will feel stable. There will be a slight fold in your inguinal grooves and your lower spine will curve under.

Stretching/Straightening

2. In this step, there are two opposite actions: opening the kwa and straightening your spine. (Figure 4-12c).

   From the perspective of the kwa, the tailbone drives forward and upward to stretch open the kwa; from the perspective of the spine, the tailbone drives downward to straighten and stretch the lower (lumbar) spine. When these two combine, the tailbone drives forward with a slight downward action, which opens the kwa deeper than in the previous exercises. This motion happens as you simultaneously shift your weight onto the balls of your feet and straighten your lumbar spine, which adds a little extra pressure in your feet and stretches your psoas muscles that bit deeper.

   (a) Adhere to the 70-Percent Rule and be mindful not to apply too much force.

   (b) Maintain your knee alignments and make sure your knees feel comfortable.

3. Relax to release the extra pressure in your legs and feet, and bring your weight back onto the arches of your feet. This action brings you back to the neutral position (Figure 4-12d).

Important Points

- Always maintain your knee alignments and never use so much force that you could strain your knees or your lower spine.

- When done correctly, the movement should be smooth, easy, comfortable and pleasant on the body, creating flexibility and increasing blood circulation.

- If your temperature rises a few degrees, it is not only normal, but also a sign that you are on the right track. Increased blood and qi flow through gentle, repetitive, slow-motion exercise creates a felt sense of heat and is one of the many benefits of qigong.

The Kwa Is the Leader and the Engine

When practicing the C-curve as a standalone exercise, the movement is initiated from the mid spine. When practicing the kwa squat, the movement is initiated from the lower spine (sacrum and tailbone). When combining the two, the kwa becomes the leader. The kwa leads while the spine and the rest of the body (including the arms), follow. The kwa squat not only becomes the leader, but also the engine, both leading and powering the motion.

The kwa produces power by connecting the legs to the spine (via the psoas muscles and various other body parts), which creates a unified motion. Internal power never solely relies on one part. The aim is to integrate the whole body to produce smooth, connected power that is significantly more than any single body part can produce on its own.

COMBINE THE KWA SQUAT AND THE C-CURVE

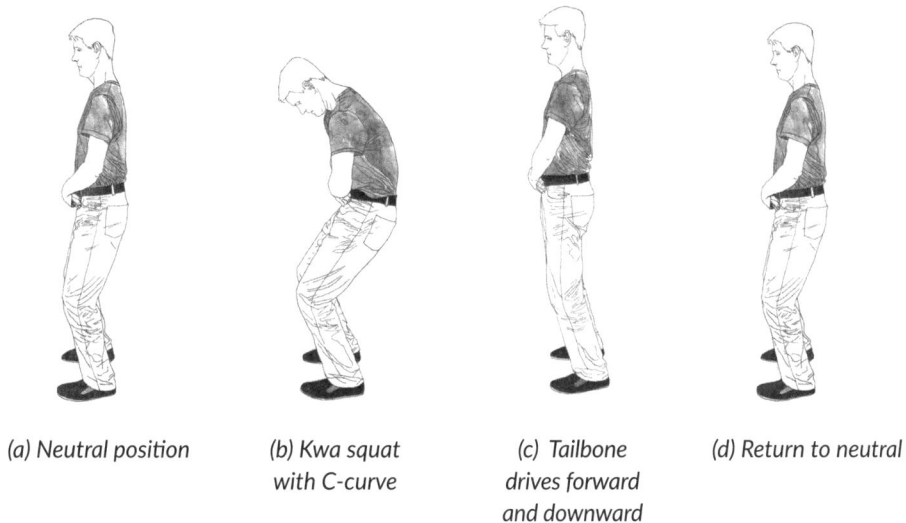

(a) Neutral position   (b) Kwa squat with C-curve   (c) Tailbone drives forward and downward   (d) Return to neutral

Figure 4-13: Combine the Kwa Squat and the C-Curve

Start in the neutral standing posture and relax (Figure 4-13a).

1. Initiate the bending action with the kwa squat and, as soon as you begin to fold in your inguinal grooves, start tucking under your tailbone, which activates the spine and the three vectors of the spine—all of which happen simultaneously (Figure 4-13b):

   (a) The tailbone sinks downward, under and forward.

   (b) The mid spine draws back.

   (c) The neck hooks forward.

2. Initiate the stretching action by driving your tailbone forward and downward to open your kwa, which straightens your spine and drives your head up (Figure 4-13c). The opposite actions of the lower spine driving down and the upper spine lifting up allows you to maintain some of the opening in the back of the spine while stretching open the front of your spine.

3. Relax into the neutral position while softening your body and mind before repeating the exercise (Figure 4-13d).

Important Points

- The movement of the kwa engages motion in the three parts of the spine with the C-curve and straightening actions, thereby activating the whole spine.

- You want the kwa squat and all three sections of your spine to move as one unit rather than disconnected pieces. Just to achieve this level of practice takes time and focus.

- On the bend, the full C-curve is complete (via the stretch in the posterior/back part of the spine) at the moment the kwa finishes bending. Your weight will end up on your heels.

- On the stretch, the spine becomes straight and elongates (via the anterior/front of the spine) at the moment the kwa finishes stretching open. Your weight will end up on the balls of your feet.

- At the end of each round, spend a few seconds softening to neutral to release your nerves and refocus for the next round. Your weight will be on the arches of your feet. It is better to do a few accurate movements while remaining present rather than many sloppy repetitions.

REVIEW

In this chapter you learned and combined two critically important aspects of Heaven and Earth Qigong—the kwa squat and the C-curve—which require time, energy and practice to develop. Continue practicing these components individually and in unison in order to refine your technique, access and release tensions from your body, open up your system and reap the full range of potential benefits from qigong training.

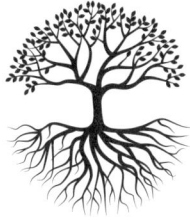

CHAPTER 5:

COMPLETING THE BASIC HEAVEN AND EARTH FORM

HOW TO ASSEMBLE THE BASIC COMPONENTS

First you learned the arm movements and the weight-shift pattern of Heaven and Earth Qigong, then joined them together. Next you learned how to do the kwa squat and the C-curve, then joined them together. Now we will unify the two streams to complete the basic Heaven and Earth form with some of the essential internal content. Hereafter any additional content is all about adding depth and nuance to your form in order to achieve higher states of practice by increasing qi flow for health and healing, martial arts and meditation.

This process follows the Taoist Principle of Separate and Combine, where each component is teased out, broken down into smaller, more easily digestible pieces and practiced individually to hone your skill set before seamlessly recombining them back into one whole.

In Heaven and Earth Qigong, the primary four components are:

- The arm movements
- The weight shift
- The kwa squat
- The C-curve.

Apart from the fact that your mind must be able to focus on all four components at the same time, the biggest challenge is joining the weight shift and the kwa squat. However, if you have sufficiently practiced all four components, independently and in pairs, you are likely to find the combination process much easier because your body and mind will be familiar with the territory.

If you struggle with the next set of instructions, or you experience major discomfort or pain of any kind, stop practicing the combined exercises and spend more time on the previous two streams until you have them down pat. If you find you cannot practice without pain or discomfort, you should seek out guidance from a qualified teacher who can correct your mistakes or show you how to make the necessary personal adjustments. Qigong training does not normally cause pain—or even significant discomfort. Spend time practicing the component exercises while carefully following the instructions and adhering to your 70-percent range of motion in body, mind and qi.

JOINING THE ARM MOVEMENTS AND WEIGHT SHIFT WITH THE KWA SQUAT AND C-CURVE

From the perspective of the arms, the weight:

- Shifts forward as the arms rise up.
- Shifts backward as the arms descend.

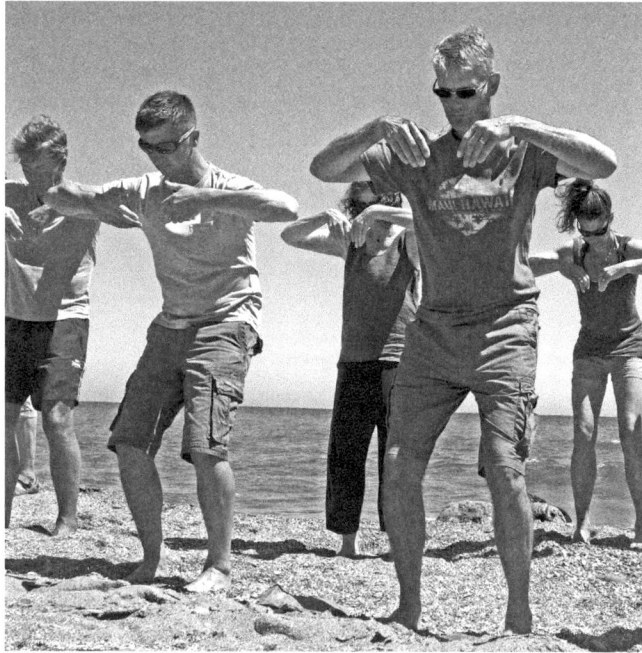

PHOTO BY JACKIE SMITH

Completing the first C-curve in
Heaven and Earth Qigong, Crete, 2019

From the perspective of the kwa squat, the weight:

- Shifts backward during the bending phase.
- Shifts forward during the stretching phase.

Now you will learn how to join these two components from the perspective of the six-phase sequence, stretch-bend-stretch-bend-stretch-release, with which you are already familiar.

The first time you join these components together, simply combine the kwa squat with the C-curve and the weight shift, and leave out the arm movements. This will allow you to focus on unifying these two important and seemingly conflicting components. Once you are familiar with the motion, add your arms. The following instructions are the same whether or not your arms are involved.

Figure 5-1: The Marriage of Heaven and Earth Qigong—Basic Form (Front View)

MACROCOSMIC ORBIT

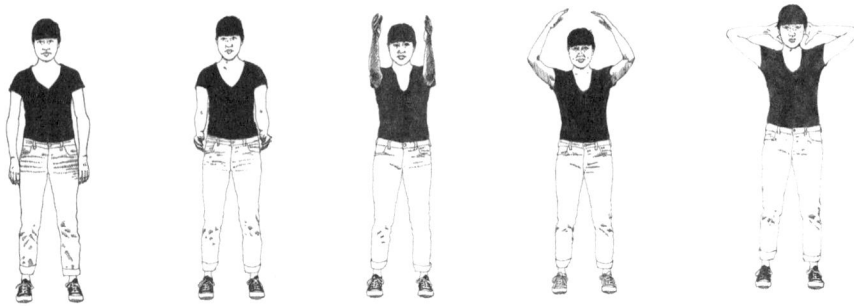

(a) Neutral posture   (b) Step 1   (c) Step 2   (d) Step 3: Midpoint   (e) Step 3: Endpoint

First-Phase Stretch ⟶

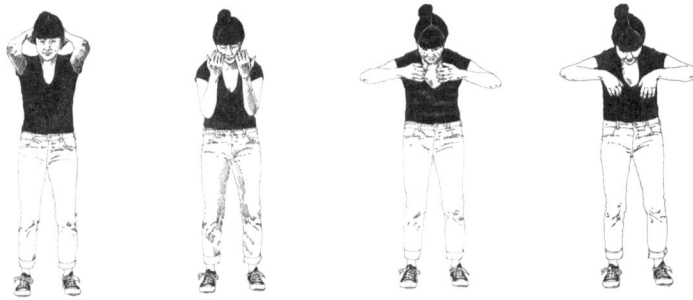

(f) Step 4   (g) Step 5   (h) Step 6   (i) Step 7

Second-Phase Bend ⟶

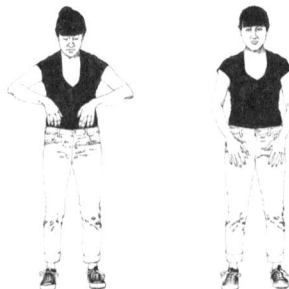

(j) Step 8: Midpoint   (k) Step 8: Endpoint

Third-Phase Stretch ⟶

MICROCOSMIC ORBIT

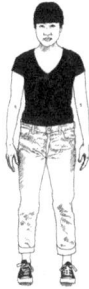
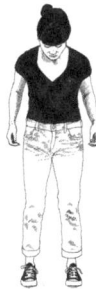
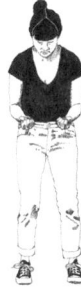

(l) Step 9   (m) Step 10   (n) Step 11

Fourth-Phase Bend ———————————————————————————⟶

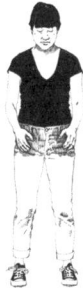
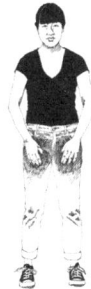

(o) Step 12   (p) Step 13

Fifth-Phase Stretch ———————————————————————————⟶

NEUTRAL

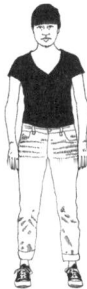

(q) Step 14

Sixth-Phase Release ———————————————————————————⟶

Macrocosmic Orbit

First-Phase Stretch - From the perspective of the weight shift, you move forward because your arms are going up. From the perspective of the kwa, your weight is also going forward because you are stretching open. The two elements come together naturally to form a perfect match, so there is no real catalyst for igniting any strain or tension by combining these two techniques. This is a pure yang movement: forward, upward and stretching open. See Figure 5-2.

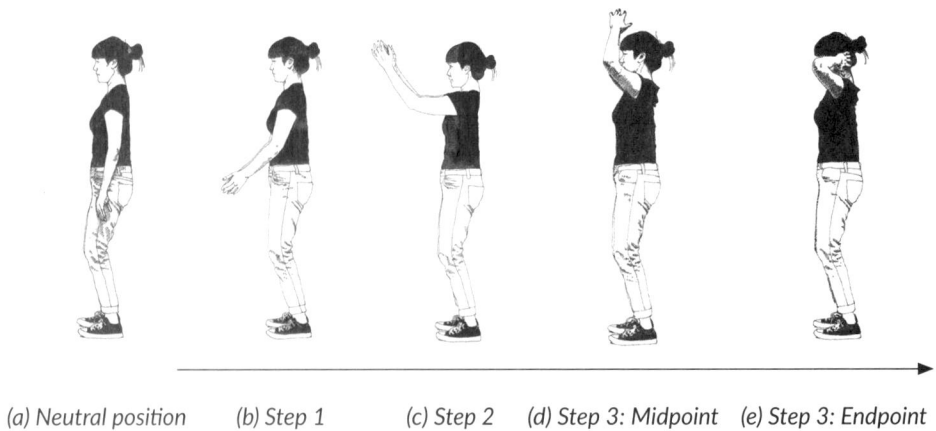

(a) Neutral position   *(b) Step 1*   *(c) Step 2*   *(d) Step 3: Midpoint*   *(e) Step 3: Endpoint*

Figure 5-2:
Macrocosmic Orbit—First-Phase Stretch

Second-Phase Bend - From the perspective of the kwa, your weight naturally wants to shift backward onto your heels, but from the perspective of the weight shift and arm movements, you will only go backward onto the arches of your feet—not all the way back to your heels (Figure 5-3).

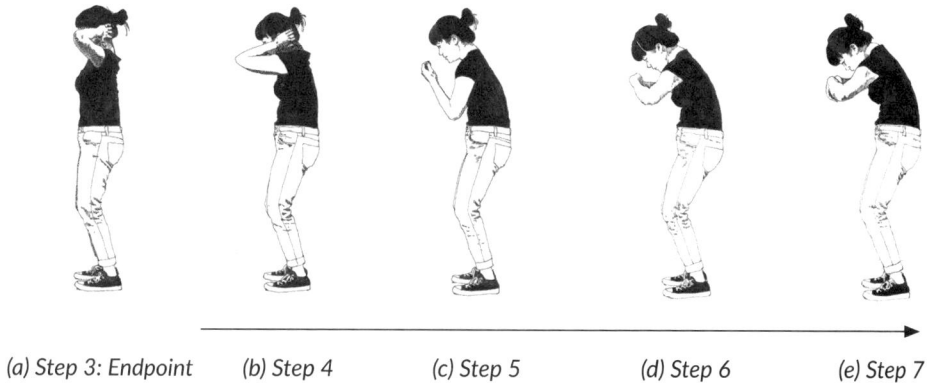

| (a) Step 3: Endpoint | (b) Step 4 | (c) Step 5 | (d) Step 6 | (e) Step 7 |

Figure 5-3: Macrocosmic Orbit—Second-Phase Bend

So you have somewhat of a conundrum:

- Since your arms are not significantly going up or down, the aim is to energetically balance the upward and downward flows, which allows you to focus on other internal techniques that will be presented in subsequent chapters.

- While the kwa is indeed the leader and the primary generator of qi during the movement, the weight shift acts as the controller, guiding the body's motion to generate the correct flow of qi. The kwa then supercharges that flow. So you bend in your kwa, yet arrive on the arches of your feet with a small internal adjustment.

- Simply drop your weight onto your arches and bend to the degree that is comfortable for you in the moment. In time and with regular practice, you will create more internal space and be able to bend your kwa and C-curve your spine progressively more.

- Your knees never push beyond your toes. Do not force your body to bend into your arches and thereby pressurize your knees. Take your time, feel your body and adhere to the 70-Percent Rule.

Third-Phase Stretch - Now you have two opposing forces: your kwa is stretching open and wants to drive forward; while your arms are going down, so your weight wants to shift backward onto your heels (Figure 5-4).

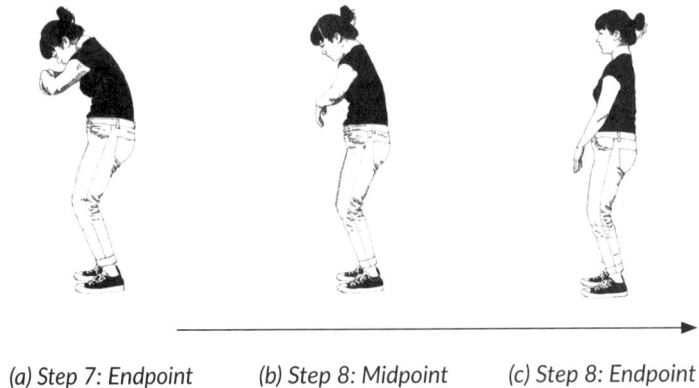

(a) Step 7: Endpoint   (b) Step 8: Midpoint   (c) Step 8: Endpoint

Figure 5-4: Macrocosmic Orbit—Third-Phase Stretch

- Since the weight shift is the controller, it wins the day and your weight shifts backward onto your heels while your kwa stretches open. There is no risk of over-pressurizing your knees because, if you stretch open as you go backward, you elongate throughout your legs and do not condense them (as done in the previous bend). The concern here is more about disconnecting from your kwa by pulling back and locking your knees, which would transform the practice into a purely external exercise.

- Consider the kwa squat and recall that your knees must remain bent and still in space to maintain the connection, which should be easy enough for you to do by now. Therefore, as your weight shifts backward, do not allow your knees to lock and simply stretch open your kwa. This is achieved by *intending* to leave your knees still in space as you shift backward, which will take the stretching open of your kwa deep into your body.

- If you find this exercise difficult, go back and practice the kwa squat separately to learn how to stabilize your knees, maintain the internal connection within your kwa and keep your psoas muscles engaged.

Microcosmic Orbit

Fourth-Phase Bend - This phase is where you must pay special attention and feel your body as you practice. If there is a glitch in the system, it is likely to be at this point and, more accurately, the glitch will be due to tightness or excess tension in your body. If your body is relatively soft and open, you will not experience any issues, so practice carefully and train sensibly. See Figure 5-5.

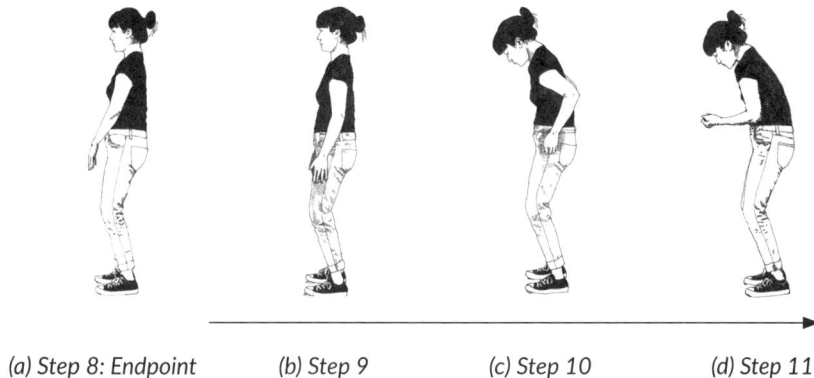

(a) Step 8: Endpoint   *(b) Step 9*   *(c) Step 10*   *(d) Step 11*

Figure 5-5:
Microcosmic Orbit—Fourth-Phase Bend

Step 10 depicts the beginning version; ideally, intermediate practitioners circle their forming fists up to the height of their midriff, between the bottom of the ribs and the top of the hip bones

From the perspective of the kwa bending, your weight wants to shift backward; from the perspective of your arms rising, your weight wants to shift forward onto the balls of your feet to raise energy. If you have internally opened in the last stretch, you will have the space to bend because your weight shifts forward as you do so. If not, there will be two opposing forces, which could generate pressure in your knees or lower back, or drive your knees forward and beyond your toes. Neither action is permitted in qigong. Be mindful and move slowly as you bend in your kwa.

- Again the weight shift is the controller and wins the day, so your weight shifts forward onto the balls of your feet and you bend in your kwa—*to the extent that you can*. The kwa is not really the issue, instead it is the lower spine tucking under and forward. While shifting your weight forward, there is a tendency for the tucking action to cause the knees to also push forward. Do not allow your knees to inch forward beyond your toes.

- Practice slowly and carefully. Feel your body (lower spine and knees) and only move as far as is comfortable for you. If you practice correctly, over time you will open your body, stretch out your tissues and joints, and create more internal space. This is how to achieve a deeper motion without straining your system.

NO SPACE TO MOVE?

In neigong training, there is always an ideal, but also a fudge or adjustment that assists in the learning and early training process to prevent damage and allow the people who are less internally open to make progress. If you find you do not have the space to bend and shift forward while maintaining your knee alignments, in the beginning, you may lean forward a bit more on this phase (by folding in your inguinal grooves) than on the previous C-curve. The main aim is to activate the bubbling-well points—just behind the balls of the feet (to be covered in Chapter 15)—without applying undue pressure through the lower spine or knees. Over time, as your body opens, try to lean forward less to become more vertical in the C-curve.

Practice sensibly and do not go for the ideal or force your body, mind or qi in any way. Chasing benefits either causes injury or builds up internal resistance to training—both of which prevent you from achieving your goals.

Fifth-Phase Stretch - Similar to the third-phase stretch, the kwa stretching open would direct your weight forward, while your arms descending and fists opening would direct your weight to shift backward along the soles of your feet to finish on your heels. In this phase, you want your weight to shift backward while your arms descend and extend, and your kwa stretches open—all without locking your knees. The feeling is almost identical to the third-phase stretch. The only difference is that you are beginning from the balls of your feet instead of your arches, which makes the weight shift slightly larger. See Figure 5-6.

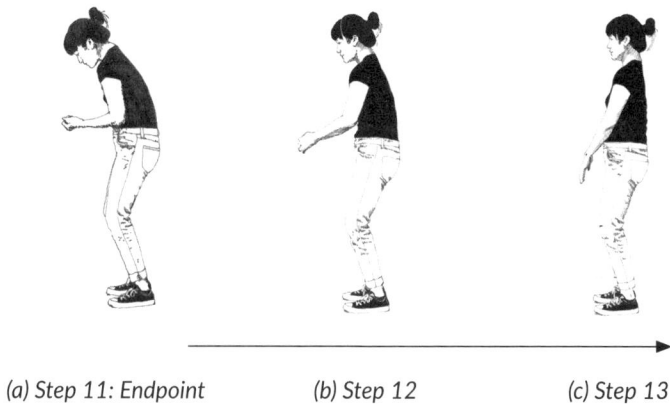

(a) Step 11: Endpoint   *(b) Step 12*   *(c) Step 13*

Figure 5-6:
Microcosmic Orbit—Fifth-Phase Stretch

Neutral

Sixth-Phase Release - At the end of the stretch-bend-stretch-bend-stretch cycle, simply relax, release and settle into the neutral position. The rising and falling energies are in balance, so you let go onto the arches of your feet in preparation for the next round. Softening and relaxing into neutral allows you to gain the space to stretch open once again on the next repetition. See Figure 5-7.

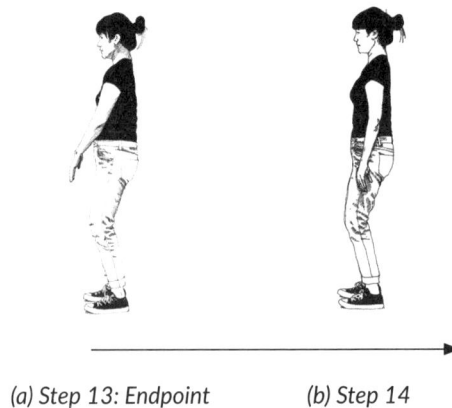

(a) Step 13: Endpoint   *(b) Step 14*

Figure 5-7:
Neutral—Sixth-Phase Release

REVIEW: SIMPLIFIED INSTRUCTIONS

Start in the neutral posture (Figure 5-8a).

MACROCOSMIC ORBIT

First-Phase Stretch (Steps 1-3) - Shift your weight forward onto the balls of your feet as your arms stretch up, while simultaneously stretching open your kwa and your spine (Figure 5-8b-e).

Second-Phase Bend (Steps 4 7) - Shift your weight backward onto the arches of your feet as your arms bend, while simultaneously bending in your kwa and bowing your spine (Figure 5-8f-i).

Third-Phase Stretch (Step 8) - Continue shifting your weight backward onto your heels as your arms stretch downward, while simultaneously stretching open your kwa and straightening your spine (Figure 5-8j-k).

MICROCOSMIC ORBIT

Fourth-Phase Bend (Steps 9-11) - Shift forward onto the balls of your feet as your arms bend, while simultaneously bending in your kwa and bowing your spine (Figure 5-8l-n).

Fifth-Phase Stretch (Steps 12-13) - Shift backward to your heels as your arms stretch downward and your fists open, while simultaneously stretching open your kwa and straightening your spine (Figure 5-8o-p).

NEUTRAL

Sixth-Phase Release (Step 14) - Shift onto the arches of your feet as you release everything simultaneously into the neutral position (Figure 5-8q). Settle and allow yourself to completely let go before starting the next repetition. Take a few breaths if your breathing has become erratic, and let your inhale-exhale cycle become smooth and easy.

Repeat as many repetitions as you like as long as you do not force, strain or push yourself toward any external goal. Only do what is comfortable for you and allow your stamina to grow over time with this deep, internal practice.

Figure 5-8: The Marriage of Heaven and Earth Qigong—Basic Form (Side View)

MACROCOSMIC ORBIT

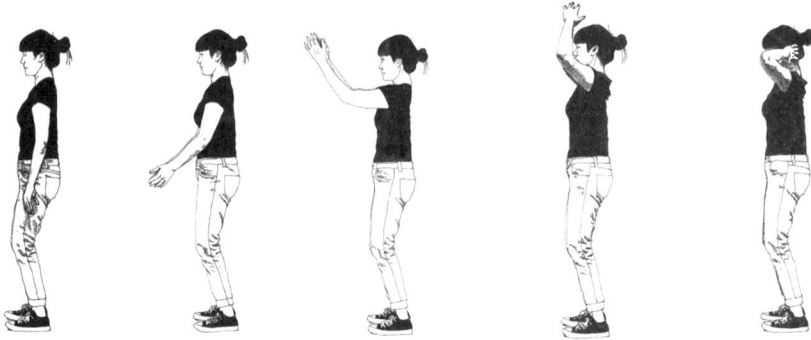

(a) Neutral posture   (b) Step 1   (c) Step 2   (d) Step 3: Mipoint   (e) Step 3: Endpoint

First-Phase Stretch ——————————————————————→

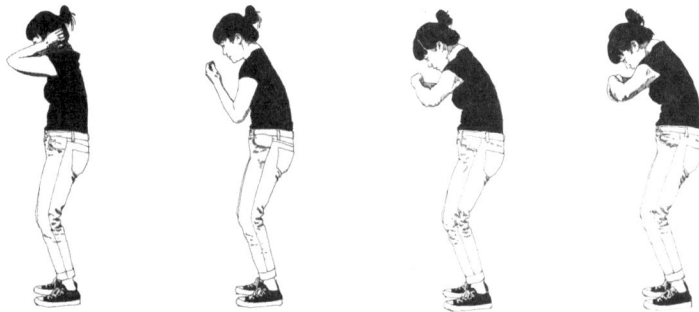

(f) Step 4   (g) Step 5   (h) Step 6   (i) Step 7

Second-Phase Bend ——————————————————————→

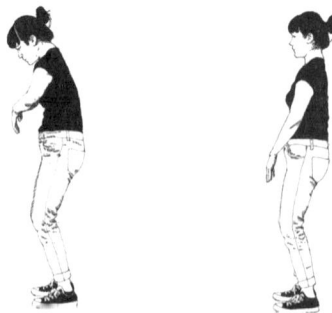

(j) Step 8: Midpoint   (k) Step 8: Endpoint

Third-Phase Stretch ——————————————————————→

MICROCOSMIC ORBIT

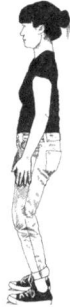 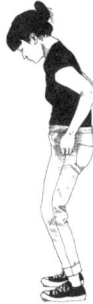 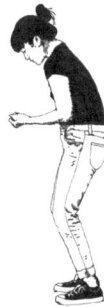

(l) Step 9 *(m) Step 10* *(n) Step 11*

Fourth-Phase Bend ────────────────────────────────────▶

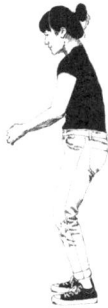 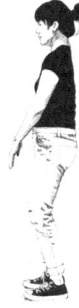

(o) Step 12 *(p) Step 13*

Fifth-Phase Stretch ──────────────────────────────────▶

NEUTRAL

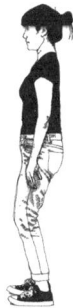

(q) Step 14

Sixth-Phase Release ──────────────────────────────────▶

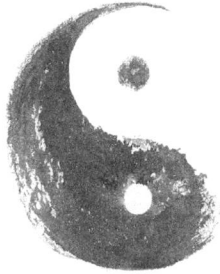

ESSENTIAL NEIGONG— BRINGING THE FORM ALIVE

Neigong techniques covered in this section:

- Bending and stretching the body
- Energetically penetrating the legs
- Taoist breathing
- Turning and twisting the body's soft tissues
- Balancing yin and yang.

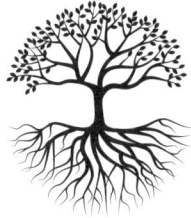

CHAPTER 6:

BENDING AND STRETCHING THE BODY

EXTERNAL VERSUS INTERNAL MOVEMENT

Now that you have learned the basic structure of the Marriage of Heaven and Earth Qigong, the aim is to bring alive your practice by imbuing your form with qi. Many qigong sets are taught in an external, follow-me fashion by both Chinese and Western teachers alike—without inclusion of the mechanics and internal principles for developing qi in the body—which is, after all, the purpose of qigong. Movement can indeed generate some qi, but practicing choreography alone would be like only learning a few letters of the alphabet: you could join the letters together to form some small words and not much more. The instructions in Section One were aimed at helping you learn the foundational mechanics and basic internal aspects of Heaven and Earth. From here forward what you will learn is based on the deeper internal processes that enable the form to become a qi-development paradigm rather than solely a mechanical external exercise, however sophisticated.

The neigong material presented is derived from and fundamental to Taoist qi arts from China, including qigong, tai chi, hsing-i, bagua, qigong tui na, Taoist yoga and Taoist meditation. They are efficient containers for neigong, but the choreography of the forms themselves is not the point of practice: it is to develop qi, which wakes up the body and mind. For example, tai chi imbued with neigong versus tai chi lacking internal content are two different practices. Once you learn neigong techniques, you will naturally discover ways to integrate them in all forms of exercise, including external martial arts and other sports.

However, learning internal methods for mobilizing and cultivating qi can be challenging, especially in the beginning. You do not know what you do not know and your eye might not be able to detect the associated and some-times obscure or relatively invisible motions. The instructions in this text will go far to give you some ideas about how neigong is applied in Taoist qi arts—not just in Heaven and Earth Qigong, but all energy arts.

> Using the same form movements, neigong becomes *shengong* when practitioners develop the skill to penetrate beyond their body and its qi to uncover, strengthen and release blockages in the deeper spiritual aspects of themselves.

Taoist philosophy posits that, through regular, deep neigong and meditation practices, you can become healthier—more flexible, resilient and vital—even into old age. What is responsible for this seemingly impossible phenomenon is the progressive learning, training and integration of ever-more profound layers of neigong, which release bindings, activate the dormant areas of the body and develop strong, naturally flowing energy. Qi governs how cells and all the systems of the body function *and* powers all aspects of the phys-ical body, both the conscious and the subconscious. Therefore, when qi is stagnant and blocked, optimal functioning is downgraded; when qi consis-tently flows strongly over time, all functions of the body can be upgraded. In Heaven and Earth, the systematic process of cultivating the many threads and unique weaves of refined neigong begins with bending-and-stretching,

Taoist breathing, twisting and other qi techniques, such as energetically penetrating the legs with the tailbone.

BENDING-AND-STRETCHING NEIGONG: THE FIRST LEVEL OF LENGTHENING

At the very foundation of qigong motion is bending-and-stretching neigong, a method of activating the soft tissues of the body through relaxation. This is in stark contrast to the Western model of reciprocal inhibition, which is based on tensing and releasing muscle groups in opposition to one another to activate the body. For instance, the bicep muscle is responsible for bending the elbow and drawing the hand toward the body; the triceps muscle, on the other side of the upper arm bone (humerus), extends the hand away from the body and straightens the arm. Even though only one muscle or group of muscles is tensed at a time while its opposite relaxes, a residue of tension in the body's soft tissues is left behind and builds over the years if not released.

Bend-and-stretch techniques are unique in that they activate *both* sets of muscles during *both* the bending and stretching halves of the cycle through relaxation, which releases tension from the body's tissues. During the bending phases, energy is stored in the tissues. During the stretching phases, that energy is released, thereby lengthening or elongating all the muscles involved in the action. This continuous cycling of bending/storing and stretching/releasing is responsible for breaking the habit of reciprocal inhibition and expelling long-term, accumulated tensions embedded deep in the tissues, as well as initiating rejuvenation processes in those tissues. Over time and with ongoing qi practice, the body becomes more supple, relaxed and springier, and blood and qi circulate more powerfully through-out the entire body—the holy grail of Chinese medicine.

You have already initiated bending and stretching in your hands, fingers and forearms (see Chapter 2). In the beginning, you were only introduced to the hands to tag the difference between stretching and bending. Now you will learn how bending and stretching is applied to the whole body.

As you bend, you will flex the arms and legs to varying degrees. As you stretch, you will extend and lengthen, but not fully straighten the limbs as that would cause you to disconnect from your spine and the insides of your body. Disconnection can dramatically reduce blood and qi flow.

ACTIVATING BENDING AND STRETCHING

PRELIMINARY EXERCISE: INITIATE THE RYTHYM

To initiate the bending-and-stretching rhythm, begin in the neutral standing posture, then raise your arms up in front of you with your palms facing down.

1. Gently extend your elbows in front of your body to take the slack out of your shoulders and the soft tissues between your shoulder blades and your spine, but do not stretch them (Figure 6-1a).

    (a) Your palms face down, your fingertips lightly extend out from your elbows and your elbows remain bent.

    (b) Adhere to the 70-Percent Rule and be sure to remain soft and relaxed.

2. Activate your kwa with the squat and, as you do so:

    (a) Bend and stretch your arms in sync with your legs. The aim is to activate all the soft tissues of the limbs in unison, from your spine to your fingertips, and from your spine to the tips of your toes.

    (b) As you bend in your kwa squat, sink your elbows down to create a bend in your arms and "load" the tissues as you would if you pushed down on a lightly stretched out bungee cord. See Figure 6-1b.

3. As you rise up from the squat, release and extend your hands forward to stretch your tissues—without straightening your arms, hands and fingers (Figure 6-1c).

4. After the stretch, slowly release back to neutral (Figure 6-1d).

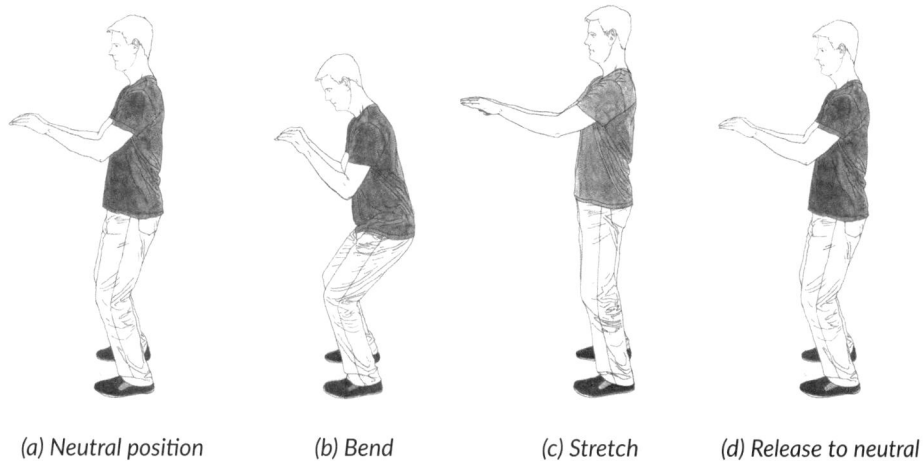

| (a) Neutral position | (b) Bend | (c) Stretch | (d) Release to neutral |

Figure 6-1:
Bend-and-Stretch Preliminary Exercise

Be sure to bend and stretch your hands and fingers in sync with the rest of your body.

This preliminary exercise, when practiced correctly and with relaxation and fluidity, will activate and engage all the tissues of your limbs. Once this occurs, the bend-and-stretch rhythm will sink deeper into your body: first by activating the tissues in your torso and, later, by sinking deeper toward your organs.

Preliminary exercises are used to wake up and activate specific neigong threads which, when alive, can more easily be woven into the structure of Heaven and Earth—or any form of qigong you practice. This process is precisely how you weave in layer upon layer of neigong techniques into any given exercise, especially one like Heaven and Earth with so little external motion in comparison to most qigong and internal martial arts forms.

In order to weave in the internal neigong content that follows, you need an experiential contrast to the bending/storing and stretching/lengthening halves of the cycle. This will allow you to contact and "grab" your tissues with your mind, and then move them as directed. Practice this preliminary exercise regularly, so that eventually you can embody progressively more advanced aspects.

BENDING AND STRETCHING IN HEAVEN AND EARTH QIGONG

Always begin in the neutral standing posture and take a few minutes to relax (Figure 6-2a).

MACROCOSMIC ORBIT

First-Phase Stretch

Steps 1-3 - As your arms ascend, in a wave-like action:

- Stretch out your soft tissues from your spine through your shoulders, down your arms to your fingertips to whatever degree you can do comfortably.
- Simultaneously stretch open your kwa and shift your weight forward (Figure 6-2).

Coordinate the timing of the stretch so that it finishes when your fingers touch your occiput.

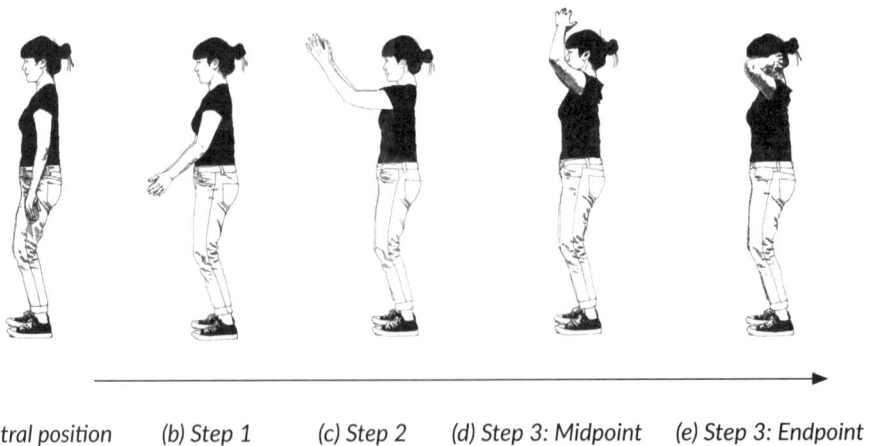

(a) Neutral position   (b) Step 1   (c) Step 2   (d) Step 3: Midpoint   (e) Step 3: Endpoint

Figure 6-2:
First-Phase Stretch

Because this stretch begins from the neutral position rather than a bent position (as in the third-phase and fifth-phase stretches), you will not have much space to move. In fact, the elasticity of the tissues of your upper back, shoulders and arms is what allows the stretch to last the entire movement. However, you must be mindful not to raise your shoulders. This means you must be conservative as you begin to stretch, but do not let it fade out or become dormant either. This balancing act is what generates a smooth, continuous stretch. Finding the balance point can be challenging, even for more experienced practitioners.

Remember: Even though the first-phase stretch, step 3 (Figure 6-2d-e) contains a physical bending of the elbows, it is still considered a stretch because the elbows are stretching sideways, away from the spine, while the fingertips stretch toward each other to contact the occiput.

Second-Phase Bend

Steps 4-7 - Release the previously stretched tissues as you simultaneously and progressively cup/bend your hands and fingers, allowing energy to be stored in the tissues of your arms (Figure 6-3).

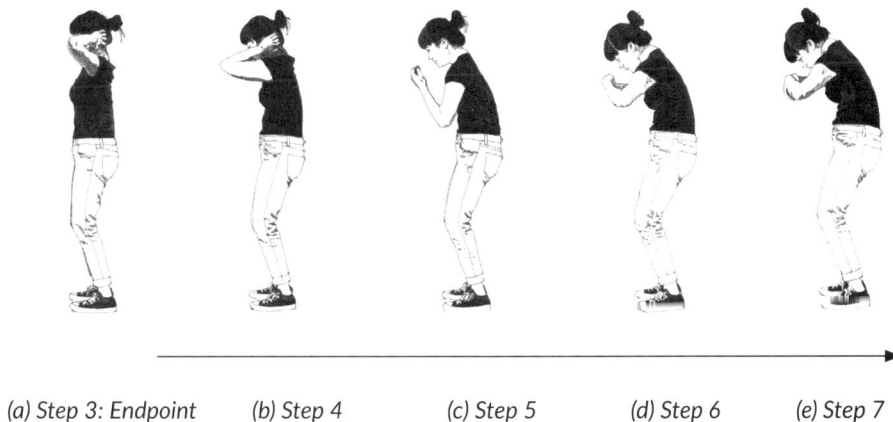

(a) Step 3: Endpoint   (b) Step 4   (c) Step 5   (d) Step 6   (e) Step 7

Figure 6-3:
Second-Phase Bend

Third-Phase Stretch

Step 8 - As you stretch up and out of the C-curve/kwa squat, release the stored energy in your arms, which propels your arms downward. As they sink downward, in a wave, stretch from your upper back and down your arms, all the way to your fingertips. See Figure 6-4.

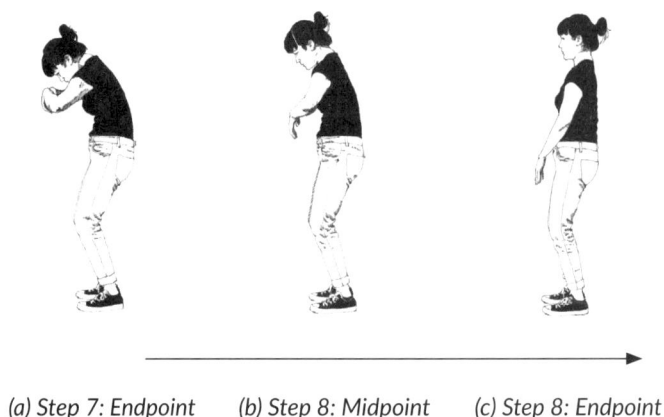

(a) Step 7: Endpoint   (b) Step 8: Midpoint   (c) Step 8: Endpoint

Figure 6-4:
Third-Phase Stretch

Maintain a minimum of one fist width distance between your hands and torso at all times and do not lock your elbows (as explained in Chapters 1 and 2). This stretches open the tissues in your neck and allows you to sink your chest into your belly.

Through correct practice of the two-part Heaven and Earth movement, you will develop many opposing forces in the body. Here, the spine rises while the arms and the tissues on the chest stretch downward. This motion opens the body on a profound level by generating internal space, creating the foundation to later embed deeper pulsing and lengthening techniques into the form. The better you perform bending-and-stretching and all other techniques presented in this section, the better prepared your body will be to receive more profound opening-and-closing techniques—the primary *modus operandi* of Heaven and Earth Qigong.

MICROCOSMIC ORBIT

Fourth-Phase Bend

Steps 9-11 - As you release the previous stretch, simultaneously and pro-gressively squat/curve your spine, while circling your hands to the top posi-tion and bending your arms, hands and fingers to store qi in your soft tissues (Figure 6-5).

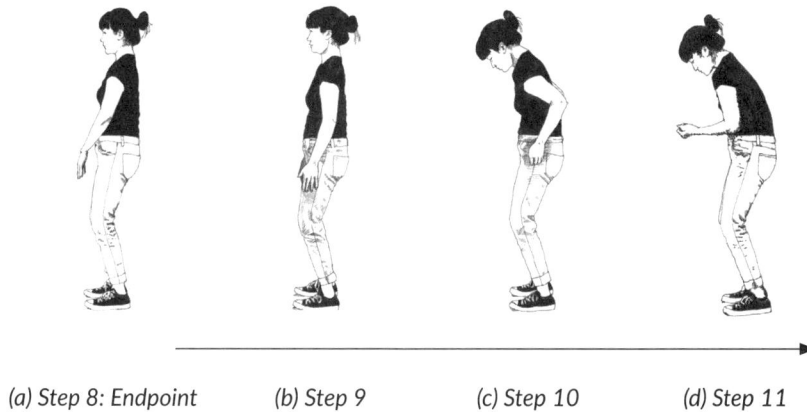

| (a) Step 8: Endpoint | (b) Step 9 | (c) Step 10 | (d) Step 11 |

Figure 6-5:
Fourth-Phase Bend

Note: Step 10 depicts the beginning version; ideally, intermediate practitioners circle their forming fists up to the height of their midriff

Fifth-Phase Stretch

Steps 12-13 - As you release the stored energy in your arms and begin to stretch, your elbows drive forward as your weight shifts backward and the space between your shoulder blades opens by default. The arms advancing and descending initiate a wave-like action from the shoulders, down the arms to the fingertips. As your hands descend and circle downward and backward, your chest will naturally sink into your belly as your spine rises. See Figure 6-6.

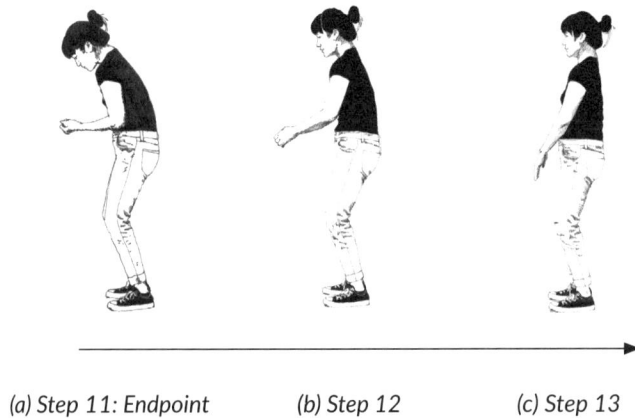

(a) Step 11: Endpoint   (b) Step 12   (c) Step 13

Figure 6-6:
Fifth-Phase Stretch

NEUTRAL

Sixth-Phase Release

Step 14 - As should always be done when letting go to neutral, release your tissues, joints, nerves and all effort from your body, and relax onto the arches of your feet (Figure 6-7). This step is critical because if you do not release and allow your body to return to neutral, you will not have any room to stretch in the first phase of the next repetition. Let your breathing become steady and even.

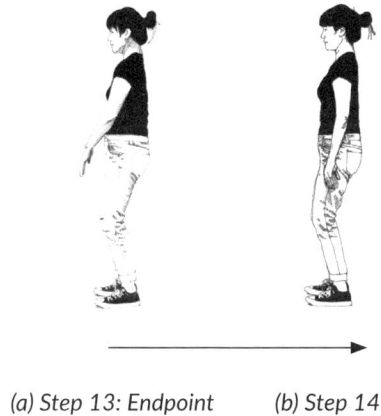

(a) Step 13: Endpoint   (b) Step 14

**Figure 6-7:
Sixth-Phase Release**

A PROGRESSIVE METHODOLOGY

Every dedicated practitioner wishes to improve at a good rate, but an over-enthusiastic outlook has a tendency to push the body beyond its natural capacity. Be patient and gentle with yourself by allowing your soft tissues to develop more elasticity over time. When you do, your nerves will release the tense and shortened tissues in which they are housed, and actually open up your body more quickly than can be done with force. Qigong, like tai chi, is a soft art.

A Word to the Wise: Bending and stretching the soft tissues is far easier in the arms than in the legs, so spend the time you personally require to embody upper-body techniques before attempting the exercises that follow. If you already practice Heaven and Earth regularly or, once you have practiced the material presented in the previous sections for a minimum of six months, continue onto bending-and-stretching techniques for the legs.

Doing one thing well is better than doing many things poorly.

BENDING AND STRETCHING THE LEGS: INTERMEDIATE PRACTITIONERS

In both the arms and legs, stretches in the soft tissues should always follow the direction that the qi flows. At this stage, you are not trying to move through your torso directly, but referred stretches may occur there. For example, as you extend your arms out of your back in the first-phase stretch, over time the middle and lower back tissues become engaged. Eventually arm stretches link into the gluteal muscles on the back of your pelvis, without the shoulders raising at all. In this way, the arms begin connecting to the legs.

MACROCOSMIC ORBIT

First-Phase Stretch

In one clear wave:

- Stretch from your feet and your ankles, through your legs, to your hips and the back of your pelvis.
- Simultaneously stretch from your spine to your fingertips (Figure 6-8).

The stretch in the legs will naturally extend and connect to your arms once you have made the link between your arms and your buttocks, and you can activate the tissues of your whole back via your arm motions.

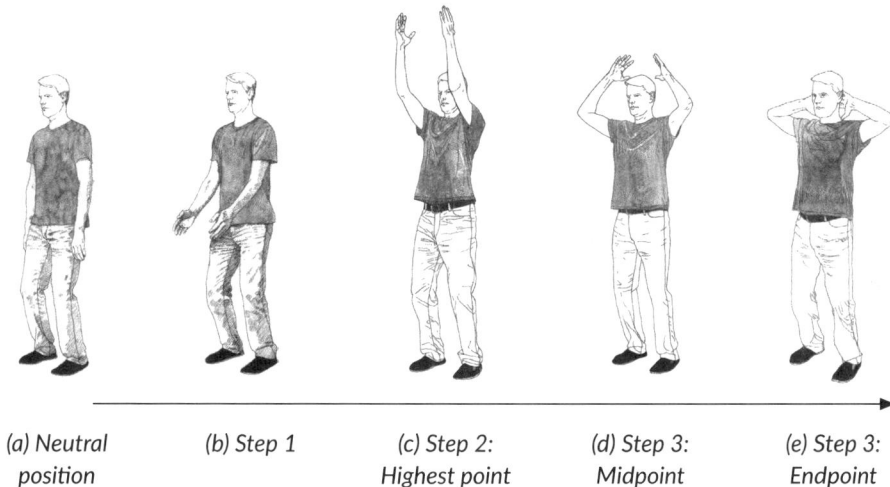

| (a) Neutral position | (b) Step 1 | (c) Step 2: Highest point | (d) Step 3: Midpoint | (e) Step 3: Endpoint |

Figure 6-8:
First-Phase Stretch—Intermediate Practitioners
The higher your hands go up, the more your shoulder should sink down

Remember the 70-Percent Rule: The optimum position is for your fingertips to arrive vertically above the crown of your head, but most people can only raise their fingertips to where they can reach the top of their forehead without tensing or raising their shoulders. Only raise your arms 70 percent as high as is possible for you without igniting any sense of strain or distorting your alignments.

Second-Phase Bend

As you bend all your limbs, store energy in both your arms and your legs (Figure 6-9).

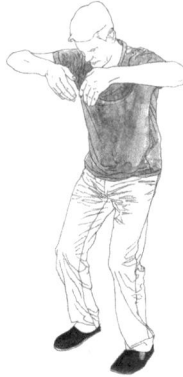

Step 7: Endpoint

Figure 6-9:
Second Phase Bend—Intermediate Practitioners

Third-Phase Stretch

While extending, release the stored energy in your arms and legs, which will cause your muscles to:

- Stretch from your pelvis down your legs to your feet.
- Simultaneously stretch from your upper back, down your arms to your fingers (Figure 6-10).

When your arms stretch out properly, your chest will sink into your belly, which naturally joins the stretch down your legs.

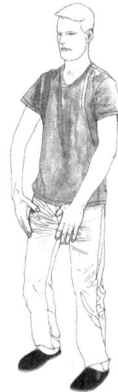

Step 8: Endpoint

Figure 6-10:
Third-Phase Stretch—Intermediate Practitioners

MICROCOSMIC ORBIT

Fourth-Phase Bend

Bend and store energy as in the second-phase bend (Figure 6-11).

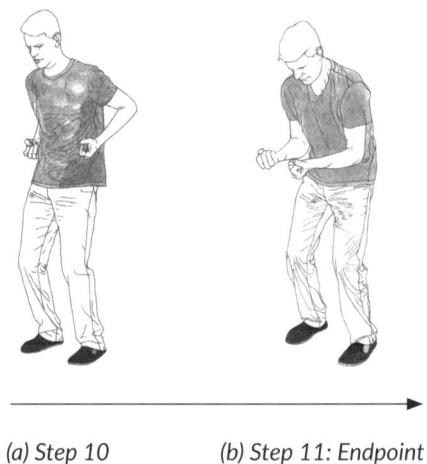

(a) Step 10   *(b) Step 11: Endpoint*

Figure 6-11: Fourth-Phase Bend—Intermediate Practitioners

Fifth-Phase Stretch

Release and stretch down as in the third-phase stretch (Figure 6-12).

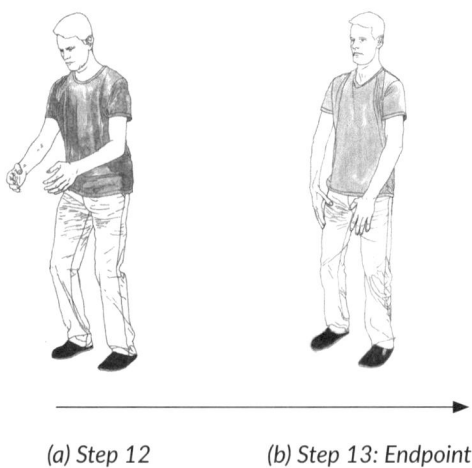

(a) Step 12   *(b) Step 13: Endpoint*

Figure 6-12: Fifth-Phase Stretch—Intermediate Practitioners

NEUTRAL

Sixth-Phase Release

Smoothly transition into a total release (Figure 6-13).

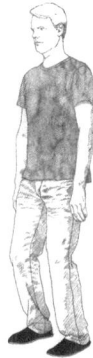

Step 14: Endpoint

Figure 6-13:
Sixth-Phase Release to Neutral—Intermediate Practitioners

REVIEW

This is the basic bending-and-stretching rhythm of the Heaven and Earth form, which is the precursor to lengthening the yang and yin meridians to be covered in Chapter 19. This technique must be fully alive to release stagnant qi and physical blockages, and to gain fine control over your soft tissues in preparation for more advanced stages to come. Each layer is built upon the previous, so moving through the layers too quickly will simply slow down your long-term development.

"Nature does not hurry yet everything is accomplished."
—Lao Tzu

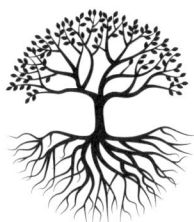

CHAPTER 7:

ENERGETICALLY PENETRATING THE LEGS

This exercise establishes a string of energetic connections between your spine and the channel that runs along the centerline of each foot, between the heel and the bubbling-well point (see Figure 7-1 on the next page). The aim is to forge the connection before starting the Heaven and Earth movement and to maintain that connection throughout the entirety of your practice. In so doing, you will dramatically increase qi flow in your spine, legs and whole body, especially the ascending and descending currents of qi.

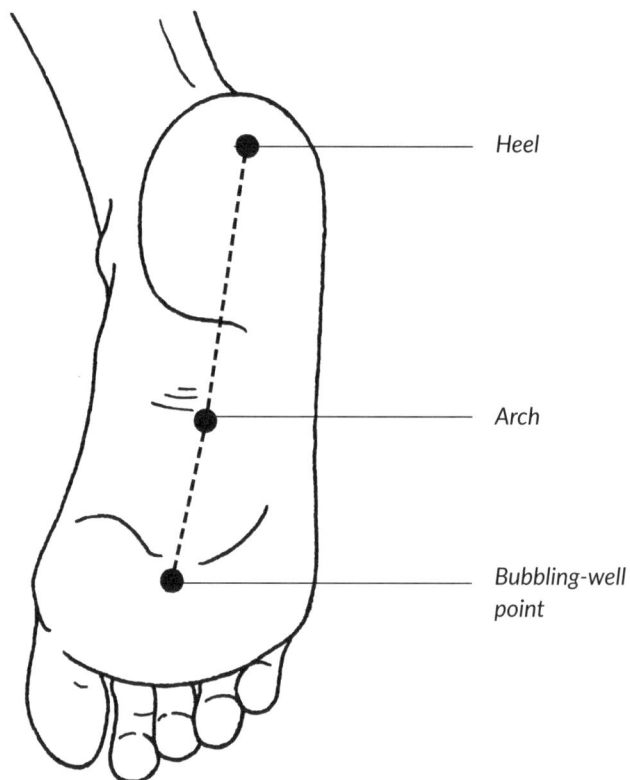

Figure 7-1:
The Centerline of the Foot

As always there are layers to this process and, until you can achieve the first method, you should not attempt the second method as you will not be able to stabilize the foundation required to achieve higher-level qi practice.

HOW TO PENETRATE THE LEGS WITH THE TAILBONE

EXERCISE ONE: FORGE THE CONNECTION

Stand in the neutral standing posture and take a moment to bring your legs, torso, spine, neck, head, shoulders and arms into alignment with a sense of your spine rising while everything else sinks down.

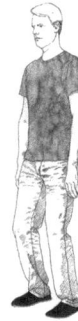

1. Put your focus on your tailbone and the back of your pelvis. Begin to relax your lower back muscles and lumbar vertebrae, allowing your sacrum and tailbone to sink. This is possible because the psoas muscles that enable the ability to stand do not connect to the sacrum or tailbone, but rather the lumbar spine. The buttocks (gluteal) muscles at the back of the pelvis are not required to remain upright either and therefore can soften, release and sink. This action draws out the lower back muscles, which releases tension and opens up the lower spine. With this, as the psoas elongates to help lift the spine, the back of the pelvis, sacrum and tailbone can sink down from the bottom of the spine—without the torso losing height.

2. As you progressively release your lower back and drop your sacrum and tailbone downward, gently direct the increasing pressure in your legs to the back of your knees. The back of the knee is a cavity designed to transfer weight from the upper body down to the foot, which prevents over pressurization in and damage to the knee.

3. As you stand longer, you want to maintain the connection to the back of your knees and drop that pressure down into the arches of your feet. The arch of the foot functions as a strong, spring-like bridge that absorbs the load of the body's weight plus anything you carry, and it transfers that pressure into the ground. These alignments are safe, functional and follow the way in which your

body is designed to operate. They also prevent injury, make the body stronger and increase power for internal arts training and daily activities.

4. Once you have established the connection between your tailbone, back of your knees and arches of your feet, stay there and continue to increase the connection for a while by holding up your body from C7 and sinking the back of your pelvis, sacrum and tailbone through your knees into your feet.

5. Once the connection is physically tangible and solid, raise the back of your pelvis and direct your buttocks backward to enable you to feel the disconnection. Notice how the pressure in your feet dissipates to some degree.

6. Next re-establish the correct, solid connection from your tailbone to your feet.

EXERCISE TWO: ADD THE WEIGHT SHIFT

This exercise and the one that follows should be practiced while continuously maintaining the connection you have established. If at any point you find you have disconnected your tailbone from your legs and/or feet, go back to the beginning and reconnect. This is important because, if you disconnect and continue on anyway, you will train your body to move without the tailbone being connected to your legs and soon the connection will be lost altogether. Naturally qi development will also be diminished, dramatically so over time; focus and patience are required to become more internal. If at any time you need a point of reference, review the material on the weight shift (in Chapter 3).

1. Establish the tailbone-to-back-of-knees-to-arches-of-feet physical connection described in the previous exercise.

2. Maintain this connection while practicing the six-stage weight shift: forward-middle-back-forward-back-middle (see Chapter 3, Figure 3-1). Be sure to move slowly!

If you set up your standing posture correctly, this exercise will now become more intense and start to open up the tissues of your legs and feet. It will also feel like you are heavier in some way and your legs will tire more quickly. This is due to the increased internal pressure from the connection of your tailbone penetrating your legs and connecting to the soles of your feet. The increase in internal pressure is precisely what engorges the blood vessels and generates the stronger circulation and deeper penetration of blood and qi in the legs.

EXERCISE THREE: ADD THE KWA SQUAT

If at any time you need a point of reference, review the material on the kwa squat (from Chapter 4).

The previous exercise was presented first since there is not any upward-and-downward motion, which makes it easier to achieve. With the kwa squat, there are two considerations:

- **On the descent** - If you drop the back of your pelvis, gluteal muscles, sacrum and tailbone, you will increase the tailbone penetration into your legs and feet.
- **On the rise** - If you stretch open your kwa correctly, your tailbone will extend down slightly while maintaining and increasing the pressure through your legs.

Note: The downward extension of the tailbone through the stretching open of the kwa is physically very small and is directed by your intent, rather than by activating a strong, muscular force. The motion of the tailbone is smooth and continuous, which allows the internal pressure to build gradually in the legs.

During the rise, if you do not keep your tailbone extending downward slightly or you rise up too much, you will unplug your tailbone from your legs and/or feet, and make the exercise an external one. Move slowly, remaining present and focused. If you disconnect, go back to the standing posture and start over.

This exercise is not easy to do continuously and you will need to practice it a lot in order to embed the technique in your system. Once you do, you will be ready for applying it in the two-part Heaven and Earth movement. First practice Heaven and Earth with only the weight shift, kwa squat and C-curve components. It will be easier for you to stay focused when you do not move your arms.

PENETRATING THE LEGS IN HEAVEN AND EARTH QIGONG

Start in the neutral standing posture with your tailbone penetrating your legs and connected to your feet (Figure 7-2a).

MACROCOSMIC ORBIT

First-Phase Stretch

Steps 1-3 - Stretch open, shift your weight forward and gently extend your tailbone down into the bubbling-well points of your feet (Figure 7-2).

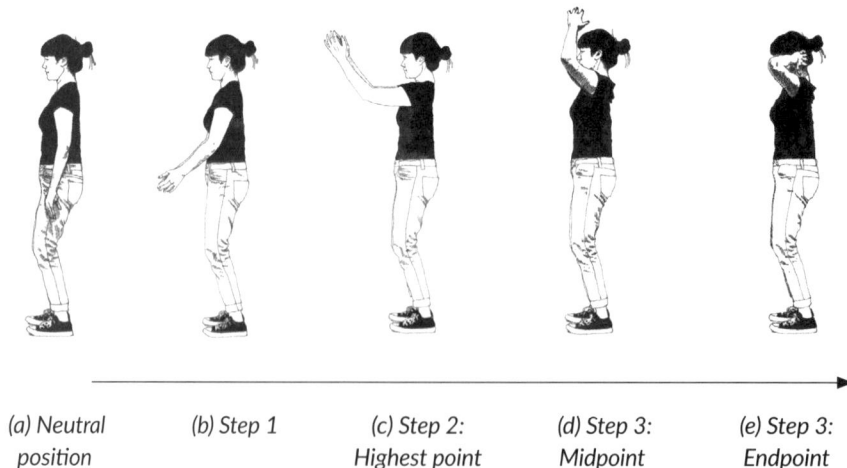

| *(a) Neutral position* | *(b) Step 1* | *(c) Step 2: Highest point* | *(d) Step 3: Midpoint* | *(e) Step 3: Endpoint* |

Figure 7-2:

Penetrating the Legs—First Phase

Second-Phase Bend

Steps 4-7 - Bend, shift your weight onto the arches of your feet and drop the pressure from your tailbone through the back of your knees into the arches of your feet (Figure 7-3).

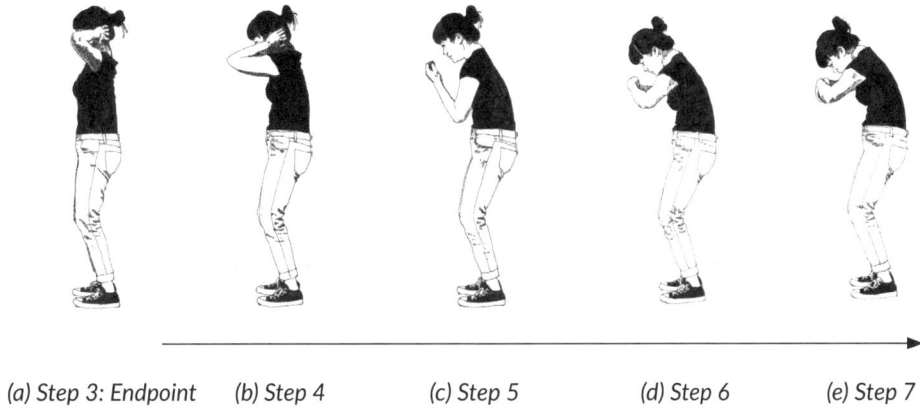

(a) Step 3: Endpoint   *(b) Step 4*   *(c) Step 5*   *(d) Step 6*   *(e) Step 7*

Figure 7-3: Penetrating the Legs—Second Phase

Third-Phase Stretch

Step 8 - Stretch open onto your heels while extending your tailbone down into your heels to create a direct pressure there (Figure 7-4).

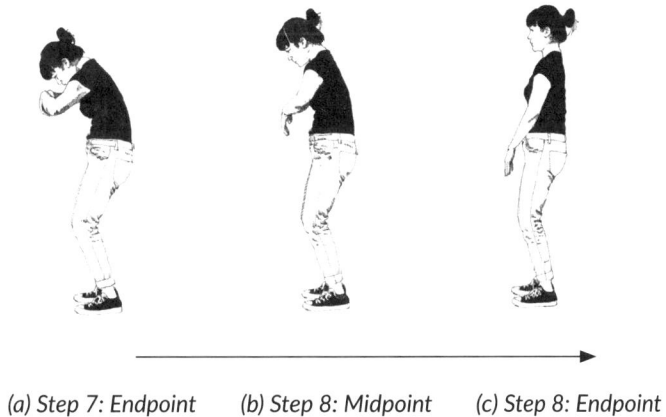

(a) Step 7: Endpoint   *(b) Step 8: Midpoint*   *(c) Step 8: Endpoint*

Figure 7-4: Penetrating the Legs—Third Phase

MICROCOSMIC ORBIT

Fourth-Phase Bend

Steps 9-11 - Bend, shift your weight forward and drop your tailbone into the bubbling-well points of your feet (Figure 7-5).

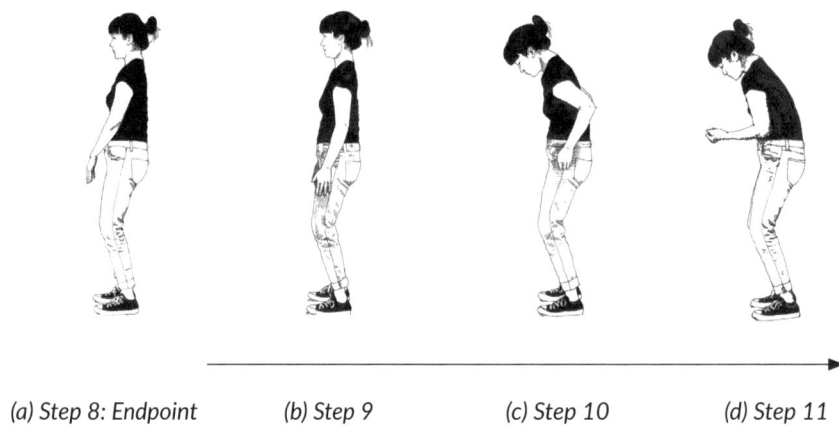

(a) Step 8: Endpoint   (b) Step 9   (c) Step 10   (d) Step 11

Figure 7-5:
Penetrating the Legs—Fourth Phase

Fifth-Phase Stretch

Steps 12-13 - Stretch and shift your weight backward while extending your tailbone down into your heels to create a direct pressure there (Figure 7-6).

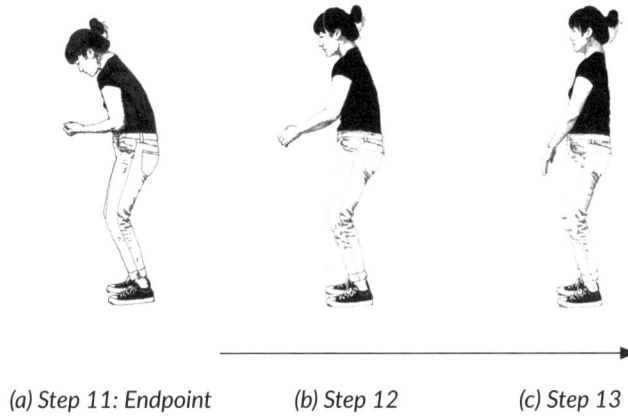

(a) Step 11: Endpoint   (b) Step 12   (c) Step 13

Figure 7-6:
Penetrating the Legs—Fifth Phase

NEUTRAL

Sixth-Phase Release

Step 14 - Release into the neutral position as you shift forward and drop your tailbone into the arches of your feet (Figure 7-7).

If for any reason you have disconnected your tailbone from your feet or legs while practicing the Heaven and Earth form, it is the sixth-stage release where you have the best chance of reconnecting. Focus and try to maintain a consistent connection between your tailbone and your feet on the next round.

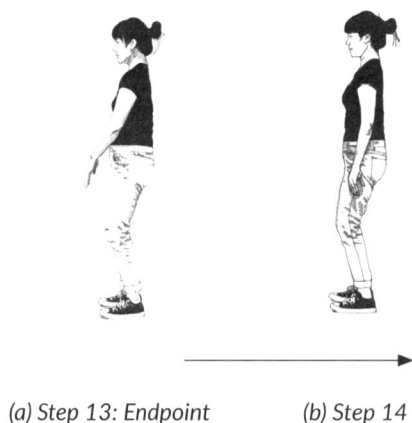

(a) Step 13: Endpoint   (b) Step 14

Figure 7-7:
Penetrating the Legs—Sixth-Phase Release

Once you have practiced this sequence and feel you have assimilated the motions, you will be ready to add the arms.

Important Points

- If your alignments do not feel comfortable, or you experience pain in your knees or lower spine during the kwa squat or when combining it with the weight shift, stop practicing and rest. Go back and practice the weight shift with your tailbone penetrating your legs for a while longer.

- If you lose the connection between your tailbone and feet while incorporating them in the Heaven and Earth form, go back to the preliminary exercises for a while. This is an indicator that you have not fully assimilated this component and you need to practice it more before moving on to a more complex practice. Take your time and be gentle with yourself.

ADDING THE ENERGETIC ASPECT: INTERMEDIATE PRACTITIONERS

Before trying to incorporate the considerations in this section, all of the material previously presented on the tailbone penetrating the legs should be fully activated and online so that it is smooth, continuously alive, fully embodied and integrated into the Heaven and Earth form.

From the perspective of choreography, all instructions are pretty much the same, except your mind's intent is looking to energetically thread your qi from your tailbone, through your legs to your feet. As you release your lower back (from the neutral position) and drop your tailbone, thread the qi that extends out of your tailbone through the perineum to the center of your hip joint, knee joint, ankle joint and on down into the channel that runs the length of the foot—from the heel to the bubbling-well point (review Figure 7-1).

The speed at which someone can feel their qi penetrate their legs varies person to person. To develop this skill, be thorough by moving slowly and working through your legs in stages.

- First practice moving qi from your tailbone through your perineum to the hips to the middle of your thighs.

- When you can move qi from your tailbone to your mid thighs with minimal effort, continue down to the center of your knees.

- When you can move qi from your tailbone to the middle of your knees comfortably—no matter how long that process takes—project your qi from your tailbone to the middle of your calves and, eventually, down to your ankles, bottom of your feet and heels/ tips of your toes.

You will very likely have to proceed incrementally, step by step, to achieve this internal qi connection. You may need several days or weeks of consistent practice to solidify each stage. If you try to extend your qi too quickly, the stream becomes extremely thin and starts to break up, which leaves gaps. Until qi flows strongly to your mid thighs, do not attempt to move down to your knees and so on. This protocol, along with the following exercises will strengthen the flow of qi and enable you to develop a deep, energetic penetration through your legs:

1. The weight shift.
2. The kwa squat.
3. The Heaven and Earth form without arm movements.
4. The complete, two-part Heaven and Earth form including arm movements.

At this stage of your development, you can physically move slightly less on the weight shift as your tailbone and energy does the work for you, while simultaneously increasing the volume of blood and qi circulating throughout your body. This fact often surprises many students because they are moving less yet gaining more from their practice and feeling tired much more quickly. The Taoist principle that sheds light on the experience is: "More on the outside, less on the inside; less on the outside, more on the inside."

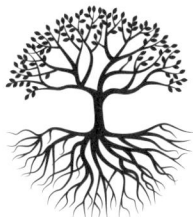

CHAPTER 8:

I KOU CHI,
ONE BREATH OF QI

TAOIST BREATHING

Taoist breathing includes two main aspects:

- What you do with your breath internally, or how you breathe.
- At which points in the form you breathe in or out.

These two aspects become the guiding aspirations with two important considerations:

- What is the ideal scenario?
- What is possible for you within 70 percent of your capacity in any given moment in time?

Of course these considerations are important for all styles and levels of practice, but are particularly so for breathing because of its direct connection to the internal organs and nervous system and, thereby, the emotions and the mind.

Pushing, forcing or straining your breathing can have profoundly negative effects on your body-mind-qi, so caution is always warranted when you try to achieve any external goal with a breathing practice. Attempt to maintain the intention of encouragement rather than expectation for safe and suc-cessful training that supports rather than undermines your health and sense of wellbeing.

Just because you achieve a certain degree of depth or range one day, does not mean you will automatically be able to repeat that level of practice on the next. Each time you come to your breathing practice, begin with a fresh mind, let your breathing be what it is and just register the quality of your breathing before trying to implement any specific techniques. In so doing, you will have the opportunity to read yourself correctly and avoid the pit-falls of the ego's expectations.

ANATOMY AND PHYSIOLOGY OF A BREATH

The lungs are responsible for the exchange of oxygen into and carbon dioxide out of the blood, yet they are not the engine of breathing. Instead, the diaphragm, a dome-shaped sheet of skeletal muscle that separates the thoracic cavity from the abdominal cavity, is responsible for causing air to enter into and exit the lungs. The diaphragm descends to draw air into the lungs and ascends to expel air out. Besides moving up and down, a healthy diaphragm also has the ability to expand from the center outward to the periphery and shrink back inward to its original position (Figure 8-1).

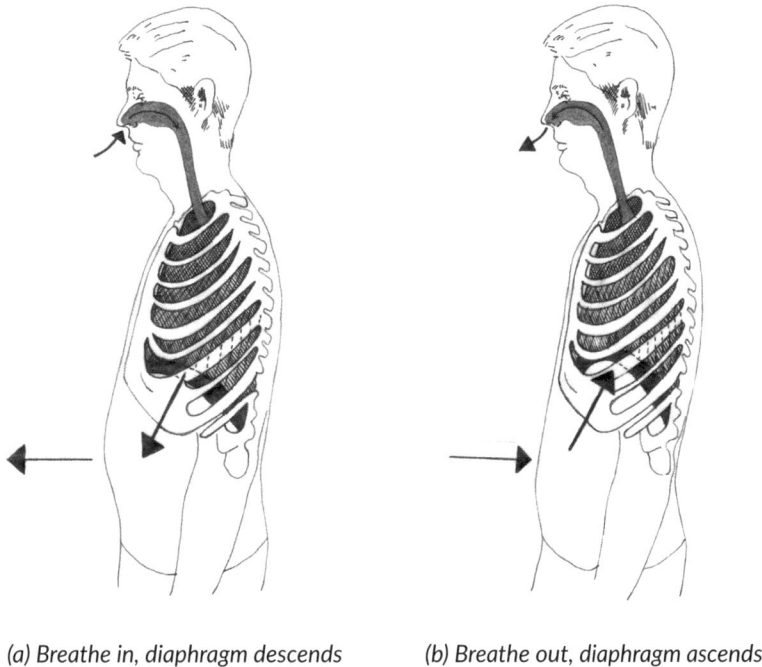

(a) Breathe in, diaphragm descends   *(b) Breathe out, diaphragm ascends*

Figure 8-1:

Natural Breathing Exercise

In addition to enabling air to enter into and exit the lungs, the diaphragm, through a series of ligaments, membranes and other soft tissues, can slightly stretch and release the anatomy within the abdominal cavity. The nature and quality of this motion has an incredibly positive effect on health and vitality because it:

- Generates movement within and between your internal organs.
- Creates internal pressures within your intestines and digestive valves, which aid bowel elimination (peristalsis).
- Causes fluids to move up and down the abdominal cavity.
- Increases nerve flow into and away from the abdominal cavity.

If your breathing becomes strong enough, you can also benefit from:

- Blood and qi being driven up into the brain and released back down to the internal organs.
- Better communication between the brain and the abdominal cavity via the nerves.

All of these processes synchronize with and benefit from the diaphragm smoothly and continuously descending and ascending.

HOW TO BREATHE: THREE-PART EXERCISE

Besides serving as a relaxation technique, the first goal of Taoist breathing is to fully engage the diaphragm, which creates referred pressures that massage the lower internal organs. However, you must keep your chest still in space and not allow it to rise. When the chest rises, the movement of the diaphragm becomes restricted, which limits the degree to which the internal organs can be contacted and exercised.

All of the breathing exercises presented in this chapter can be done while standing in posture or sitting upright. When sitting, be sure to align your spine, torso, neck and head, and maintain these alignments throughout your practice session—just as you would during standing.

Note: Taoist breathing is usually done through the nose, unless you have a medical reason or illness that prevents you from doing so. Also, do not direct incoming air below your lower tantien, which can imbalance your qi.

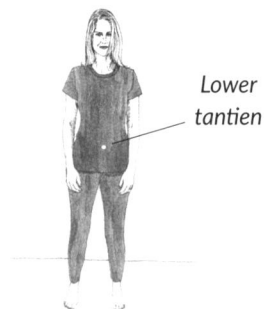

Lower
tantien

PART ONE: BREATHE AND ACTIVATE THE DIAPHRAGM

To start, simply breathe in through your nose while expanding your diaphragm downward and not allowing your chest to rise. Focus on filling your belly (between the solar plexus and the lower tantien) on the in-breath and relaxing your belly on the out-breath. With practice you can engage, open, release and soften the internal organs in your abdominal cavity. Do not be in a rush to move on to the next stage of practice as you will need a full breath and relaxed intent to move forward without igniting tension. Avoid dissipating the good progress you can make from this simple component practice alone.

PART TWO: BREATHE INTO THE LIVER

In the second part, breathe into your belly as in the first part but, once your belly is engaged in its expansion, guide some of the in-breath sideways into your midriff and floating ribs equally on both sides of your body.

This inhalation is a one-two practice:

1. Breathe into your belly.
2. Continue to breathe into your belly and spread the inhaled air to your sides.

On the out-breath, release everything together as one unit, smoothly and slowly. In order to achieve a good result in part two, part one must be practiced to the point of increasing the capacity and length of your inhale-exhale. If you only have a 2-3 second in-out-breath, you cannot possibly fill your belly and your sides. Increasing your breathing capacity can and usually does take time.

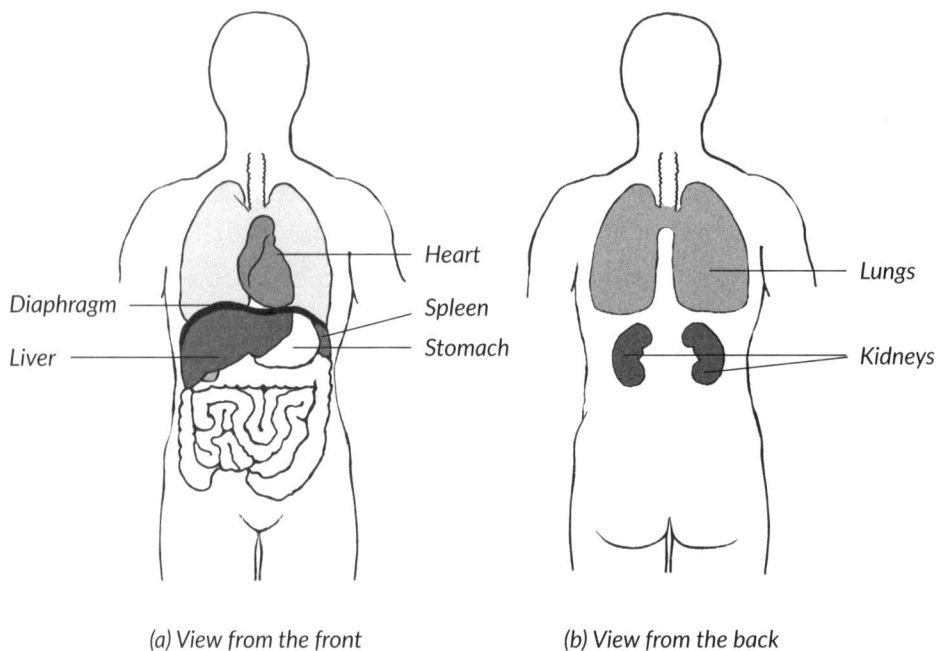

(a) View from the front   (b) View from the back

Figure 8-2: Internal Organs of the Human Body

When you breathe into your belly, the front of your diaphragm will descend. As you breathe into the midriff area, the sides of your diaphragm descend and it is here that the liver is directly engaged. Yes, you will also engage your stomach and spleen on the left side of your body, but the main event is moving the liver. The liver is associated with the Wood Element and Heaven and Earth is a Wood Element qigong. However, from a practical and physical perspective, you are always looking to create a balanced inhale-exhale and balance in all aspects of practice for that matter. The balance between the in-out breaths and the left-right sides of your body is precisely what yields integration. Integration is what allows two separate aspects to become uni-fied as one, like pouring water into water.

Practice this breathing exercise until you feel you have embedded it in your system and increased your breathing capacity to some degree, at which point you will be ready to move on to part three.

PART THREE: BREATHE INTO THE KIDNEYS

Once your belly and sides are engaged and online, you are ready to target your kidneys. The kidneys are situated directly under the back of the diaphragm, on top of the psoas muscles, so they benefit greatly from breathing and kwa squat/C-curve practices.

The kidneys are important to health and wellbeing for many reasons. If your kidneys do not move, qi becomes stagnant and diminishes. In Taoist medical theory, the kidneys are considered the essential battery pack of life because they activate the circulation of qi throughout the internal organs.

In part three, you will need a deeper breath to access the back of your diaphragm because of the one-two-three nature of the inhalation half of the exercise. It works like this:

1. Breathe into your belly.
2. Continue breathing into your belly and spread the incoming air to your sides.
3. Continue breathing into your belly and sides, and then spread the incoming air to your lower back.

The area you want to engage is between your diaphragm and the top of your sacrum—your lower back (around your lumbar spine).

On the out-breath, release everything together as one unit—smoothly, evenly and slowly—and in equal length to the in-breath.

The reason for the step-by-step inhalation is that if you do not fully engage and open each piece, one by one, you will leave many small spaces untouched by the breath. When this happens you cannot fully engage, release tension from or revitalize the contents of the abdominal cavity. Conversely, completely releasing everything together affects the whole on a profound level. By definition a partial release implies that something is being held onto and not allowed to relax. Release everything in unison—slowly, smoothly and evenly.

INTERMEDIATE CONSIDERATIONS

There are many ways of looking at more advanced components and higher levels or deeper techniques, but the crux of the matter always comes down to integration. If you have practiced the above instructions for sufficient time, you will have opened up your breathing capacity and the internal spaces inside your body, while increasing and balancing the length of your in- and out-breaths. If you do not feel confident that you have achieved this level of practice, continue practicing the three-part breathing exercise and leave the following instructions for another day. If you do feel confident that you have embedded the fundamentals of Taoist natural breathing in your system, this next section is for you.

Move the Diaphragm as One Integrated Whole

The purpose of the previous practices is to activate the various parts of your diaphragm, along with your internal organs and glands that lie beneath. Now the focus shifts to moving your diaphragm as one integrated whole.

First breathe into the center of your diaphragm and encourage it to both descend as one unit and expand out to its extremity, in all directions. Your breathing should be long and deep, allowing the time and space needed for this more advanced exercise. The descending, expanding diaphragm must spread evenly throughout your lower organs and in a smooth and balanced manner in order to be fused within the Heaven and Earth form.

BREATHING IN STILLNESS VERSUS MOVEMENT

Breathing well while sitting, standing or lying down is very different to breathing well while moving. When you are still, your diaphragm is only affected by your inhale-exhale cycle and the internal tensions you carry. When you start to continuously bend and stretch your tissues in various directions, the space in which your diaphragm has to move internally shifts

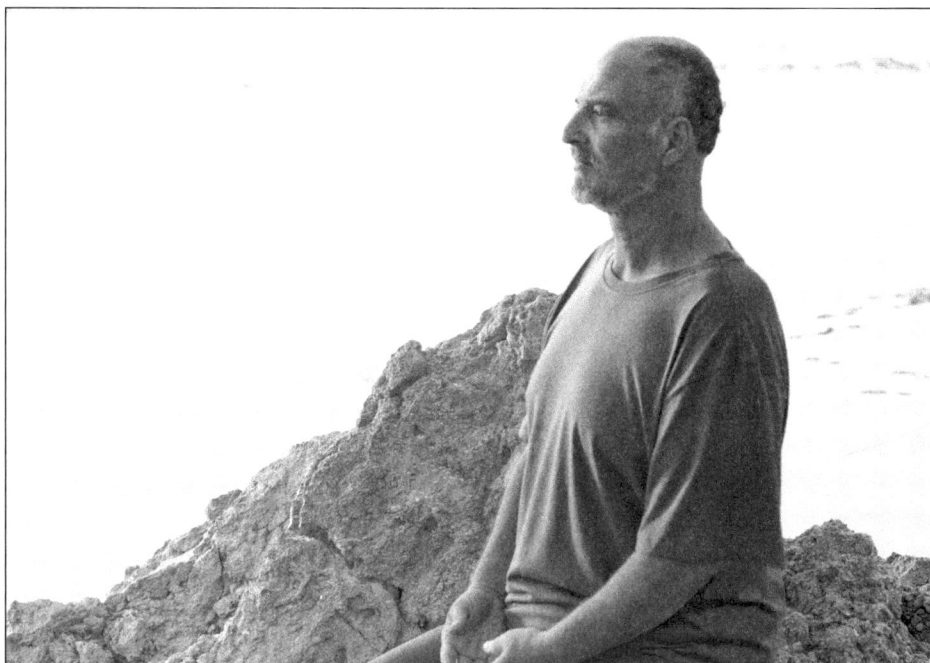

Master Frantzis breathing in meditation

and changes. Through a series of anatomical connections, primarily fascia and ligaments, the diaphragm is directly connected to all the bodily tissues between the head, chest, abdomen and pelvis. The movement of the diaphragm, therefore, does much more than only control the breathing process.

Some parts of the form will encroach on your internal space, whereas others will open up more internal space and support fuller breathing. You might be surprised by how much your breathing changes in the form. Most students find that, in the beginning, their breathing tends to become dramatically restricted during moving practice. Eventually breathing techniques within Heaven and Earth can release bindings, and increase the length and depth of your inhale-exhale cycle.

If you only practice breathing in meditation, it is unlikely that your breathing will initially become full and alive in movement. Practicing breathing in Heaven and Earth can be a huge benefit to meditators by engaging the soft tissues of the body much more deeply than only sitting, standing or lying down. This deeper activation is precisely what enables you to contact and gain access to the tensions that are hidden within your body and slowly release them over time. Then, when you go to sit, you will find you have greater range of motion in your breathing, which you can use to elongate your breath in order to enter into more profound states of consciousness and stillness. This is just one of the ways that Heaven and Earth can support and upgrade meditation practice.

BREATHING IN HEAVEN AND EARTH QIGONG

In the instructions that follow, the ideal method is presented first to make crystal clear the goals of developing a breathing practice. However, few students achieve the ideal without copious practice and using some intermediary steps to get there.

In neigong, the first rule is not to strain or force the body-mind-qi by allowing an overambitious ego to take over control. After all, creating stress and tension is the opposite goal of qigong. Practice what you can do easily, and only increase the demands on your body slowly. Regardless of how experienced you may be, always start with a few rounds of Heaven and Earth while letting your breathing pattern do what it wants and just noticing what that is. In this way, you can get a feel for how your breathing pattern is affected by your movements in the moment and gauge what is appropriate for you to practice accordingly.

The following instructions are the same whether you are using the three-part breathing pattern or the more advanced, integrated breathing pattern.

MACROCOSMIC ORBIT

The ideal scenario is to take one full breath for this part of the movement—that is, one inhale and one exhale. The in-breath begins at the moment you move your body from the neutral standing posture and start the first stretch or, more accurately, you will initiate the first stretch at the moment an out--breath ends and an in-breath is initiated.

1. **Breathe in** during the first-phase stretch and second-phase bend until your fingertips point down with your elbows wide and high (Figure 8-3a-i).

2. **Breathe out** during the third-phase stretch (Figure 8-3j-k).

Figure 8-3: Macrocosmic Orbit—One In-breath and One Out-breath (Ideal Method)

MACROCOSMIC ORBIT

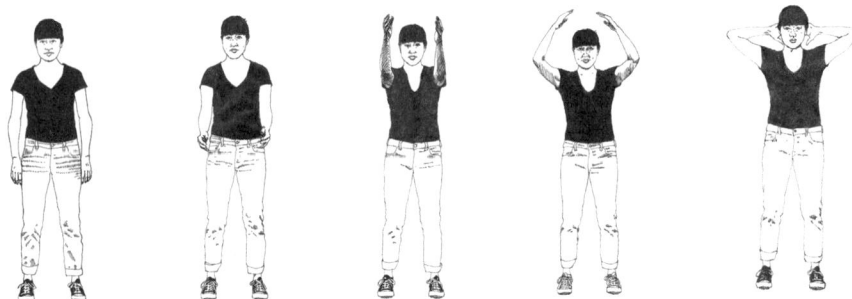

(a) Neutral posture   *(b) Step 1*   *(c) Step 2*   *(d) Step 3: Midpoint*   *(e) Step 3: Endpoint*

First-Phase Stretch: Breathe in ————————————————————————————→

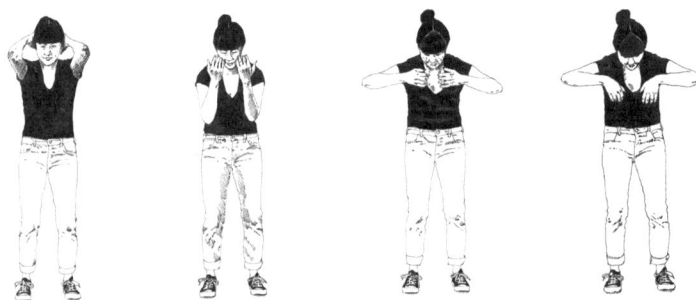

(f) Step 4   *(g) Step 5*   *(h) Step 6*   *(i) Step 7*

Second-Phase Bend: Continue breathing in ————————————————————→

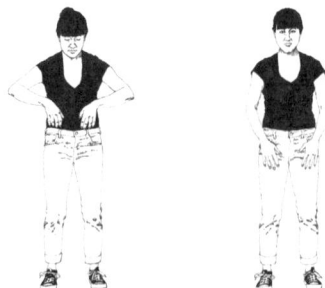

(j) Step 8: Midpoint   *(k) Step 8: Endpoint*

Third-Phase Stretch: Breathe out ————————————————————————→

MICROCOSMIC ORBIT

Just as in the macrocosmic orbit, the ideal is one breath for the microcosmic orbit.

1. **Breathe in** during the fourth-phase bend (Figure 8-4a-d).
2. **Breathe out** during the fifth-phase stretch (Figure 8-4e-f).

Figure 8-4: Microcosmic Orbit—One In-breath and One Out-breath (Ideal Method)

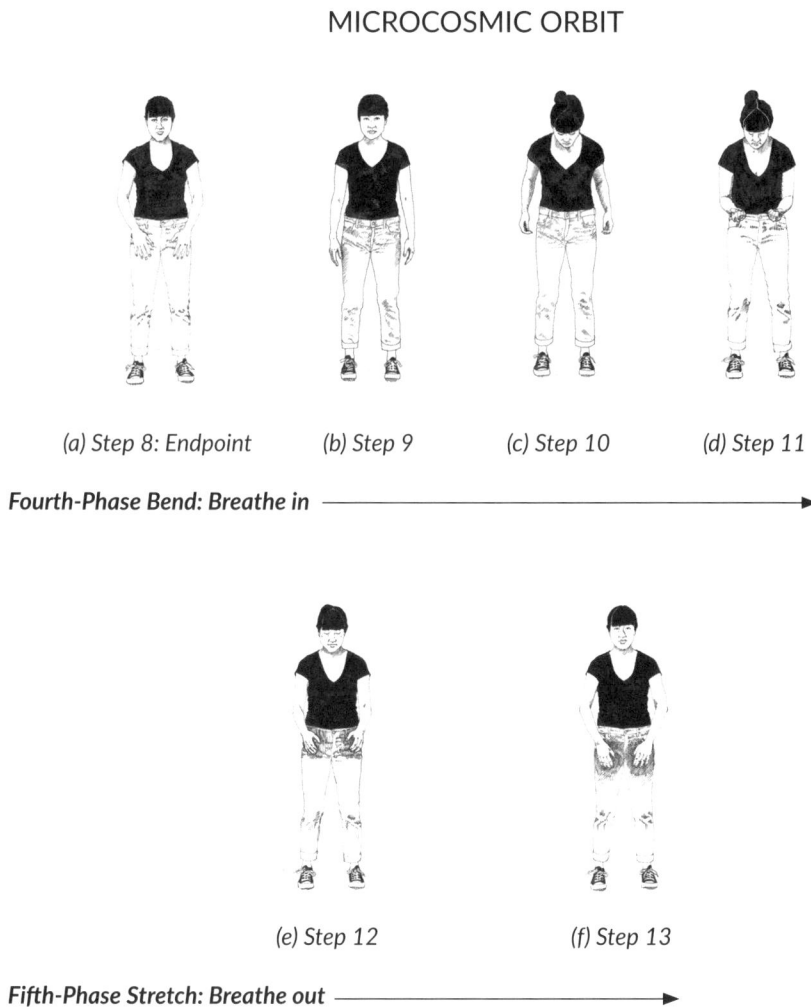

MICROCOSMIC ORBIT

(a) Step 8: Endpoint   *(b) Step 9*   *(c) Step 10*   *(d) Step 11*

Fourth-Phase Bend: Breathe in ⟶

(e) Step 12   *(f) Step 13*

Fifth-Phase Stretch: Breathe out ⟶

NEUTRAL

Release and let go into neutral during the sixth phase (Figure 8-5), allowing your breathing pattern to do what it wants. Your body may take one, two or three short in-out breaths during this phase. This is a safety mechanism to allow any tension created from moving and breathing to dissipate before it can compound and become locked in your system in the following repetitions.

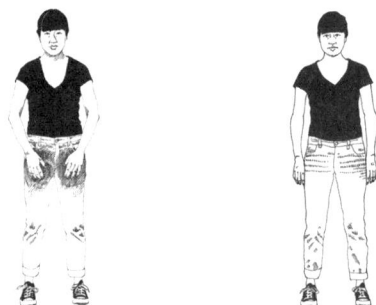

(a) Fifth-phase stretch: Endpoint   (b) Sixth-phase: Release to neutral

Releasing breaths ————————————————————→

**Figure 8-5:
Release to Neutral and Let Go of the Breath**

During the let go, notice if you have pushed yourself in any way and register what adjustments need to be made in order to maintain a relaxed, gentle intent and soft operation of your body.

You will notice that the first in-breath is long, slow and deep—much longer than the other in- or out-breaths in the form and therefore the most difficult. In the beginning it is very common to need an intermediary step or two to prevent strain.

ADJUSTMENT ONE: ADD AN EXTRA BREATH

Adding an extra breath within the macrocosmic orbit will make the breathing pattern more accessible for many practitioners.

1. Start with an in-breath as before, but this time only breathe in during the first-phase stretch.
2. Changeover and breathe out during the second-phase bend, step 4 as your elbows come forward.
3. Breathe in for the rest of the second-phase bend.

The rest of the Heaven and Earth movement and breathing pattern remains the same.

ADJUSTMENT TWO:
ADD MORE THAN ONE EXTRA BREATH

As previously mentioned, you cannot expect your breathing capacity to be the same every time you practice. Some days you will not be as open as you are normally or your breathing is restricted for whatever reasons, and you will require additional adjustments. The following instructions will help you if both of the previous breathing patterns are unobtainable even for a short period of time, for example when you have a serious cold or flu.

The main technique that can be easily applied to Heaven and Earth is adding extra breaths. If you add more breaths, you remove the strain; however, there arc a lot of possibilities here, so the following instructions will help guide you through the options.

The first rule of thumb is to only add what is needed. Adding more breaths than is required does not help you in the long run as it makes your inhale-exhale cycle very short. Instead, try to time your breathing so that you key into specific points along the way, such as:

- Beginning the first-phase stretch with an in-breath; then finishing with an in-breath too.

- Completing the second-phase bend with an in-breath, so that the third-phase stretch begins with an out-breath.

- Completing the fourth-phase bend with an in-breath, so that the fifth-phase stretch begins with an out-breath.

- In between these points, take as many breaths as you need, so that you prevent stress and strain.

- Elongate the release to neutral, so that you can take several breaths and allow your breathing to settle.

If you achieve these points, it will help to circulate qi, especially when:

- Bringing qi up your body on the first-phase stretch and fourth-phase bend.

- Sinking qi down your body on the third-phase and fifth-phase stretches.

If you find you are using this method on a regular basis, it is a strong indicator that you need to work on breathing as a separate practice. The Principle of Separate and Combine can save the day and allow you to continue your progress rather than relying on these adjustments many years into your training. Breathing practice is easy to incorporate into daily activities and is better done regularly rather than once in a blue moon. Short, regular practice sessions are also better than long practices a couple of times per week to establish a rhythm, which can then be elongated to improve and build on the foundation you have created.

CIRCULAR BREATHING

Before attempting circular breathing, first become very familiar and comfortable with the three-part breathing exercise with special focus on integrating the three parts into one whole.

Most people subconsciously hold their breath at the end of both the inhale and exhale, which creates a momentary freeze in the anatomy within the torso, nervous system and mind. It also interrupts qi flow, which, over a lifetime, can be extremely detrimental to health and wellbeing. Taoists practice circular breathing because they strive to follow universal law. This starts with the fact that all things in the natural world are in perpetual and continuous motion, including the stars and galaxies above us, the interior of the planet below our feet and all the living things in our environment.

The main points to consider when practicing circular breathing are:

- Aim to keep your airways open without closing the back of your nose or throat at any time.
- Aim to keep your diaphragm continuously moving, however slowly, which will keep the anatomy moving inside your thoracic and abdominal cavities, as well as support uninterrupted nerve flow.

The easiest way to wrap your mind around circular breathing (no pun intended!) is to recognize you must create a smooth changeover from the out-breath to the in-breath and the in-breath to the out-breath.

If you watch a pendulum swing or a wave climb up a beach, you will notice a slowing down as each reaches its zenith or peak, and then a momentary suspension before each returns in the direction from which it came. If you look very carefully, however, you will notice that the suspension point is not really a stop, but rather a circular changeover as the upward energy is overcome by gravity and so the return begins.

The metaphor of the wave is actually more relevant to breathing: the rising wave moves up the beach and becomes thinner and thinner as it does so; eventually it disappears into the sand before reappearing on its descent. Likewise, when your lungs become nearly full, air intake reduces to a fine thread and breathing slows down until the changeover. Then, on the out-breath, the thread grows again until breathing slows and once again begins reducing at the end of the out-breath. The aim is not to cut that fine thread, but instead keep it alive during the transitions, even if air is moving in or out imperceptibly slowly from an outside point of view. The thread grows and shrinks as air gradually fills the lungs and empties. Although there may be moments where it appears that breathing has stopped, internally air is always moving in or out of the lungs as guided by the action of the diaphragm. The airways at the back of your nose and throat always remain open.

If you stop or hold your breath, you cut the continuous passage of air (whether in or out), but also nerve signals, blood circulation, fluid movement through the soft tissues and organs and, by way of these, the flow of qi in your body. Circular breathing, on the other hand, aids and drives the flow, allowing you to experience the health and healing benefits associated with mobile, active, flexible and fully alive insides.

Increased blood circulation through deep, circular breathing also:

- Includes that which goes into and out of the brain, boosts venous return, and enables the lungs to oxygenate the blood more fully.
- Allows the blood to sink into and penetrate the internal organs from the strong pulsation of the abdominal cavity, which is generated by the motion of the diaphragm.

Eventually circular breathing can affect all the systems of your body—including the primary circulatory, nervous and musculoskeletal systems—from the bottom of your feet to the crown of your head, and back down again. For this reason, circular breathing is one of the most powerful tools for fostering health and wellbeing. You will need to be able to work up to at least 10 minutes of focused circular breathing in order to carry it into and maintain it during a typical Heaven and Earth practice session. With sustained and regular practice, you can breach the subconscious barrier and change your body's breathing pattern to circular breathing, which can yield incredible health benefits over your lifetime.

TRAINING EXERCISE: SLOW DOWN YOUR BREATHING

There are many ways to slow down your breathing, but a simple, effective method is by using a straw. As previously stated, Taoist breathing is usually done exclusively through the nose, unless you have a medical condition or illness that prevents you from doing so. For this reason, using a straw and thereby breathing through the mouth is only practiced as a temporary training exercise. Since the straw restricts airflow in and out of the lungs in a given timeframe, it will aid you in slowing down and elongating your breath.

Ideally, you would start with a straw that has a large diameter and later progress to a thinner straw when you feel comfortable using the larger straw. Starting with a straw that is too thin can increase the struggle—a little bit of struggle is good, but a lot creates tension—the opposite goal of Taoist practices in general.

From the neutral standing or sitting posture:

1. Begin by relaxing for a few minutes, which will naturally lower your heart rate and thereby slow down your breathing.

2. Softly close your lips around the straw and keep your mouth relaxed.

3. Breathe in and out in a deliberate pattern, regulating airflow so that you do not ignite any sense of tension.

4. As you continue to breathe through the straw, notice that you cannot suddenly breathe in or out as the airflow is governed by the diameter of the straw. Use this governor to recognize how your body reacts to the inability to speed up when airflow is restricted.

5. Continue breathing with the intent to create a pattern that is smooth, slow, continuous and easy to maintain.

6. Once you have balanced the in- and out-breaths reasonably well, you can focus on making the changeovers from in-to-out and out-to-in smooth, circular and longer.

This practice will help you regulate your breathing and tune in to the subtleties of circular breathing which, when active, will begin to give you an increased sense of presence and subtle motion. Of course this awareness has great value in terms of improving your control over all other neigong threads, as well as the choreography of any forms in which you train.

ONE BREATH OF QI

Heaven and Earth Qigong is the ideal exercise for learning Taoist breathing. This is because expanding and deepening the breathing process is essentially an opening mechanism, which is bound to both the Wood Element and the process of opening-and-closing. Therefore, a major objective of Heaven and Earth, a Wood Element qigong, is to get your entire body to breathe. Initially the focus is on physically linking the breath (that is, the diaphragm moving up and down, and thereby causing air to enter into and exit the lungs) to the bending and stretching of the arms and legs in Heaven and Earth, so that your movements synchronize with and power your breathing. This process can create an incredible amount of internal space. Traditional Wood Element practices call for developing the ability to expand the breath, until ultimately you can make space for a much larger breath inside your body—not just of air, but of qi. That is to say, the practitioner absorbs qi from the air they breathe, which the Chinese call *i kou chi* or "one breath of qi."

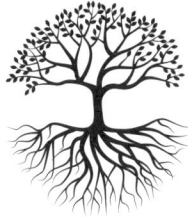

CHAPTER 9:

TURNING AND TWISTING THE SOFT TISSUES OF THE BODY

Turning techniques soften and release the body's soft tissues (skin, fascia, muscles and tendons) by expelling superficial tensions, whereas twisting techniques penetrate the body much more deeply and, thereby enable access to and the release of more entrenched and accumulated tensions. Twisting actions not only loosen up the tissues, but also the blood vessels and the nerves, yielding greater flexibility and better functioning. For this reason, twisting the tissues is an important neigong component, adding depth to movements, building power and supercharging various other neigong threads. Twisting techniques build on bending-and-stretching and turning techniques, and take soft-tissue development to the next level.

Imagine a cloth soaked in water with the soft tissues represented by the cloth and the fluids (specifically blood, lymph and interstitial fluid) represented by the water. If you take the water-soaked cloth and press it between your hands and stretch it out (as in bending-and-stretching techniques), some of the water will be expelled from the cloth (equivalent to the movement of fluids within the soft tissues). However, if you wring out the cloth (equivalent to twisting the soft tissues), much more water is expelled from the cloth (as the fluids are flushed through the tissues). The wringing/twisting action dramatically increases fluid movement and releases the nerve pathways which, in turn, increase qi circulation.

Twisting actions also loosen the muscles, so they do not become fused to the bones. Muscles are attached to bones at insertion points via tendons. Aging, stress and blunt-force trauma reduce mobility, causing the fascia on the underside of the belly of the muscles that lie along the bones to also form unwanted attachments. Twisting actions roll the muscles left and right, loosening and releasing stuck tissues. These attachments, when left unattended, not only reduce flexibility and range of motion, but can also lead to many other internal limitations, such as reduced blood and nerve flow. Over time restrictions that impede circulation can cause or exacerbate cardiovascular problems, such as high-blood pressure, restricted arteries and poor venous return. Twisting the soft tissues is therefore an essential part of maintaining health, enabling the body to feel open, free and alive, as well as adding power to internal martial arts forms.

TURNING AND TWISTING TECHNIQUES

Turning and twisting are different.

- **Turning** - occurs when the bones and muscles of a limb rotate in or out in concert with one another.
- **Twisting** - occurs when the rotation of the muscles is greater than that of the bones in either direction. In refined twisting, the muscles literally roll around the bones to some degree.

To get a direct experience of the difference, try the following two exercises.

TURNING EXERCISE

In the following exercise, you will turn one arm at a time.

1. Start in a seated position at a dining-room-style table or armchair, where your elbow tip can rest on a surface in order to prevent it from moving. Keep a bend in your elbow with your palm facing upward. This is the beginning position (see Figure 9-1a).

2. Gently rotate your palm to face downward and then upward. Be sure to keep the tip of your elbow still in space and in contact with the surface at all times. See Figure 9-1b-e.

3. Repeat the rotation several times, making sure the motion is smooth and even without igniting any sense of strain or tension.

4. Repeat steps 1-3 on the other arm.

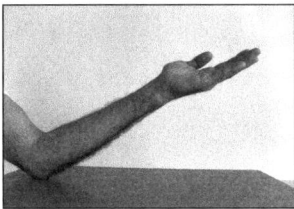

(a) Neutral position   (b) Begin turning the   c) Continue turning the
                                  palm downward   palm downward

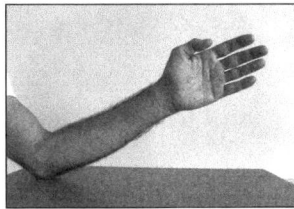

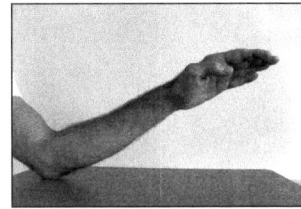

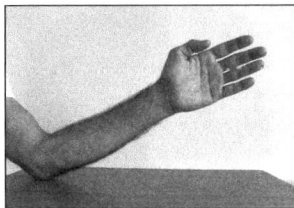

(d) Palm changes direction to turn upward   (e) Continue turning the palm upward

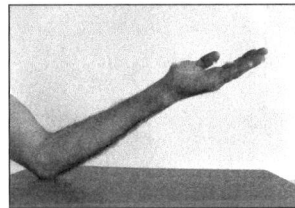

Figure 9-1:
Turning

TWISTING EXERCISE

To twist:

1. Repeat steps 1-3 from the turning exercise but, this time, when your palm is turned down and reaches its natural endpoint of rotation, put a little extra twist into your forearm muscles. In other words, when the bones run out of range, persuade your muscles to continue a little farther in the same direction, so that they rotate around the bones themselves—without moving the tip of your elbow. This creates a twist in the tissues of the forearm and wrist, and turns the palms a bit farther. See Figure 9-2a-d. *Important:* Do not force the twist as it will degenerate into tensing. When you twist, blood and qi flow increase; when you tense, they decrease.

2. Repeat step 1 to twist your palm, but in the opposite direction. As the bones run out of rotation, twist your soft tissues so that they rotate around your bones—again, without moving the tip of your elbow and turning your palm all the way up. See Figure 9-2e-h.

3. Repeat the twisting exercise while paying special attention to relaxing and softening after each twist and especially as you change to the opposite direction. Be sure not to force your body beyond its natural comfortable range.

4. Repeat steps 1-3 on the other arm.

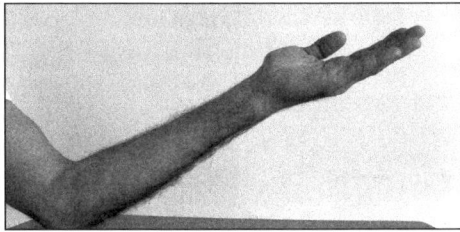

(a) Neutral position, palm up

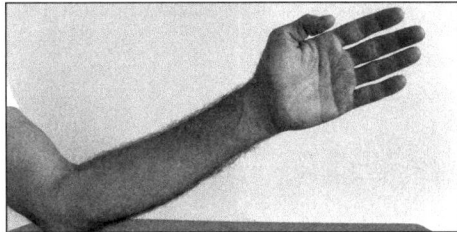

(b) Start turning the palm downward

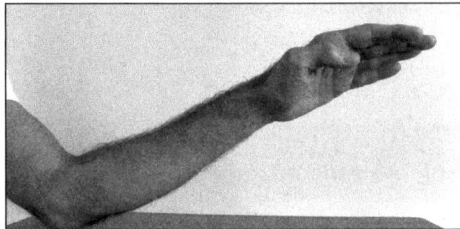

(c) Continue turning the palm downward

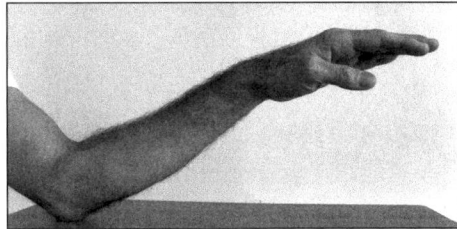

(d) Twist the muscles until the palm faces directly downward

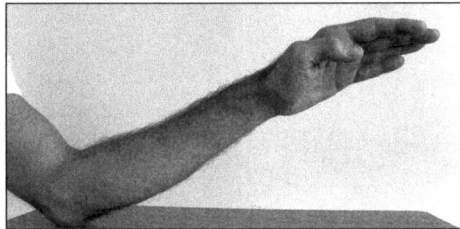

(e) Release the twist, palm changes direction

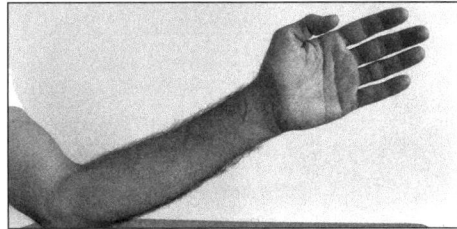

(f) Begin turning the palm back

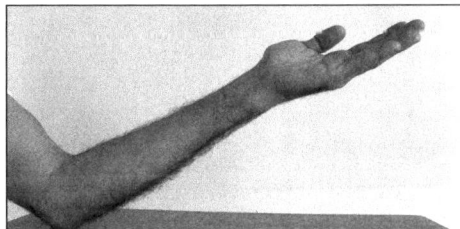

(g) Continue turning the palm upward

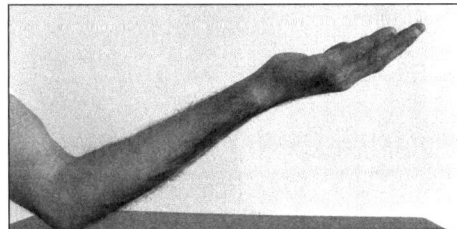

(h) Continue and twist the palm to face directly up

Figure 9-2: Twisting

Turning is soft, light and empty; twisting is stronger, which rotates the palm of the hand farther. Never force your body to twist into the bones themselves or you may strain your tissues or damage your bones.

When you have control over twisting your forearms, move on to twisting the tissues of your upper arm, allowing all the soft tissues of your whole arm to twist in and out together—without moving the tip of your elbow at all.

Once you have a tangible understanding of the difference between turning and twisting while sitting, you can apply your experience in standing, with your arms parallel and at shoulder height. Since your elbows are free from contacting any surface, you can develop skill with maintaining a sense of your elbow tips sinking down without a prop. When you feel you can keep your elbows still in space while twisting, you can move on to integrating twisting within your Heaven and Earth form.

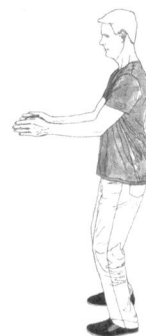

FROM HEALING TO HIGH-PERFORMANCE

Turning is the beginning version and twisting is the intermediate version. Since turning requires less effort and is softer on the body, it can also be applied when you are ill, injured or exhausted to generate a sense of comfort and wellbeing. By contrast, twisting accesses and stretches open deeper layers of soft tissues and makes the Heaven and Earth form more demanding. So this pair of techniques spans both ends of the spectrum, from healing to high-performance.

If you have been following the instructions so far, the form has been built using turning techniques. Next we will upgrade the Heaven and Earth movement by adding twisting.

Before we get to the sequence of the form, it is important to understand that it is not about the direction in which a limb turns that defines whether it is an inward or outward twist, but whether the twist aids the body expanding and opening out (an outward twist) or condensing and gathering in (an inward twist). An outward twist naturally pairs with a stretch and an inward twist naturally pairs with a bend, incorporating subtle details that transform the quality of movement within qigong.

There are several layers to twisting. Two of these will be covered to offer a beginning and an intermediate option.

TWISTING IN HEAVEN AND EARTH QIGONG: BEGINNING METHOD

As always, begin in the neutral standing posture (Figure 9-3a).

MACROCOSMIC ORBIT

First-Phase Stretch

Step 1 - Twist your arm muscles outward to roll under the tips of your elbows as your arms come forward and become parallel with each other (Figure 9-3).

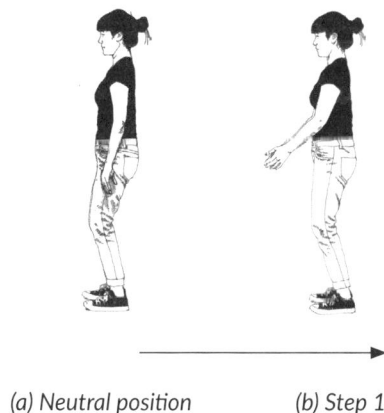

(a) Neutral position   (b) Step 1

**Figure 9-3:
Step 1—Twist Out**

Step 2 - As your arms rise while remaining parallel to each other, simply maintain the twist created in step 1. Refrain from twisting farther, which creates a tendency to turn the palms too much, whereby they face behind you (incorrect) rather than toward each other (correct). See Figure 9-4.

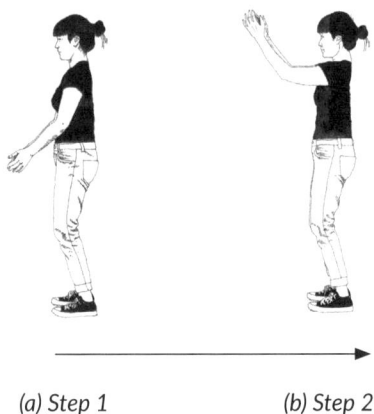

(a) Step 1   (b) Step 2

Figure 9-4:
Step 2—Maintain the Twist

Step 3 - Again, twist outward as your hands come over your head to your occiput (Figure 9-5).

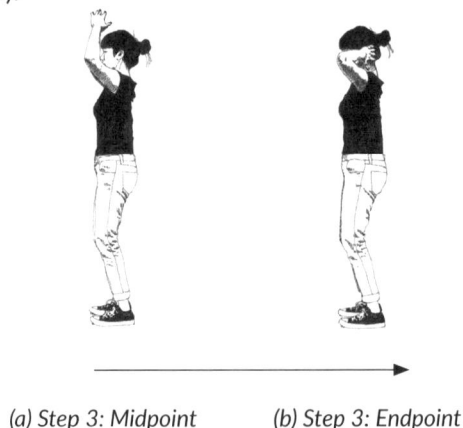

(a) Step 3: Midpoint   (b) Step 3: Endpoint

Figure 9-5:
Step 3—Twist Out

Second-Phase Bend

Step 4 - Release the outward twist and begin to twist inward as your elbows come around to and arrive in front of your shoulders (Figure 9-6).

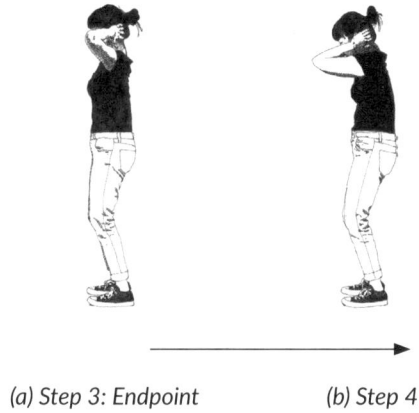

(a) Step 3: Endpoint   *(b) Step 4*

Figure 9-6:
Step 4—Twist In

Step 5 - Continue to twist inward as your hands come over your head (Figure 9-7).

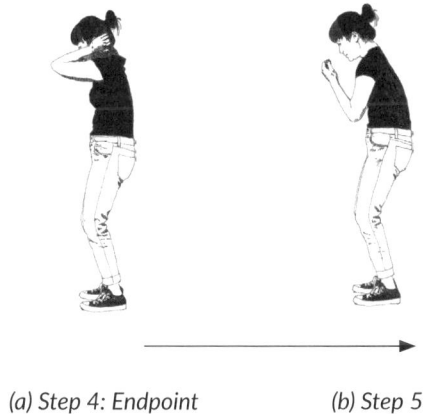

(a) Step 4: Endpoint   *(b) Step 5*

Figure 9-7:
Step 5—Continue to Twist In

Step 6 - Release the inward twist and twist outward as your elbows open out to the sides and upward (Figure 9-8).

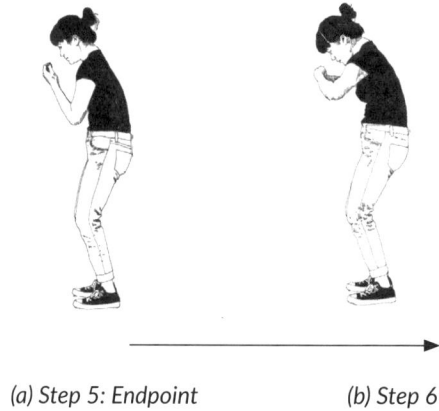

(a) Step 5: Endpoint   *(b) Step 6*

Figure 9-8:
Step 6—Twist Out

Step 7 - Release the outward twist and twist inward as your fingers drop (Figure 9-9).

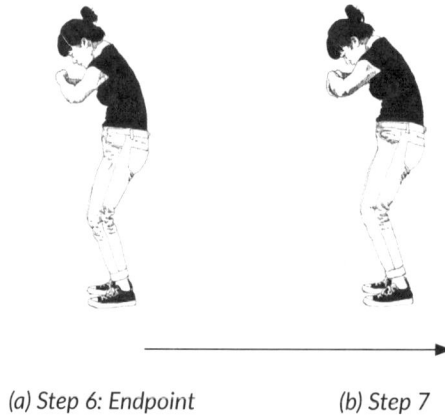

(a) Step 6: Endpoint   *(b) Step 7*

Figure 9-9:
Step 7—Twist In

Third-Phase Stretch

Step 8 - Release the inward twist and twist outward as your hands drop down in line with your left and right channels. Your palms face your body for the entirety of the downward motion (Figure 9-10).

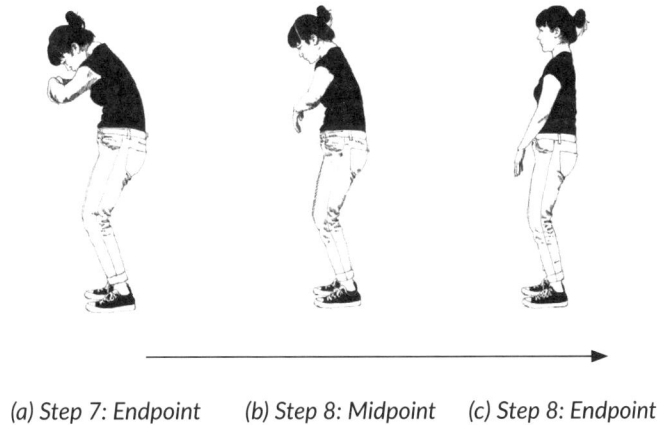

(a) Step 7: Endpoint   (b) Step 8: Midpoint   (c) Step 8: Endpoint

Figure 9-10:
Step 8—Twist Out

MICROCOSMIC ORBIT

Fourth-Phase Bend

Step 9 - As your hands come to the outside of your thighs, release the outward twist (Figure 9-11).

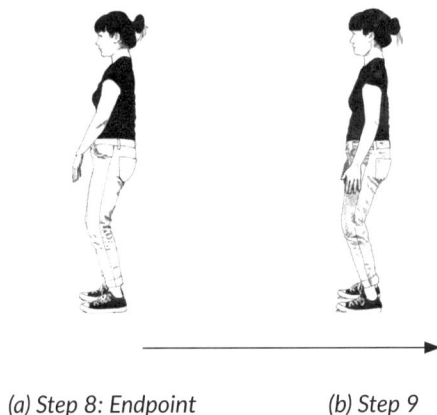

(a) Step 8: Endpoint   *(b) Step 9*

Figure 9-11:
Step 9—Release

Steps 10 and 11 - Twist inward as your hands circle backward, upward and forward to the top of the circle (Figure 9-12).

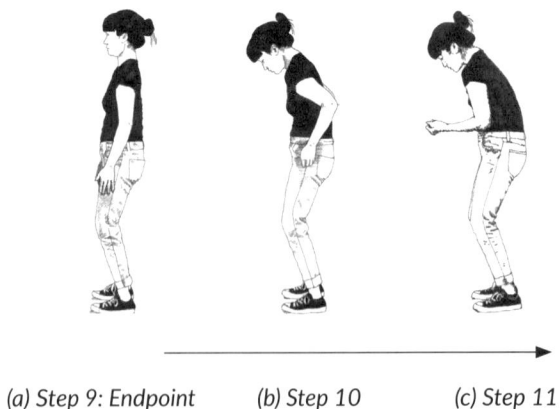

(a) Step 9: Endpoint   *(b) Step 10*   *(c) Step 11*

Figure 9-12:
Steps 10 and 11—Twist In

Fifth-Phase Stretch

Steps 12 and 13 - Release the inward twist and twist outward as your hands circle forward, downward and backward to the bottom of the circle (Figure 9-13).

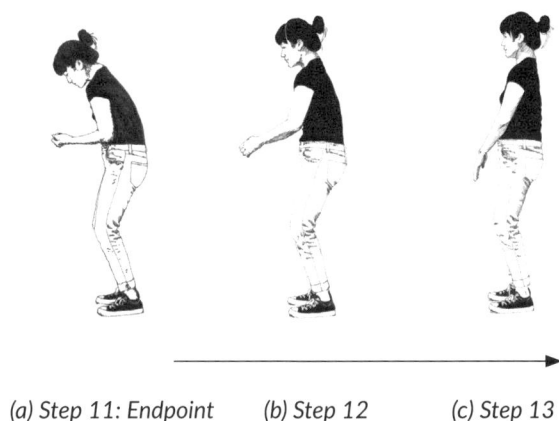

(a) Step 11: Endpoint   *(b) Step 12*   *(c) Step 13*

Figure 9-13:
Steps 12 and 13—Twist Out

NEUTRAL

Sixth-Phase Release

Step 14 - Release the outward twist to neutral (Figure 9-14).

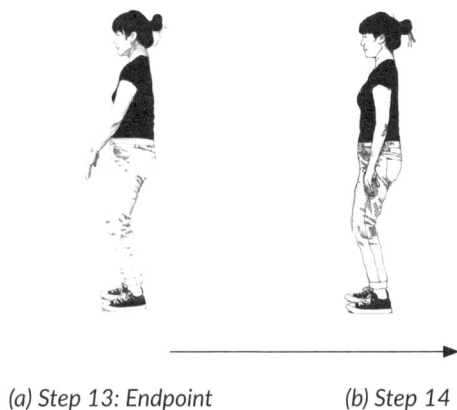

(a) Step 13: Endpoint   *(b) Step 14*

Figure 9-14: Step 14—Release to Neutral

Important: The arms twist outward on the fifth-phase stretch at the end of the form and again on the first-phase stretch on the next repetition. Therefore, the let go to neutral in between these two outward twists is essential or you will not have any space to continue twisting.

Make sure you have embodied the correct quality and sequence of twisting with this beginning method before moving on to the intermediate method.

INCREASE THE DEPTH AND INTENSITY OF THE TWIST: INTERMEDIATE PRACTITIONERS

MACROCOSMIC ORBIT

Although the bulk of the pattern remains the same as the first twisting method for the macrocosmic orbit, two subtle yet defining points increase the intensity and depth of the twist:

- In the first-phase stretch, the twist becomes continuous, running through steps 1-3 until your fingers reach your occiput (Figure 9-15).
- In the first-phase stretch, step 2, the main issue is continuing the twist—without turning your bones whatsoever—so that your palms remain facing each other.

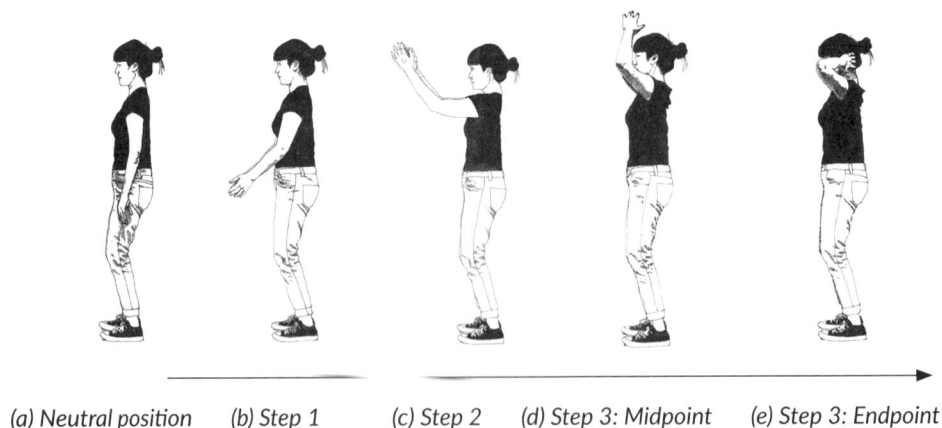

(a) Neutral position   *(b) Step 1*   *(c) Step 2*   *(d) Step 3: Midpoint*   *(e) Step 3: Endpoint*

Figure 9–15: First-Phase Stretch—Twist Out (Intermediate Method)

The rest of the macrocosmic orbit is practiced the same as in the beginning method.

MICROCOSMIC ORBIT

The microcosmic orbit is done entirely differently as the aim becomes to wind up the muscle groups of your arms in one direction and then release them in order to ignite the reversal and rotation back in the opposite direction (Figure 9-16).

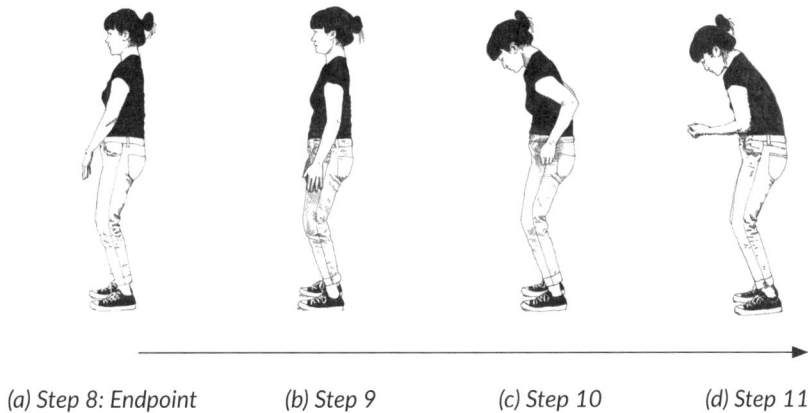

(a) Step 8: Endpoint	*(b) Step 9*	*(c) Step 10*	*(d) Step 11*

Figure 9-16:
Fourth-Phase Bend—Twist In

- In the fourth-phase bend (Figure 9-16), once again twist your muscles inward, but this time increase the twist all the way to the top of the circle to the extent that the soft tissues of your arms feel as though they want to reverse. If you use force, the tissues will simply tense and go hard, which prevents the natural reversal. Conversely, if you do not twist enough, you will not generate the spring-back action that creates the reversal. You will have to practice a lot while paying close attention to the quality of the inward twist and staying within your body's comfortable, 70-percent range.

- When you get the quality and timing just right during the fourth-phase bend, your arm muscles will naturally and without effort unwind and let go at the moment you shift into the fifth-phase stretch. This letting go of the twisted muscles, along with the releasing of the in-breath to the out-breath, is what starts to yield a very yin quality to the stretching action in the fifth-phase stretch.

As you develop the twisting action in both the macrocosmic and microcosmic orbits, they travel deeper into your body. This depth penetrates lengthwise (through the shoulders), both front and back into the torso, and deeper toward (but never into) the bones. This double action is common in neigong and serves as a sign that practice is doing its job: expelling tension, connecting up the body via the soft tissues and opening the pathways through which qi travels to bring about true integration. When one part moves, all parts move.

ABOUT TWISTING THE LEGS

Twisting the legs relies upon the ability to twist the arms well and yet is activated and practiced through a very different methodology. There are many safety concerns when twisting the tissues of the legs. If done incorrectly, twists can destabilize the sacrum and, thereby, the entire spine. For this reason, twisting the legs is not included in this book and should only be learned once all of the essential and foundational components of Heaven and Earth have been integrated to the point that you could turn them on like a light switch. For the weeks and months that follow, practice twisting in your arms frequently—until all ambiguity is lost and a concrete, physical sensation of twisting is alive and available to you on-demand.

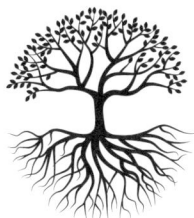

CHAPTER 10:

THE YIN-YANG DICHOTOMY AND GROWING YOUR CAPACITY

YIN AND YANG ENERGIES

Yin and yang is the concept of opposing forces or energies. They are two sides of one coin, or two halves of any natural phenomenon in the manifest realm, such as night and day, female and male, rest and activity, and so on. Each neigong thread or internal process, system and substructure of the body can be expressed by these opposites. The principle of yin and yang is so fundamental to Taoist thinking that it lies at the very bedrock of their philosophy and outlook in all aspects of life.

At one level, Heaven and Earth, like all neigong practice, is actually just the oscillation between opposites. Some parts of the form call for manifesting yin energy while others call for yang energy. Heaven and Earth is quite literally a study in how to create flow between yin and yang. For instance, bending is yin and stretching is yang, while opening is yang and closing is yin. These

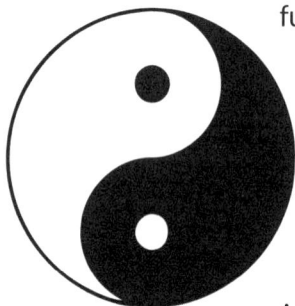

fundamental threads of neigong are woven together to form an internal arts cloth. All techniques are governed by the same universal principles that give rise to the natural world in which we live and reality as we experience it, including the myriad of dichotomies. These laws are manifested through yang and yin energies, opposing forces that come into existence, accumulate, grow, reach their potential and flip to their opposites in a never-ending cosmic dance.

USING STEPPING STONES

From the perspective of Heaven and Earth Qigong, the interplay between yang and yin manifests a form that is smooth, fluid and constant. As you stretch open and expand to your maximum comfortable capacity, your body naturally calls for the flip to bend, shrink and smoothly recoil, and the cycle repeats *ad infinitum*. As you systematically isolate each and every part of your physical body and its qi through ongoing qigong practice, play with the yang and yin aspects of your body to expand their range to your maximum potential while adhering to the 70-Percent Rule. In so doing, you open up, engage, strengthen and integrate all parts of your body, which enables you to "move all parts" and, with dedicated training over many years and decades, move all parts extremely well.

Each of us brings to training a collection of tensions within ourselves due to illnesses, injuries, bad posture, over or under activity, aging, trauma or just bad luck. Parts of you may be stuck, stagnant, closed down or completely dormant. Initially the purpose of training is to awaken, open up, heal and bring more life to your body and qi in order to restore health and vitality, and cultivate consciousness. This is one of the reasons why Heaven and Earth both begins and ends on a stretching/opening movement. Each round slowly and progressively opens up your body and allows you to release bindings, tensions and qi blockages trapped inside you. With ongoing practice and, as neigong threads become alive and embedded in your body, more internal space is created for your muscles, blood vessels, nervous system, internal organs, glands and metabolism to function optimally. Then the range of yin-yang motion within your form increases dramatically, allowing you to cultivate vibrancy and more qi.

As discussed in Chapter 8 on breathing, there is always an ideal method for training, but normally students must take many detours before any ideal is actually appropriate for them. You must acknowledge where you are in the here and now, and then make some adjustments according to the needs of your body-mind-qi. Then, as you shed a certain degree of the tensions and bindings that hold you back from reaching the ideal, you can once again adjust and move closer to embodying the technique in its ideal form. It is called practice because training will never be perfect and should not be expected to be. Paradoxically you aim for perfection, as any art can always be improved upon, but you never have the delusion that you can achieve it.

WHAT IS MY CAPACITY?

All things considered, the one limiting factor is capacity. You continually ask the question: What is my capacity for any specific aspect or technique? For example, you may open and close well, but twist your tissues poorly, or vice-versa; you may be able to inhale well, but exhale poorly, or vice-versa. As you practice, you will discover and rediscover what works well and that which does not. The focus in the Water tradition is always on playing to and strengthening your weaknesses to create more balance. Western culture is designed to play to people's strengths. However, chains break at the weakest links, and balance and integration can never be achieved by ignoring some parts of yourself, whether related to your body, mind, qi or any combination thereof. Lasting satisfaction comes from feeling whole, at ease with life and awake from deep within oneself.

CONTINUE MOVING LIKE THE COSMOS

The ego's drive to achieve satisfaction in the manifest world can sometimes push the body, mind or qi to do more than is within that person's capacity. What do you do if this happens to you? Forget any ideals and accept the limitations created by the restrictions that you carry, until eventually you can transcend them.

As you cycle through the various neigong threads and endless yin-yang flips, key into the endpoints and transition before you reach your maximum. As you run out of space on one half of the cycle, transition to the opposite, whether or not you are at the designated/ideal part of the form. It is true that the internal content will be out of sync with the form, but this temporary state of being is better than forcing your body beyond its capacity or allowing your form to become completely disconnected. Either way, qi flow will diminish and neigong practice is meant to do the opposite: that is, to circulate, balance and cultivate your qi.

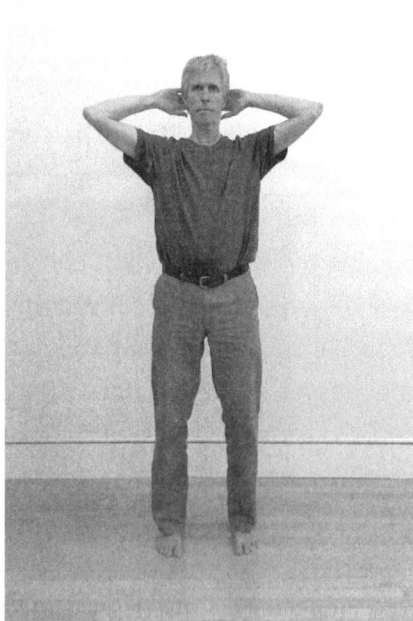

Bill Ryan, Senior Student of Master Frantzis
moving into the first close of the form

By switching to the opposite when you reach your maximum comfortable capacity (while adhering to the 70-Percent Rule), your qi continues to flow and develop. The parts that are out of sync are only temporarily so, until you can increase your capacity or slow down any particular internal aspects enough to last the allotted timeframe. This is just another form of capacity; the capacity to move continuously and slowly while remaining internal.

Throughout this text, both the ideal and next-best scenarios are presented to help dedicated students through the pitfalls of training to build their capacity in the fastest time and most efficient manner possible. Sometimes even the next-best options are difficult to achieve and, when this happens, the rule of thumb is to never strain your body-mind-qi and never lose the body's fundamental internal connections. Add in extra yin-yang cycles to whatever neigong threads require adjustments and find a pattern that works for you. Do not inhibit the flow between yang and yin, and when either becomes full, allow it to naturally flip to its opposite—without hesitation or inertia—and continue moving like the unending flow within the cosmos itself.

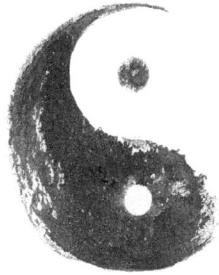

OPENING AND CLOSING
THE JOINTS OF THE BODY

The joints covered in this section are:

- Wrists, hands and fingers

- Elbows

- Shoulders and shoulder blades

- Ribs

- Toes, feet and ankles

- Knees

- Hips/kwa.

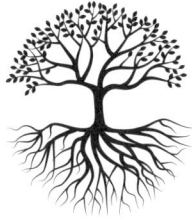

CHAPTER 11:

KAI HE GONG, OPENING-AND-CLOSING NEIGONG

Whereas many qi practices—such as those within Shaolin kung fu, karate, tae kwon do and other external martial arts—use fairly linear motions, qigong uses circular ones. Circular movements have an edge over linear ones when practiced for health and healing for several reasons. For a start, they are designed to root out and release physical tension, which yields relaxation. Relaxing and letting go stimulates blood and qi flow, which triggers production of body fluids—e.g. synovial, lymph, interstitial and blood plasma, to name a few—thereby increasing their volume and circulation.

> In Chinese medicine, "blood" is actually a blanket term, which encompasses all of the body's circulatory fluids.

All fluids play essential roles in maintaining the health of your body in one way or another, from cushioning your joints each time you move via synovial fluid to protecting your body against infectious disease with white blood cells, which are transported via blood, lymph and interstitial fluid. So stimulating production of these fluids is of high importance to health and longevity, which happens to be a specialty of qigong in general and opening-and-closing techniques in particular.

WHAT IS OPENING-AND-CLOSING NEIGONG OR "PULSING"?

The Chinese term for Marriage of Heaven and Earth Qigong is *Kai He Gong* or "Open-and-Close Practice/Skill"; it is considered a practice when the student is in the learning phases and a skill once the practitioner becomes an adept.

There are two basic components to opening-and-closing neigong (also known as "pulsing"), which are:

- Opening and closing all the body's joints, cavities, internal organs, glands and subtle energy anatomy.
- Lengthening out and in along the yang and yin surfaces of the body, which is how pulsing is applied to the body's soft tissues— that is, opening and closing the muscles, fascia, tendons, ligaments and blood vessels. (Lengthening methods will be covered in Chapter 19.)

The aim is to wake up, amplify and integrate these two fundamental components to deepen your Heaven and Earth practice. The more refined your skill is with pulsing and lengthening, the freer your body becomes, the more efficiently your immune system functions, the more qi you generate, and the more strongly you can connect to and draw upon the non-physical energies of Heaven and Earth.

PULSING THE JOINTS

At the most fundamental level, opening-and-closing techniques are initiated in the joints of the body to stimulate blood and qi flow. The pulse is a center-to-periphery and periphery-to-center action: the central point is the middle of the joint, where an energy gate is located; the soft tissues that surround and encapsulate the joint are considered the periphery.

> *Energy gates* are major relay stations of the body, where the strength of qi moving through the system is regulated. Master Frantzis covers energy gates in depth in his book, *Opening the Energy Gates of Your Body Qigong* (see the Bibliography).

In the beginning, opening-and-closing actions are linear or circular at best. When the entire skeletal frame and all the cavities get involved, pulsing edges toward the spherical. Through this method, the energies of Heaven and Earth are not only contacted, but so too are the energies of the practitioner's environment. This book will cover how to pulse the joints only. Practicing more advanced methods for pulsing, such as with the cavities and beyond, is counterproductive until you can fully activate the pulse via your mind's intent. That is to say you can open and close each and every individual joint of your body—separately or in unison with all others—at will and without any external motion whatsoever.

A Word to the Wise: You need some understanding of human anatomy to be able to correctly and precisely locate and pulse the joints of the body. As extensive anatomy illustrations would be exhaustive in a how-to text of this depth, the authors recommend obtaining a comprehensive anatomy book and keeping it on hand for reference as you both study and train neigong techniques, especially before pulsing or working with a partner. See the Bibliography for recommendations. The best neigong teachers have a solid grounding in anatomy and physiology.

Synovial Joints

All the major joints of the body and the bulk of the joints covered in this text are synovial joints, except for the shoulder blades, ribs, AH joint, AC joint, and the joints between each pair of the hand bones (metacarpals) and foot bones (metatarsals). A synovial joint is where two or more bones connect and which are surrounded by a synovial capsule, a dense fibrous sac that envelopes the joint and contains synovial fluid. On the inside surface of the capsule is the synovial membrane, which secretes fluid that lubricates the joint. During the pulsing process, the synovial membrane becomes activated, generates a capillary action and begins to deliver more fluid to the localized area. The fluid fills up the joint and thereby suspends it in a healthy, open position.

This activity helps prevent wear and tear or damage to the joint, including serious conditions such as osteoarthritis. This ailment is due to the ends of the bones becoming too close together and continually rubbing against one another during activity. The continual movement of fluids also helps to prevent unwanted calcium-deposit buildup on the ends of the bones that make up the joints. This condition can be extremely painful and limiting in terms of range of motion, and can ultimately lead to more severe problems, such as crystallization of the synovial fluid itself.

About Fluid Production in the Body

Some people have contested the claim that pulsing can increase the quantity of fluids in the joints or, if it can, postulate it would take years of dedicated training. However, think of a twisted ankle which, after injury, swells up within 24 hours. The body delivers a large quantity of interstitial fluid around the ankle to protect it from further damage, flood the site with nutrients and white blood vessels to aid repair, and remove waste material, such as dead cells, as a result of the impact.

> So if your body can respond to an injury in this way—without movement— then why could it not respond similarly and with the same efficiency to a highly refined therapeutic motion?

Synovial, interstitial, lymph and cerebrospinal fluids are derivatives of blood plasma. The body distributes fluid when and where it is required. Since pulsing activates the synovial membranes with its gentle, continual open-and-close rhythm, fluid is drawn out from the body's reserves—the blood. The more you pulse, the more fluid is deposited in the activated joints. A signal is sent back to the central nervous system to retain more fluids from what you eat and drink to prevent the blood supply from drying up. In the beginning, the overall effect is limited but, in time, the body responds to the higher demand for fluids from ongoing, regular internal exercise and progressively increases fluid production. Small gains can be made each and every time you train with even a short 20-minute pulsing session opening up all the joints and strongly circulating blood and qi.

This does not mean that you will increase the fluids in your joints forever, which would blow them up like balloons filled with water. More accurately, opening-and-closing techniques stimulate, circulate and balance fluid pro-duction and distribution in the body. Since many people lack sufficient fluid in their joints due to stress, tension and sedentary lifestyles, they benefit from an increase in fluid production. However, for disorders such as rheuma-toid arthritis that can cause excess fluid in the joints, pulsing can be applied to reduce the excess fluid and support overstretched tissues returning to a natural state, as well as other rebalancing effects in the body's systems.

Apply a Soft Application

Opening-and-closing techniques are non-invasive and incredibly yin, so they require a soft application. When you attempt to pulse a joint—whether in your own body or someone else's—use a gentle intent and move slowly, continuously and in a balanced, rhythmic manner. If you apply too much pressure when training the following hands-on techniques with a partner, their nerves will harden and the tissues around the respective joints will tighten. These protective mechanisms prevent access to the pulse, which relies on relaxation, as what you are actually attempting to do is tune into and amplify the natural pulse, not generate it *per se*.

Until you have manifested pulsing in your body or have had a skilled, quali-fied instructor induce the correct feeling in your body by pulsing your joints for you, you will be grasping around in the dark trying to find the light switch.

This phase can be frustrating, but worse is to overlay experiences of other practices you might have done in the past and project them onto the concept of pulsing. Opening-and-closing techniques are unique and not found in any other exercise or health system of which the authors are aware. Avoid making false comparisons and instead focus on directly experiencing how the pulse feels and operates in your body-mind-qi, and observe the results.

Find a Qualified Teacher

In the following section, you will learn the specifics of how to mechanically open and close the joints of your body. The main purpose of pulsing is to open up the joints, and engage the fluid within any synovial joint and the subtle energy of both the fluid and the joint itself, which most likely cannot be learned from a book alone. If your motion is too big, too small, too fast, too slow, too superficial or too hard, you will not be able to pulse and will only move the flesh—which is not the purpose of these techniques. Study the instructions carefully, then experiment with a willing training partner and especially on yourself to begin to get the big picture. Watching videos about pulsing is, frankly, more helpful than a text because at least you can see the motion. At some point you will need the assistance of a skilled, competent teacher in order to glimpse the depth, layers and profound nature of this neigong component. The information that follows is meant to support live training in order to clarify the protocols and prevent any misunderstandings.

Only a minute minority of the population will have the proprioception and physical ability to watch someone pulse and accurately replicate the motion in their own body. These are the increasingly rare physical geniuses—the one in a million—and even they have to practice to embody deeper and more profound layers of pulsing. Partner exercises are a method to learn, directly experience and cultivate the understanding and embodiment of pulsing techniques. For this reason, the bulk of this section is dedicated to exercise sets for you and a training partner. Your personal progress will rely, to a large extent, on you and your partner's ability to *feel* your body (kinesthetic sense), adhere to the instructions and practice accurately.

WITHOUT OPENING AND CLOSING, THERE IS NO TAI CHI

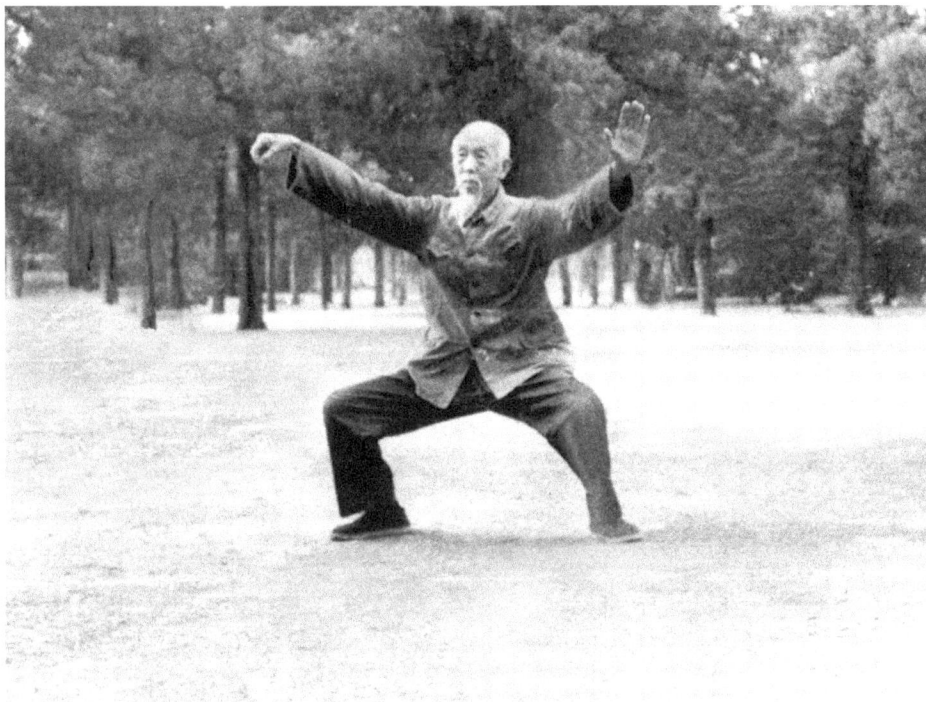

Wu Style Tai Chi Taoist Lineage Holder Liu Hung Chieh,
who transmitted the lineage to his disciple, Bruce Frantzis

Genuine tai chi masters have always said, "Without opening and closing, there is no tai chi." Yet until the 1990s, the tai chi community in the West knew nothing about the basic neigong techniques for pulsing and directly moving qi. Nobody talked or wrote about them, and certainly nobody taught them. There are still many misconceptions in almost all tai chi and martial arts schools. Within the Water tradition, opening-and-closing and complementary techniques for directly moving qi are not only exceptionally important and openly taught, but are essential for achieving higher states of practice and qi development.

SIX STAGES OF PULSING A JOINT: OPENING AND CLOSING THE WRIST

Note: This text uses both Latin and layman's terms for medical professionals and ordinary folk. The nature of the body part will not change, regardless of what you call it!

Certified Heaven and Earth Qigong Instructors: Master Frantzis recommends the following sequence for systematically and progressively teaching pulsing in a class format.

STAGE ONE: LOCATE AND UNDERSTAND THE ANATOMY OF THE JOINT

Pulsing the Wrist

The best place to begin learning how to open and close is with the wrist, a fairly large joint that is not too big or too heavy. Most people have a reasonable degree of dexterity and control over their wrist, so the tissues around the bones are relatively flexible. (Although, sadly, this is becoming less so due to continual overuse of keyboards and smartphones.) The wrist has a relatively large range of motion in comparison to many other joints, such as those in the lower body, and so requires a minimal amount of strength and sensitivity.

Before attempting to pulse a joint for the first time, the wise student will become familiar with the specifics that comprise and surround that particular joint to ensure safe and efficient training. For the purpose of pulsing, the focus is on the soft tissues that connect the bones together (ligaments) and the surrounding soft tissues that encapsulate the joints (synovial capsule, tendons, muscles, fascia and skin)—all of which are quite elastic in nature and normally move a lot with the correct momentum.

Each time you work with a new partner or student, take time to locate and feel the joint you plan to target, as there are many individual variations.

In the case of the wrist joint, unlike most joints, the structure is quite complex with eight small bones (carpals) situated between the two forearm bones (radius and ulna), and five hand bones (metacarpals). This structure gives the wrist its flexibility.

STAGE TWO:
FIND THE BEST POSITION AND HAND HOLD, AND PROPERLY ALIGN THE JOINT

When pulsing in your own body, there are various positions that are optimal for activating and engaging specific joints of the body, which will be explained in the exercises that follow. When pulsing a partner, there are generally one or two good positions for initiating the pulse.

The larger the surface contact between your hands and your partner's body part, the better you can adhere to their fascia and, thereby, the less effort or pressure you will need to open up their joint. The less effort and pressure you use, the more relaxed you both can become, the more you can feel and the greater the range of motion you can create in your partner's joint.

Holding your partner's joint in a soft and gentle way allows your partner to relax, which is ideal. Conversely, if your hands are tight and tensed, your partner's joint will also tense and, thereby, prevent the full range of motion required for the next stage.

Always make sure the joint on which you are working is properly aligned so that, when pulsed, the internal pressures generated will be spread evenly over the entire joint. If a limb is positioned or held incorrectly and pulsed, one side of the joint is likely to shut down while its opposite will be overstretched, both of which can cause damage if done repeatedly.

Partner Exercise: Prepare to Pulse the Wrist

In the case of the wrist, when holding your partner's hand and forearm, use a light yet firm contact, and make sure your fingers and hands do not add resistance to the joint by directly contacting it in any of the following exercises.

1. Hold your partner's forearm with a gentle intent.

2. Locate their wrist by running your fingers gently yet firmly over their joints, so you can recognize the end of their forearm, the beginning of their hand and their wrist in between.

3. Use a yin intent as you make adjustments to your grip. Take time to properly align the joint before moving on to the two-beat cycle (to be explained in the next section). In the case of the wrist joint, when viewed from the side, the receiver's middle finger should directly bisect the middle of their own forearm and not lean off-center, which causes a bend in the wrist. When viewed from above, their fingers should bisect their forearm and the center of their elbow joint (Figure 11-1).

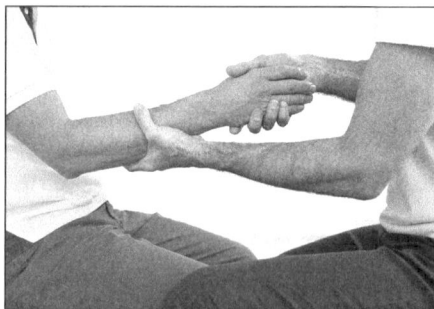

Neutral position

Figure 11-1:
Pulsing the Wrist—Hand Hold

STAGE THREE: THE TWO-BEAT CYCLE

Feeling (kinesthetic sense) is your primary feedback driver for whether you are successfully opening a joint: too little pressure and you will only move the skin and the joint will remain closed; too much pressure and you might cause discomfort or even harm. The space between the bones must become larger and all the tissues connected to and surrounding the joint must elongate in order for it to open. This is a perfectly natural phenomenon as pulsing rhythms occur in the human body whether or not you tune into or amplify them. Usually young people have a much larger range of motion, which diminishes as their fluids dry up from their body closing down—as a result of aging, stress, trauma, illness or injury. All you are attempting to do is reinstate or amplify the range of the natural pulse in yourself or a training partner in order to bring back the full range of motion possible in the moment.

Since most people's joints are closed down rather than too open and floppy, always begin with an open and finish with an open-release to allow any accumulated tension to dissipate and generate more internal space in the joint. This is one aspect that helps to generate the energy of the Wood Element—growth and expansion.

One Pulses, the Other Receives

All of the exercises in this section are for you and a training partner and, as such, are designed to be completed with reciprocity. Once you and your partner have been through one pass of any instruction set, switch roles: the receiver becomes the pulser and the pulser becomes the receiver. In this way, both parties experience having their joints pulsed, run through the handoff procedure to take over the pulse on their own and practice pulsing within Heaven and Earth Qigong. The ideal points at which to swap roles are included in the instruction sets that follow.

The person activating the pulse (the "pulser") does all the work while the person receiving the pulse (the "receiver") continuously lets go and absorbs the experience throughout the entirety of the exercise. The receiver is in charge of what the pulser does by way of feedback. For instance, if the pulser pulls too hard, moves too fast or too slowly, or is out of sync, the receiver will coach them through the adjustments required for their body to let go and open up. This process helps the pulser tune into the specific range and quality of the joint, and learn how to operate within their partner's comfort zone.

Bodyworkers and Instructors: If you are a bodyworker or qigong instructor (or hope to be one someday), you want to practice pulsing on as many different training partners as possible in order to develop experience working with a range of individual variations. A teacher/practitioner should know most of the caveats and all the safety concerns about when pulsing is appropriate before pulsing on others in a position of authority. In China, the norm was to work on thousands of patients as a volunteer before a practitioner in a clinical setting would be recognized as a qualified professional.

Range of Motion: The 70-Percent Rule and the Pump

Each and every joint in your body has a comfortable range of motion, which is referred to as 100 percent of its range of motion. If you go beyond this point, you begin to strain the soft tissues and can even cause damage to the joint—or break a joint if pushed far enough. When 100-percent range of motion is discussed, the authors specifically mean to indicate how far a person can go *without major discomfort and absolutely no pain.*

However, if you open and close a joint to 100 percent of its capacity, the fluids and qi will disconnect rather than become integrated into the motion. All energy arts training relies on and is powered by internal connections in body, mind and qi. In order to link to the fluid and qi of a joint, you must operate within 70 percent of the comfortable range of motion for each individual person, for that specific joint and in that particular moment.

You could think of an old water pump or hand pump for bicycle tires. If you activate the pump all the way to the top and bottom, no traction is generated and the water does not get drawn up, or the tire does not inflate. When you back off from both ends and stay within the 70-percent range, the water or air streams out continuously. The wrist—and any other joint for that matter—functions the same way. First you must investigate where the comfortable 100-percent open position is located and, from there, back off to working within 70 percent of the receiver's comfortable range.

Partner Exercise: Activate the Two-Beat Cycle

Once you have found a comfortable posture and a firm yet relaxed grip on your partner's body, make sure to give them a few seconds to settle down and let go before beginning the next exercise.

From the correct hand hold (Figure 11-2a), use your arm that is supporting and holding the receiver's forearm to anchor their arm. Position your other hand so that you can smoothly, slowly and gently draw their hand away from their forearm to open up their wrist in the steps that follow. Normally it takes a few seconds to fully open up the joint.

1. Slowly and smoothly draw the receiver's joint out to 100 percent of their comfortable range and then release back to neutral (Figure 11-2b-c). The elongated tissues from the opening phase will naturally draw the hand back once the joint is fully opened. Fluidly transition into slowly releasing and allowing the receiver's joint to return to neutral without doing anything to push it back in.

2. Repeat step 1 a couple of times.

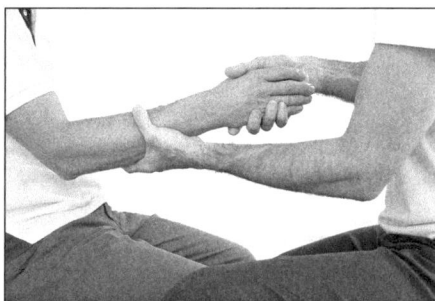

(a) Neutral position

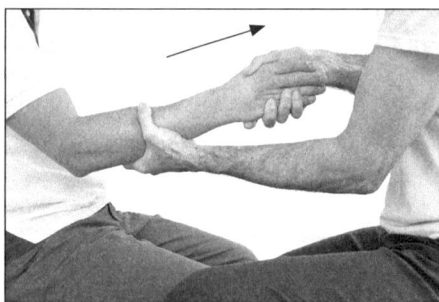

(b) 100-percent open

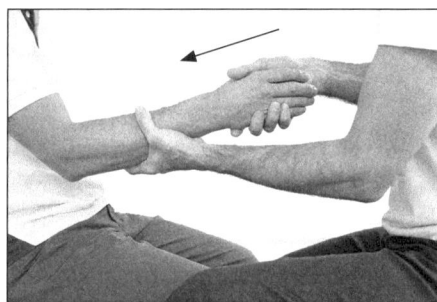

(c) Release to neutral

Figure 11-2:
Pulsing the Wrist—Two-Beat Cycle

The range of motion in a joint is not always readily visible to the naked eye. Use caution when pulsing a partner and stay focused. Arrows have been added throughout this section to clarify the direction of the movement.

3. Once you determine the 100-percent open position, back off and only open the joint to 70 percent of the joint's comfortable range; then fluidly transition into slowly releasing and allowing the joint to return to neutral—again, without doing anything to push it back in (Figure 11-3a-b).

4. Repeat step 3 a few times, until you get the hang of it. This beginning phase is referred to as the "two-beat cycle," or open-release.

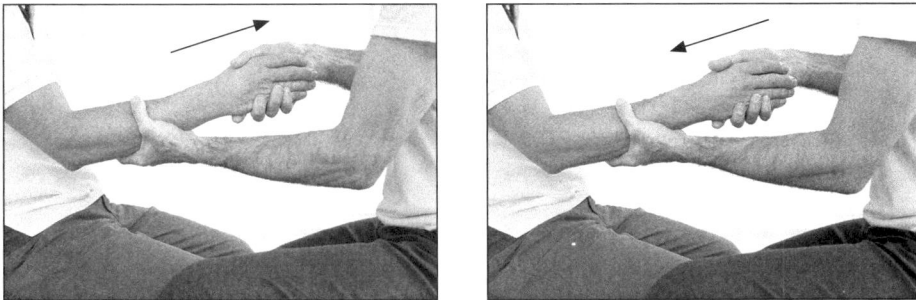

<table>
<tr><td>(a) 70 percent open</td><td>(b) Release to neutral</td></tr>
</table>

Figure 11-3:
Pulsing the Wrist—Two-Beat Cycle

Take a few seconds to both open and release the joint

Be sure to both open and release the joint smoothly and slowly. When you play the 70-percent range correctly, the receiver's body recognizes that the motion is therapeutic, not invasive, and gives up its resistances.

Repeat this open-release, two-beat cycle a dozen times or more while focusing on the quality of motion. The receiver should physically and visibly begin to relax as the wave of open-release, open-release washes away tension and the wrist becomes more elastic and open.

Through all stages:

- Stay present and pay attention to the subtle responses from your partner. If you pull too hard or too suddenly, their nerves will tighten before they scream, "Ouch!"

- The receiver is always feeling and letting the pulser know if they are being successful, and what they could do to be more so—e.g. a little less effort, a little more effort, smoother or slower. When the exercise is performed correctly, the receiver will relax, let go, become quiet and the pulser will need less and less effort to achieve the same range of motion. The receiver's arm may also become heavier as a result of their nerves releasing the bindings in their soft tissues from blood and other fluids flooding the newly opened spaces.

STAGE FOUR: CLOSE AND RELEASE THE JOINT

Partner Exercise: Close and Release the Wrist

Start with the basic hand hold (Figure 11-4).

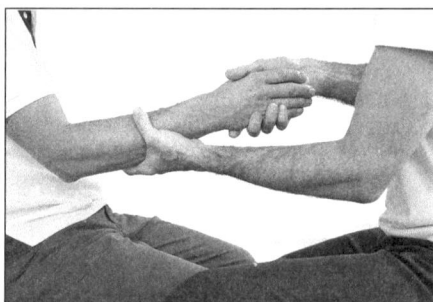

Neutral position

Figure 11-4:
Pulsing the Wrist—Hand Hold

1 Draw the receiver's joint out to 70 percent of its comfortable range, and then fluidly transition into slowly releasing and allowing the receiver's joint to return to the neutral position (Figure 11-5).

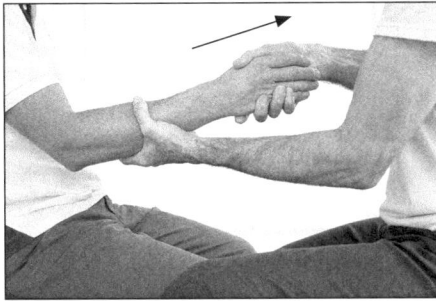

(a) 70 percent open   (b) Release to neutral

Figure 11-5: Pulsing the Wrist—Draw Open the Joint

2. Once in the neutral position, slowly and gently:

    (a) Compress the joint until you reach the 100-percent closed point by pushing your hand toward the receiver's forearm. Close the joint until you reach a natural stop without the receiver tensing, contracting or experiencing any form of pain—that is 100-percent closed within the receiver's comfortable range. See Figure 11-6a.

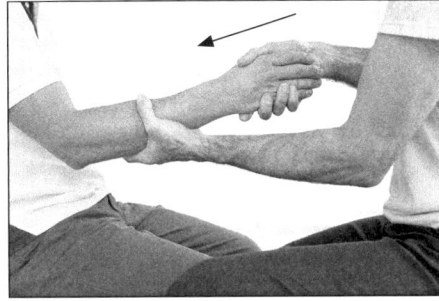

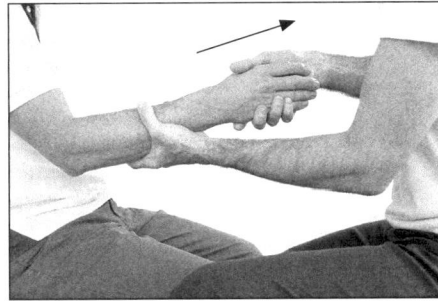

    (b) Release the joint and allow it to return to neutral (Figure 11-6b).

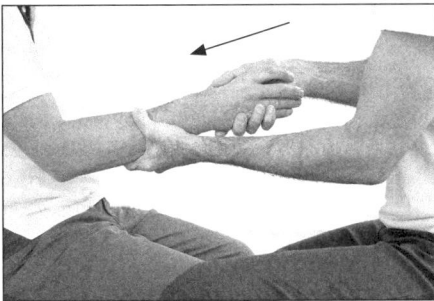

(a) 100 percent close   (b) Release to neutral

Figure 11-6: Pulsing the Wrist—Compress the Joint

STAGE FIVE: THE FOUR-BEAT CYCLE

The correct method for pulsing is to operate within 70 percent of the receiver's comfortable range (both on the open and the close), which you will learn and practice in the following partner exercise.

The four-beat cycle is:

1. Active open
2. Passive release
3. Active close
4. Passive release.

The two active beats ensure the joint opens and closes; the two passive beats ensure the operation is natural, smooth, soft and relaxing. Both aspects are critical to a clear and fluid pulse, but the passive phase allows you to follow the receiver's body in speed and range of motion. Never use force, especially on the closing half of the cycle.

When you close to 70 percent, notice:

- The thick, viscous feel on the closing half of the cycle.
- How, when you let go, the joint naturally springs open to some degree. The recoil from the close-to-neutral is normally smaller than from the open-to-neutral—unless the joint is very healthy, in which case the recoil will more or less be equal.

Remember: You are simply amplifying the natural open-and-close rhythm in your partner's body, not making them pulse.

Partner Exercise: Activate the Four-Beat Cycle

Start with the basic hand hold (Figure 11-7).

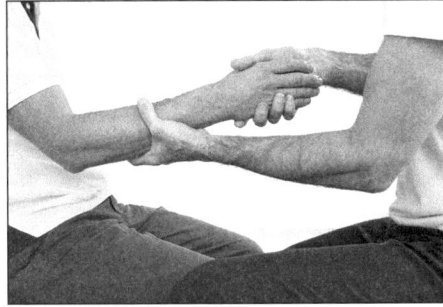

Neutral position

Figure 11-7:
Pulsing the Wrist—Hand Hold

1. Begin with an active open to 70 percent of the receiver's capacity (active open), and then fluidly transition into slowly releasing and allowing the joint to return to the neutral position (passive release). See Figure 11-8.

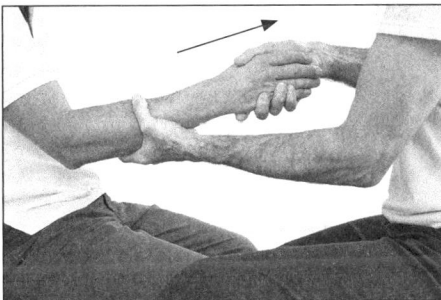

(a) 70-percent open

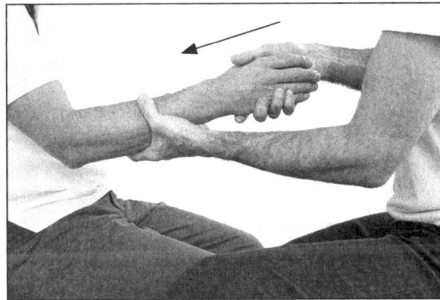

(b) Release to neutral

Figure 11-8:
Pulsing the Wrist—Four-Beat Cycle
(Active Open, Passive Release)

2. As the release begins to taper and dissipate, shift into:

   (a) actively closing the joint 70 percent (active close); then (b) fluidly transitioning into slowly releasing and allowing the receiver's joint to return to neutral (passive release). See Figure 11-9.

3. As the release from the close tapers, shift into actively opening the joint, which starts the cycle anew.

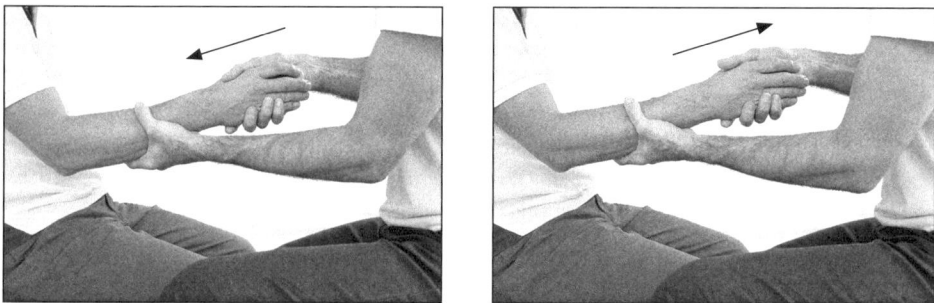

(a) 70-percent close   (b) Release to neutral

Figure 11-9:
Pulsing the Wrist—Four-Beat Cycle
(Active Close, Passive Release)

Continue this four-beat cycle while following the "Five-Point Checklist for Pulsing a Partner" that follows to amplify and bring alive the pulse in your partner.

Five-Point Checklist for Pulsing a Partner

Whenever using the four-beat cycle to pulse a partner:

- Follow the receiver's body, both in speed and range of motion, always staying within 70-percent open/70-percent close.

- Look for a smooth, continuous transition between each active-to-passive and passive-to-active phase.

- Let go of a mechanically-orientated approach, tune into the intuitive aspects of your mind and feel for the pulse, which is a never-ending transformation between yang and yin energies.

- Look for circularity in motion, not a physical circle, but a circular changeover from the out to the in and the in to the out, as practiced in Taoist breathing. Circularity prevents and eradicates inertia by removing the stops and starts.

- With your hands, monitor your partner as you pulse them through feeling their flesh and nerve responses. Observe them and adjust the pulse in order to generate maximum relaxation.

As you practice these five aspects again and again, you will slowly tune into how to pulse. Cultivating a reasonable pulse without any assistance from a partner usually takes copious training—even for the gifted. When you are on the receiving end, use the opportunity to feel without anything else cluttering up your mind. Tune into the feeling of the pulse and let your nerves absorb the experience, which should be deeply relaxing and pleasurable. Then, when you return to self-practice, you have guideposts for knowing if you are heading in the right direction or going off-track.

STAGE SIX: HAND OFF THE PULSE

Throughout Stages One to Five, the pulser contributes 100 percent of the effort required to actively amplify the pulse, while the receiver simply relaxes and tunes into the sensations of the pulse. If asked to pulse on their own, the receiver would most likely use muscular effort to get some motion going in the joint, in this case the wrist. Of course, muscular activation does not work for initiating the pulse as the muscles would contract and, thereby, close down the joint. So the handoff procedure must be done smoothly and gradually, and it must be repeated over many training sessions in order for the receiver to embody pulsing on their own.

Handoff Procedure

The purpose of the handoff procedure is to embody the pulse, so you can transition from someone pulsing you to being able to pulse by yourself without assistance.

Note: The percentages that follow correspond to a joint's range during the four-beat cycle. Therefore, 100 percent of the pulse is 70 percent of the comfortable range of the receiver's joint.

1. Once the pulser has fully activated the pulse, the receiver will begin to assist a little as the pulser backs off to 80 percent of the effort required. The receiver takes up the slack and boosts the pulse back up to 100 percent. So the pulser contributes 80 percent of the effort and the receiver contributes 20 percent of the effort to keep the pulse fully alive. The range of motion is still 70 percent of the receiver's comfortable range.

   During this handoff phase, both parties must be fully present and feedback is essential. If the receiver tries too hard, takes over more than 20 percent or engages muscular effort, the pulser guides them accordingly. Both parties will make whatever adjustments are necessary and, when both are in agreement that the split is roughly 80 percent-pulser/20 percent-receiver, they will move on to the next step.

2. Progressively, step down as follows until the receiver pulses on their own:

(a)   100-pulser/0-receiver;

(b)   80-pulser/20-receiver;

(c)   60-pulser/40-receiver;

(d)   40-pulser/60-receiver

(e)   20-pulser/80-receiver;

(f)   5-pulser/95-receiver;

(g)   0-pulser/100-receiver.

Make sure that each step is stabilized by the receiver before moving on, or the handoff will not be successful. Good communication and copious practice are the keys. Maintain contact with your partner at the end of the process for a minute or two being careful not to restrict the motion of their joint(s). This will help your partner remain focused on the joint that they are attempting to pulse.

3. Once the receiver has taken full control of the pulse and the pulser has removed their hands from the receiver's body, the receiver should sit for a minute or two and pulse the activated joint(s) on their own. Then they will let go of the pulse and feel their joint(s), comparing the feeling in their corresponding joint(s) on the side that has not been pulsed. The questions are: Is there a difference? If so, what is or are the difference(s)? Feeling for the differences will help them tune into what the pulse does to their body, which is precisely what enables a practitioner to train accurately in the future. The qualitative difference experienced can later be identified during self-practice to let the practitioner know when they are on the right track and apply their mind's intent to incrementally amplifying those signals during the weeks, months and years of training that follow.

4. Once steps 1-3 are complete and the receiver has had a moment to absorb the experience, repeat all of the instructions on the other side of the body.

Four-Point Checklist for a Self-Generated Pulse

Once the receiver has had both wrists pulsed, they attempt to pulse on their own without assistance. They stand with their hands one fist width from the sides of their thighs to initiate the pulse while adhering to the following four-point checklist.

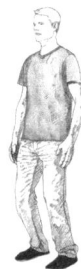

- Remember, pulsing is a yin technique, so do not try to use any obvious force or you will inhibit rather than amplify the rhythm. Gentleness leads to openness, whereas strength causes contractions that shut down the body, the nerves and the pulse. The pulse comes from inside the joint, not the surrounding muscles. When coming to the end of an opening phase, if your limbs shake or vibrate, you know your muscles have incorrectly taken over the action or you are trying too hard.

- The changeovers from open-to-close and close-to-open are smooth and circular in nature—never sudden or fast.

- The oscillation between active and passive, and the four-beat cycle are key to yielding a smooth, even and powerful pulse, which rids the body of long-term, accumulated tension and powerfully circulates qi.

- The longer you practice, look for ways to use less and less effort to maintain the pulse in your joints without significantly losing any range of motion in them. Yin training—with a focus on softness— leads to more profound levels of understanding of the Taoist philosophy "less is often more."

PULSING THE WRISTS IN HEAVEN AND EARTH QIGONG

After successfully generating the pulse in the standing posture, the receiver smoothly transitions into practicing the Heaven and Earth form (Figure 11-10) while focusing on opening and closing their wrist joints at the correct intervals. Practicing a number of repetitions directly after receiving the activation of the pulse from the pulser is precisely what maximizes the learning curve and allows the receiver to get the most benefit from the exercise.

Remember: Heaven and Earth has six phases—stretch/open, bend/close, stretch/open, bend/close, stretch/open and release to neutral.

OPENING PHASES

First, Third and Fifth Phases of Opening - Simultaneously open the wrist joints of both arms during the entirety of the first, third and fifth (opening) phases.

CLOSING PHASES

Second and Fourth Phases of Closing - Simultaneously close the wrist joints of both arms during the entirety of the second and fourth (closing) phases.

NEUTRAL

Sixth-Phase Release - In the sixth phase, release the joints and the entire body into the neutral standing posture from the previous open.

Change: Once the receiver has had a rest after solo practice, they will return the favor and pulse their partner's wrists following all of the instructions in this chapter.

Figure 11-10: The Marriage of Heaven and Earth Qigong—Pulsing the Wrist

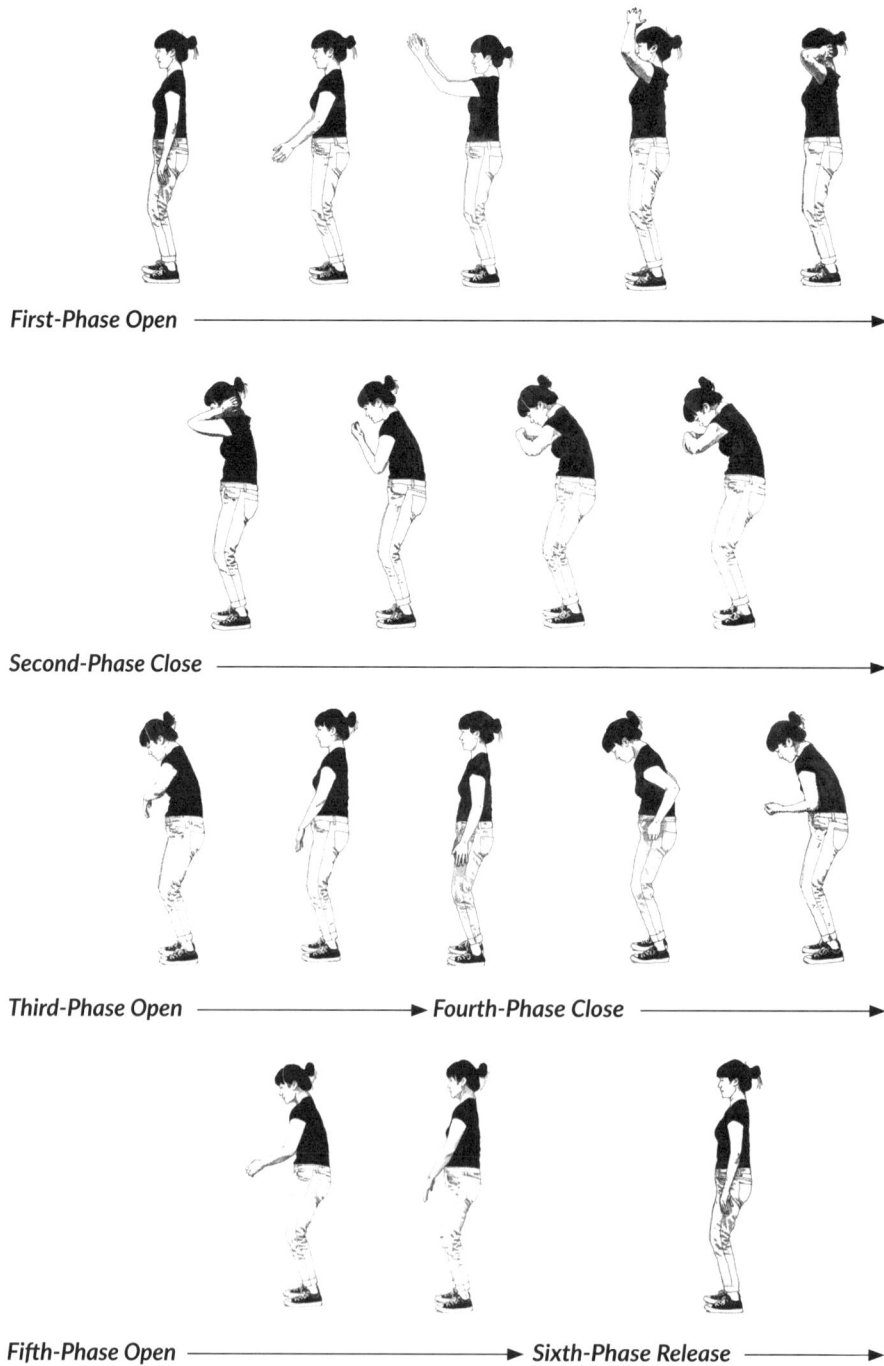

First-Phase Open ⟶

Second-Phase Close ⟶

Third-Phase Open ⟶ *Fourth-Phase Close* ⟶

Fifth-Phase Open ⟶ *Sixth-Phase Release* ⟶

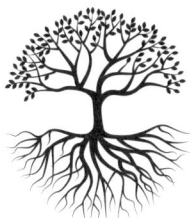

CHAPTER 12

PULSING THE HANDS AND THE FINGERS

HOW TO PULSE THE HAND

Fingers are comprised of many individual joints and each one must be activated independently before in unison with any others to ensure none are left out of the mix or operating below capacity. Just because one joint pulses well does not mean the next in the chain necessarily will too. In fact, most people will find at least a couple of joints in their fingers that are sluggish, stiff or locked up.

Before activating the fingers, the process begins with activating the hand bones, including the joints between:

- The hand bones (metacarpals), wrist bones (carpals) and finger bones (phalanges).
- The connections between the metacarpals themselves.

Each joint can be activated individually or all joints can be activated as one whole. Instructions for a whole-hand pulse follow since it is normally sufficient. In cases where people have very little space in their joints due to injury, tension or just human variation, pulsing each joint separately can be problematic. If so, live training with a Heaven and Earth Instructor who is very experienced with these methods is recommended.

ABOUT HAND HOLDS

The hand holds presented in this book are not the only way the pulse can be initiated and engaged. They have been chosen for the purposes of providing the clearest images possible, so that readers can see what is happening with these intricate and sometimes almost invisible motions. Also, due to human variation in terms of the size of the limbs/joints being pulsed and the pulser's hands, as well as differences between partner heights and lengths of limbs, you might and probably will need to make adjustments. Such adjustments are appropriate when they:

- Allow you to get a better grip with less effort.
- Help you and/or your partner relax more.
- Yield a deeper and more sustainable pulse.

PULSING THE HAND LENGTHWISE

1. Locate and Feel the Hand Bones

Familiarize yourself with the bones and joints of the hand, and feel the overall quality of the receiver's hand. Note any characteristics that are specific to the person on whom you will be working, such as the size of their hands, and whether their tissues are relatively soft and open, or tense and hard.

2. Set up the Hand Hold and Align the Joints

To pulse the receiver's hand lengthwise, with one hand, hold the end of the receiver's forearm farthest away from their torso (distal end). See Figure 12-1.

- If you grip higher up their arm (i.e. closer to their torso), as done with the wrist, you are likely to open and close the previously activated wrist joint.

- The idea is to isolate each of the joints—or, as in this case, set of joints—to the degree possible.

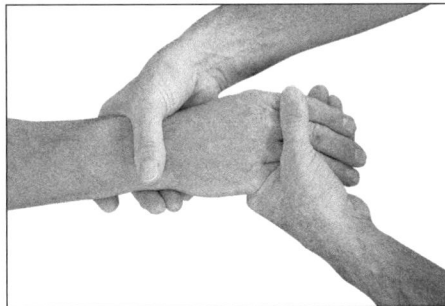

Neutral position

Figure 12-1:
Pulsing the Hand Lengthwise—Hand Hold

Your opposite hand holds the receiver's four fingers without crunching them together. The thumb and index finger of your hand act as a pincer that grabs the bones (phalanges) of the receiver's fingers, closest (proximal) to their palm. In this position, you will be able to open and close the two joints at either end of the hand bones (metacarpals).

3. Activate the Two-Beat Cycle

Once you have assumed the correct hand hold (Figure 12-1) with the joints properly aligned (which is the same alignment as the one used for the wrist), establish the two-beat cycle:

- First open the hand joints to 100 percent of the receiver's comfortable range, and then gently allow their joints to release back to neutral (Figure 12-2a-b).

- Repeat the 100-percent open, then release a couple of times, moving smoothly and slowly in order to find the full range of the receiver's joints.

- Once you have established their 100-percent range, reduce your motion to 70-percent open, and then allow their joints to release back to neutral (Figure 12-2c-d).

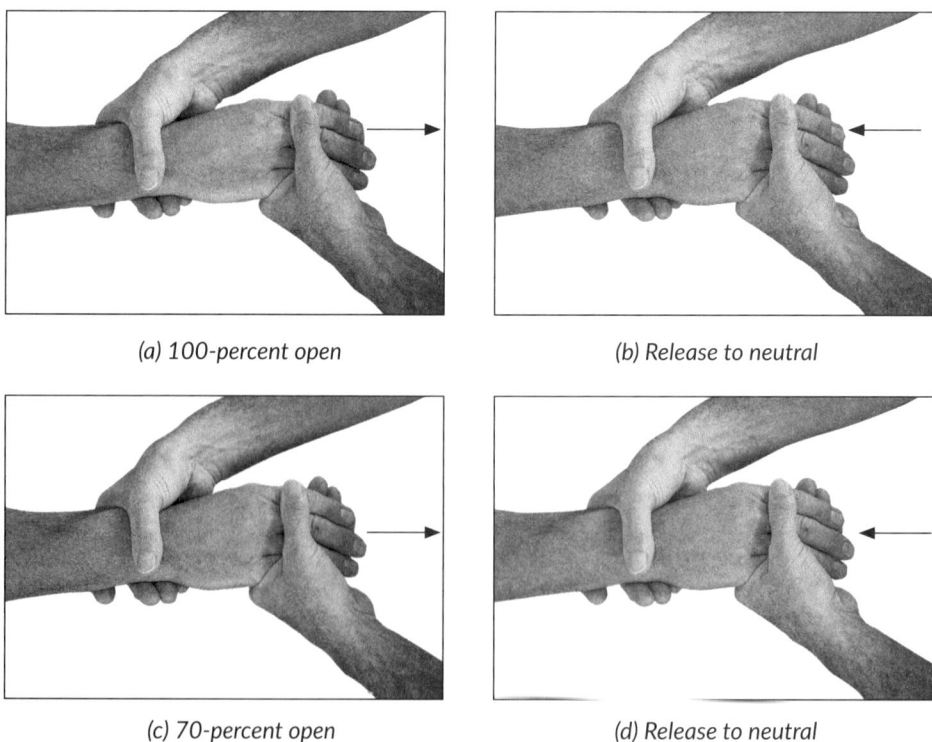

(a) 100-percent open   *(b) Release to neutral*

(c) 70-percent open   *(d) Release to neutral*

Figure 12-2: Pulsing the Hand Lengthwise—Two-Beat Cycle

Continue the two-beat cycle a dozen times or so, opening 70 percent and releasing, in order to open up their joints. This will clear out some of the tension from their hand and allow your partner to relax.

4. Close and Release the Joints

Once you have established the two-beat cycle, find the 100-percent closed position by:

- Repeating one more open-release, and slowly and smoothly transitioning into closing the receiver's joints to 100 percent of their comfortable range of motion (Figure 12-3a).
- Then allowing their joints to release back to neutral (Figure 12-3b).

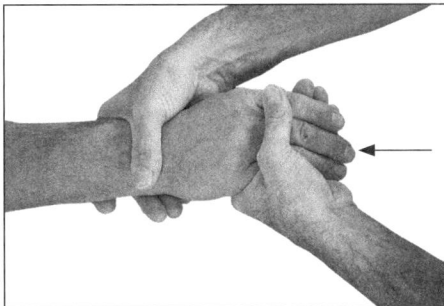

(a) 100-percent close   (b) Release to neutral

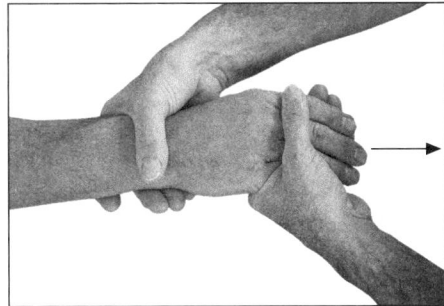

Figure 12-3:
Pulsing the Hand Lengthwise—Close and Release the Joints

5. Activate the Four-Beat Cycle

Next shift into the four-beat cycle, active open-passive release-active close-passive release (70-percent open/70-percent close) to initiate the pulse (Figure 12-4):

- Active open - open the hand joints 70 percent.
- Passive release - allow the joints to release back to neutral.
- Active close - close the hand joints 70 percent.
- Passive release - once again allow the joints to release back to neutral.

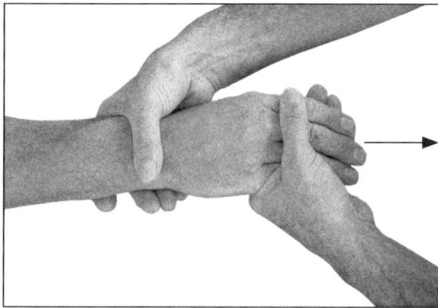

(a) Active open: 70-percent open

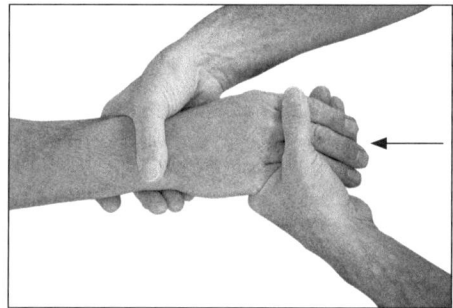

(b) Passive release to neutral

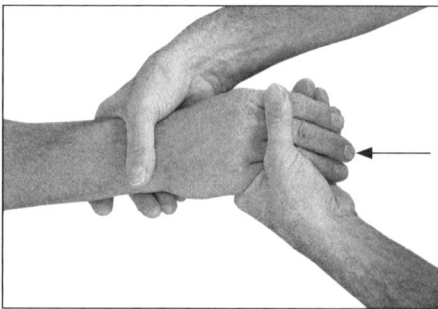

(c) Active close: 70-percent

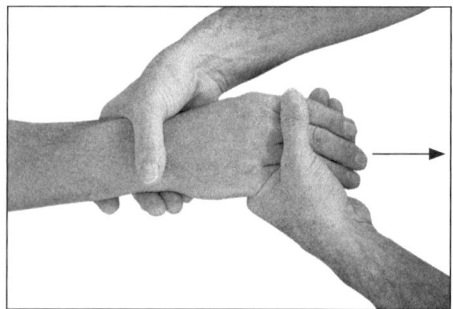

(d) Passive release to neutral

Figure 12-4:
Pulsing the Hand Lengthwise—Four-Beat Cycle

Review the "Five-Point Checklist for Pulsing a Partner" (in Chapter 11, p. 211) to generate a smooth, deep internal pulse of the receiver's hand joints.

About the Thumb: The metacarpal which connects the thumb to the wrist must be pulsed separately since it is not possible to grab the thumb at the same time as the four fingers and pulse. Apart from this variation, the method for the thumb is the same.

6. Hand off the Pulse

Follow the handoff procedure (described in Chapter 11 on p. 212) to assist the receiver with pulsing on their own.

Repeat Stages 1-6 on the receiver's other hand.

7. Practice the Self-Generated Pulse

Once both hands have been pulsed:

- The receiver stands and pulses on their own with their hands one first width from their thighs for a few minutes while reflecting on the "Four-Point Checklist for a Self-Generated Pulse" (in Chapter 11 on p. 214) to generate a deep, internal pulse. Practicing a number of repetitions directly after receiving the activation of the pulse from the pulser is precisely what maximizes the learning curve and allows the receiver to get the most benefit from the exercise in the least amount of time.

- The receiver fluidly transitions into the Heaven and Earth form, opening their hand joints during the opening phases and closing their hand joints during the closing phases.

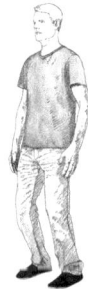

Change: Once the receiver has had a rest after solo practice, they will return the favor and pulse their partner's wrists following all of the instructions in this chapter so far.

This completes the process for pulsing the hand joints lengthwise (from Chapters 11-12). However, there is another dimension to the hand—the joints between the hand bones (metacarpals) themselves. Up until now, all techniques initiate the pulse lengthwise in the hand. Next you will pulse the hand widthwise.

PULSING THE HAND WIDTHWISE

1. Locate and Feel the Hand Bones

First you must become familiar with the hand bones, which are more prominent on the back of the hand than on the front. If you run your fingers or thumb across the back of your hand from one side to the other, you will feel a series of ridges (bones) and dips (spaces between the bones). Locate the metacarpals that connect to the little finger and the index finger. These are the two bones you will hold in order to pulse across the hand, whereby you grip your partner's hand between the heel of your thumb and your finger pads (Figure 12-5).

2. Set up the Hand Hold and Align the Joints

Misaligning the hand bones is difficult unless your partner has a major distortion in their hands, in which case take the utmost care when pulsing. The aim is to hold the bones in such a way that they cannot slip out of your grip and with the least amount of pressure, so as not to induce a tension response in your partner (Figure 12-5).

- One of your hands becomes the anchor while the other hand pulses.

- Be sure not to hold any part of your partner's hand in a way that interferes with the space between the bone you are holding and the next bone.

- Take your time to mold your hands with your partner's hand, making maximum surface contact with minimal strength. How you make and maintain contact with another person is an art unto itself.

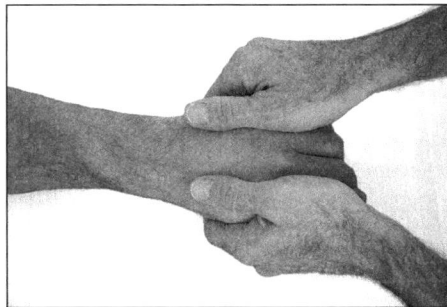

Neutral position

Figure 12-5:
Pulsing the Hand Widthwise—Hand Hold

One hand anchors the receiver's hand while the other hand pulses

3. Activate the Two-Beat Cycle

Once you have assumed the correct hand hold (Figure 12-5), establish the two-beat cycle:

- First open the hand joints to 100 percent of the receiver's comfortable range, and then allow their joints to naturally and smoothly release back to neutral (Figure 12-6a-b).

- Repeat the 100-percent open, then release a couple of times, moving smoothly and slowly in order to find the full range of the receiver's joints.

- Once you have established their 100-percent range, reduce your motion to 70-percent open, then allow their joints to release back to neutral (Figure 12-6c-d).

- Continue the two-beat cycle a dozen times or so, opening 70 percent and releasing, in order to open up their joints, clear out some of the tension from their hand and allow your partner to relax.

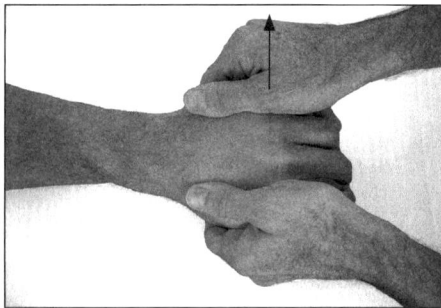

(a) 100-percent open

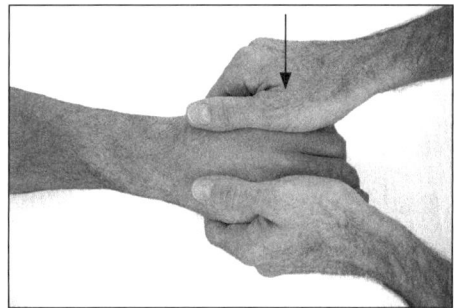

(b) Release to neutral

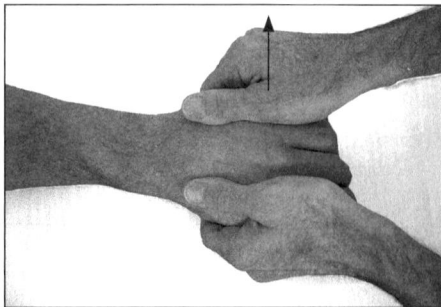

(c) 70-percent open

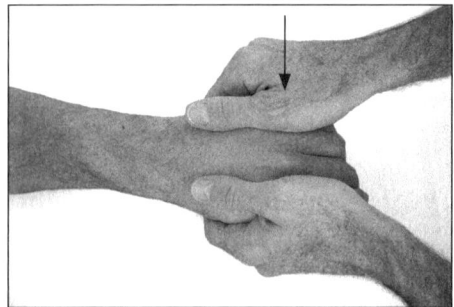

(d) Release to neutral

Figure 12-6: Pulsing the Hand Widthwise—Two-Beat Cycle

4. Close and Release the Joints

Once you have established the two-beat cycle, find the 100-percent closed position by:

- Repeating one more open-release, and slowly and smoothly transitioning into closing the receiver's joints to 100 percent of their comfortable range of motion (Figure 12-7a).

- Then allowing their joints to release back to neutral (Figure 12-7b).

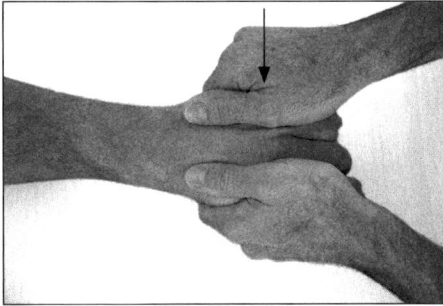

(a) 100-percent close   *(b) Release to neutral*

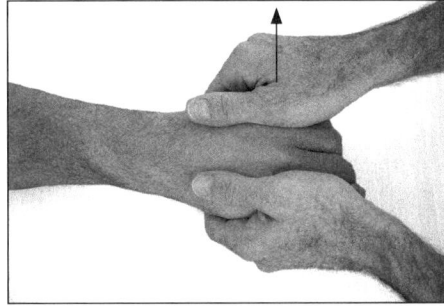

Figure 12-7:
Pulsing the Hand Widthwise—Close and Release the Joints

One hand anchors the receiver's hand while the other hand pulses

5. Activate the Four-Beat Cycle

Shift into the four-beat cycle, active open-passive release-active close-passive release (70-percent open/70-percent close) to initiate the pulse (Figure 12-8):

- Active open - open the hand joints 70 percent.
- Passive release - allow the joints to release back to neutral.
- Active close - close the hand joints 70 percent.
- Passive release - once again allow the joints to release back to neutral.

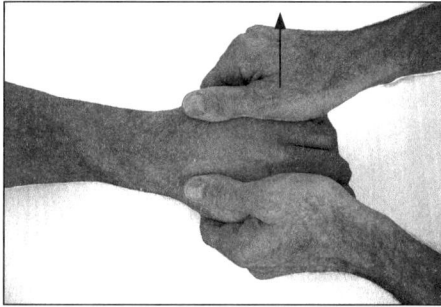

(a) Active open: 70 percent

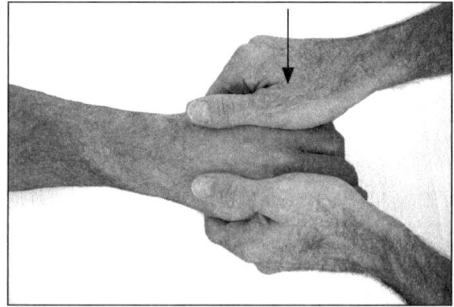

(b) Passive release

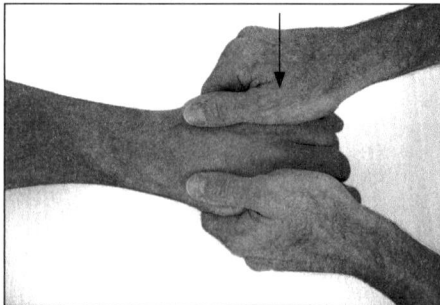

(c) Active close: 70 percent

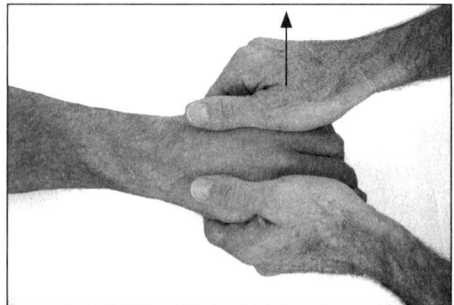

(d) Passive release

Figure 12-8:

Pulsing the Hand Widthwise—Four-Beat Cycle

Review the "Five-Point Checklist for Pulsing a Partner" (see Chapter 11) to generate a smooth, deep internal pulse of the receiver's hand joints.

6. Hand off the Pulse

Follow the handoff procedure (described in Chapter 11) to assist the receiver with pulsing on their own.

Repeat Stages 1-6 on the receiver's other hand.

7. Practice the Self-Generated Pulse

Once both hands have been pulsed:

- The receiver stands and pulses on their own with their hands one fist width from their thighs for a few minutes while reflecting on the "Four-Point Checklist for a Self-Generated Pulse" (see Chapter 11) to generate a deep, internal pulse. Practicing a number of repetitions directly after receiving the activation of the pulse from the pulser is precisely what maximizes the learning curve and allows the receiver to get the most benefit from the exercise.
- The receiver fluidly transitions into the Heaven and Earth form, opening their hand joints during the opening phases and closing their hand joints during the closing phases.

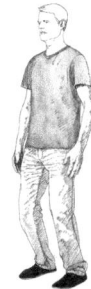

Change: Once the receiver has had a rest after solo practice, they will return the favor and pulse their partner following all of the instructions on pulsing the hands widthwise.

PULSING THE FINGER JOINTS

The finger joints are small and the range of motion is minimal, so if you attempt to pulse more than one at a time, you are likely to create motion in the joints, but not a pulse. In order to perform the exercise properly, you must pulse each of the joints of all five fingers on both hands one at a time.

1. Locate and Feel the Finger Bones

If you have been following the progression, you have already covered the joints that connect the fingers and thumbs to the hands. This leaves two joints on each finger and one joint on each thumb, which are farthest from (distal to) the palms to be pulsed.

You should be fairly familiar with your partner's hand by now, so simply feel their fingers and note any defining characteristics, especially anything out of the ordinary, such as swelling or a higher-than-normal degree of tension.

2. Set up the Hand Hold and Align the Joint

From the perspective of the alignment, the primary focus is to keep the joint slightly bent throughout the entirety of the pulsing exercise. Due to the size of the fingers and the distance between the joints, there is only one good way to pulse another person's finger joints: use the pads of your index finger and thumb to sandwich a single finger bone (phalange) with one of your hands on each side of the joint you wish to pulse (Figure 12-9). One of your hands becomes the anchor while the other hand pulses.

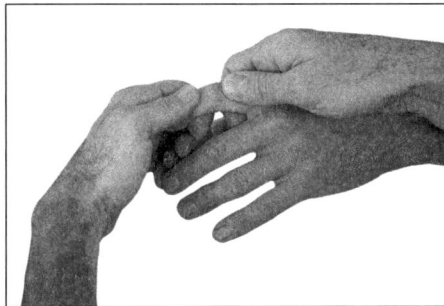

Neutral position

Figure 12-9:
Pulsing the Fingers

The hand closest to the wrist stabilizes the joint, while the other hand pulses

3. Activate the Two-Beat Cycle

The process for pulsing the fingers is similar to pulsing the hand lengthwise. Begin by holding the receiver's finger (Figure 12-9).

- First open the finger joint to 100 percent of the receiver's comfortable range and gently allow their joint to release back to neutral (Figure 12-10a-b).

- Repeat the 100-percent open, then release a couple of times, moving smoothly and slowly in order to find the full range of the receiver's joint.

- Once you have established their 100-percent range, reduce your motion to 70-percent open, then allow their joint to release back to neutral (Figure 12-10c-d).

- Continue the two-beat cycle a dozen times or so, opening to 70 percent and releasing, in order to open up their joint, clear out some of the tension from their finger and allow your partner to relax.

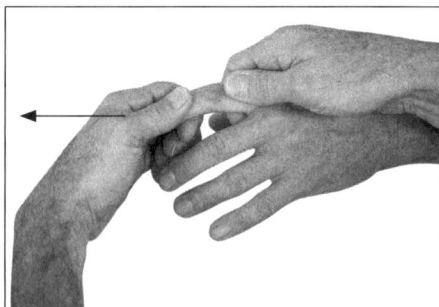

(a) 100-percent open   *(b) Release to neutral*

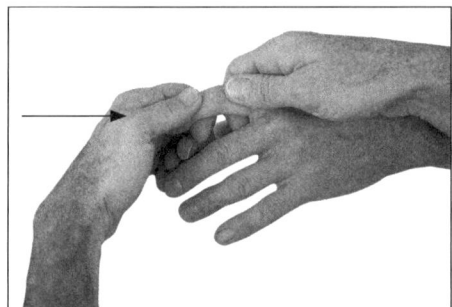

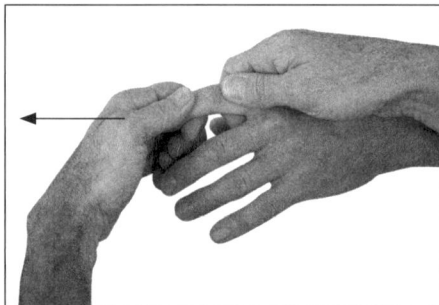

(c) 70-percent open   *(d) Release to neutral*

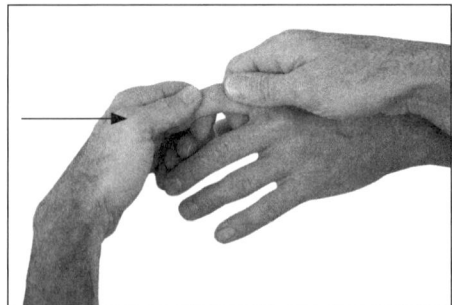

Figure 12-10: Pulsing the Fingers—Two-Beat Cycle

4. Close and Release the Joint

Once you have established the two-beat cycle, find the 100-percent closed position by:

- Repeating one more open-release, and slowly and smoothly transitioning into closing the receiver's finger joint to 100 percent of their comfortable range of motion (Figure 12-11a).

- Then allowing their joint to release back to neutral (Figure 12-11b).

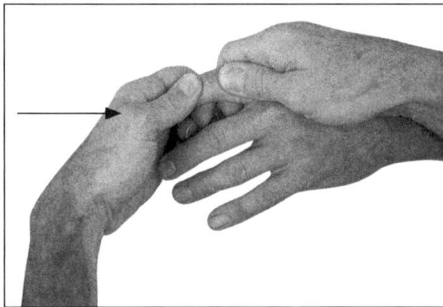

(a) 100-percent close   (b) Release to neutral

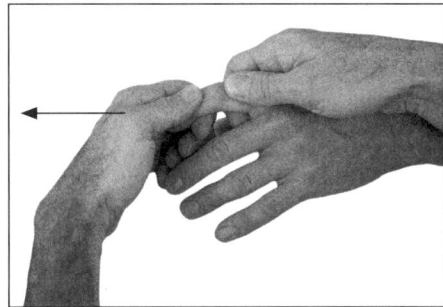

Figure 12-11:
Pulsing the Fingers—Close and Release the Joint

5. Activate the Four-Beat Cycle

Shift into the four-beat cycle, active open-passive release-active close-passive release (70-percent open/70-percent close) to initiate the pulse (Figure 12-12):

- Active open - open the finger joint 70 percent.
- Passive release - allow the joint to release back to neutral.
- Active close - close the finger joint 70 percent.
- Passive release - once again allow the joint to release back to neutral.

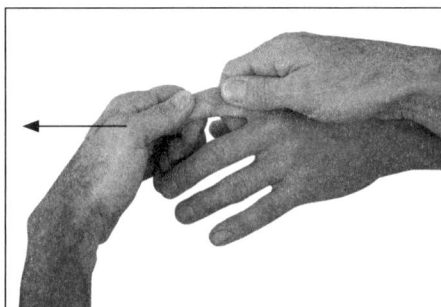

(a) Active open: 70 percent

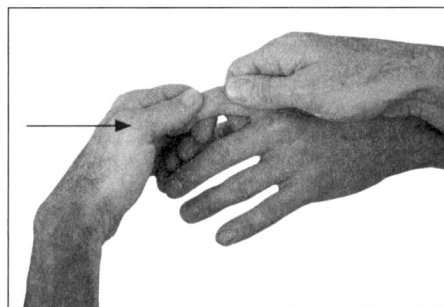

(b) Passive release

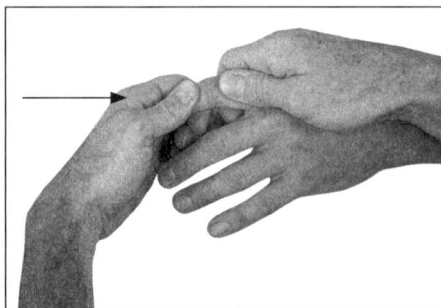

(c) Active close: 70 percent

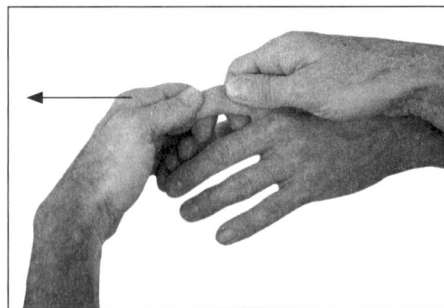

(d) Passive release

Figure 12-12:
Pulsing the Fingers—Four-Beat Cycle

Review the "Five-Point Checklist for Pulsing a Partner" (in Chapter 11) to generate a smooth, deep internal pulse of the receiver's hand joints.

Important: As there are many finger joints and the motion is very small, generally the handoff procedure is skipped. Move on to repeating Stages 1-5 on all of the receiver's other fingers on both hands.

6. Practice the Self-Generated Pulse

Once all the fingers of both hands have been pulsed:

- The receiver stands and pulses their finger joints on their own with their hands one first width from their thighs for a few minutes while reflecting on the "Four-Point Checklist for a Self-Generated Pulse" (see Chapter 11) to generate a deep, internal pulse.
- Then the receiver fluidly transitions into the Heaven and Earth form, opening their finger joints during the opening phases and closing their finger joints during the closing phases.

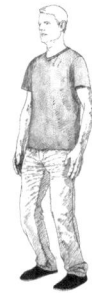

Change: Once the receiver has had a rest after solo practice, they will return the favor and pulse their partner following all of the instructions on pulsing the fingers.

JOINING THE PULSE IN THE WRISTS, HANDS AND FINGERS

Once you have been through the process of having all of the joints of your wrists, hands and fingers pulsed, and you have practiced activating the pulse in each part individually—both while standing and within the Heaven and Earth form—the aim is to join the pulses of the wrists and hands together into one seamless whole on your own.

Notice that the pulse in the palms moves in two directions: lengthwise and widthwise. Joining these two flows fully opens up the hand and initiates the pulse in the finger joints. This joining also generates a flow of qi from *lao gong* (see Figure 12-13)—an energy gate located in the center of the palm—out to the periphery (edges of the hand and fingertips) on the open and back again to lao gong on the close.

> *Lao gong* is a major energy gate that feeds qi to all the other energy gates and joints in the hands and fingers, and requires the two pulses of the hand (lengthwise and widthwise) be integrated in order to become activated to any significant degree.

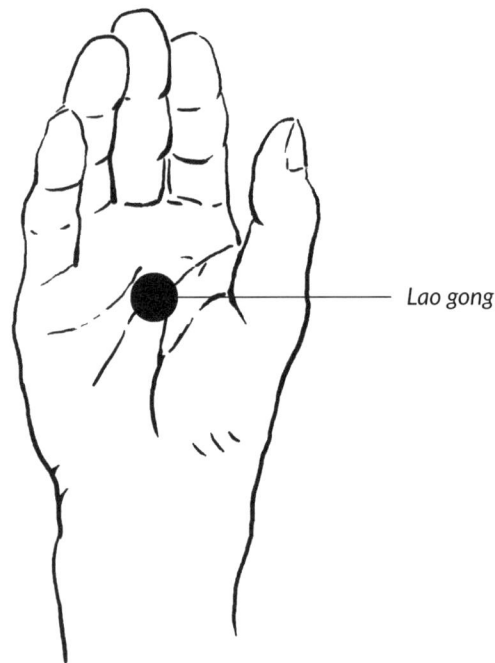

Figure 12-13

Solo Practice: Unify the Hand Pulses and Qi Flows

1. While sitting, practice pulsing your hands lengthwise and widthwise, including all your fingers, until the two become balanced and integrated.

2. Focus on moving qi from lao gong to the periphery (fingertips and edges of your hands) on the open and back to lao gong on the close.

3. Once the center-to-periphery and periphery-to-center qi flow is strong, add the pulsing of your wrists.

4. When the wrist pulse is alive, focus on moving qi from your wrists to your fingertips on the open and back from your fingertips to your wrists on the close.

5. When the flow along the length of your hand is strong and you are feeling lucky, attempt to integrate the two qi flows together. Integration is born out of balance, so when you generate even qi flows, they will naturally merge.

6. Stand and continue to pulse your wrists, hands and fingers for a minute or two, while keeping the two qi flows alive.

7. Then smoothly and fluidly transition into the Heaven and Earth form with the joined pulse and qi flows, that is:

   (a) from the wrists and lao gong to extremities on the opening phases; and

   (b) back to lao gong and wrists on the closing and neutral phases.

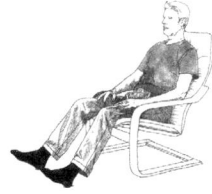

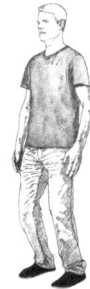

REVIEW

The classic Taoist method is to initially bring alive the pulse while sitting, keep it alive in standing practice and then, at the end of an open, release into neutral and transition into the Heaven and Earth form while focusing on your wrists, hands and fingers. During this practice, allow the pulse to dictate the length of each opening or closing phase of your form. You do not want the pulse to stop or become strained by trying to keep it going beyond its ideal, 70-percent range.

Timing is everything.

Follow the pulse and allow the speed of your physical movements to adjust to the pulse and not the other way around. You must look for the balance between range of motion and speed. If the pulse is too fast or too slow, you will disconnect from the synovial fluid within the joint and qi flow will diminish. If you move your body too slowly, you will run out of pulse before you reach the end of the opening or closing phase of the form. However, it is better to change the direction of the pulse (from close-to-open or open-to-close) than to overextend your pulse or for the pulse to stop. Therefore, in the interim period while you are learning how to pulse and developing your skill set, a small close-and-open or a small open-and-close within any designated opening or closing phase of the form is permissible to keep the pulse alive.

Eventually the pulse, whether finishing on an open or a close, should be timed to transition to its opposite at the moment you begin to transition from one phase of the form to the next. In this way, the internal content of the pulse seamlessly integrates with the six-phase Heaven and Earth exercise: open-close-open-close-open-release.

When a practitioner achieves this level of practice, the strength of their qi jumps, deeper health benefits can flourish and practice feels sublime. As you catch your flow, practice becomes more and more effortless—the first steps on the journey toward *wu wei* or "achieving without effort."

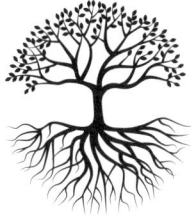

CHAPTER 13:

PULSING THE ELBOWS

A Word to the Wise: Do not attempt the exercises presented in this chapter and beyond until you have extensive experience practicing the previous pulsing exercises, both independently and with a training partner. All of the material that follows relies on a solid understanding and direct experience of pulsing both your partner's and your own hands and wrists.

ANATOMY OF THE ELBOW

The elbow joint is constructed from three bones:

- The upper arm bone (humerus).
- The two forearm bones (radius and ulna).

The elbow is a balance point and, being located in the middle of the arm (as the shoulder is the root and the wrist-hand is the tip), has a different style of operation than the joints previously covered. Even though the elbow can be pulsed similarly to the previous joints, it is easier to activate the pulse with a flexion-extension action that mimics the normal activity of the elbow during routine tasks.

HOW TO PULSE THE ELBOW

THE WATER-PUMP METHOD

In the following exercises, you will learn how to apply the water-pump method to pulsing the elbow, which differs from the instructions on pulsing the hands presented so far.

1. Locate and Feel the Elbow Bones

Familiarize yourself with the elbow joint and feel the quality of the receiver's arm. Note any characteristics that are specific to the person on which you are working, such as the size of their arm bones, and whether their tissues are relatively soft and open, or tense and hard.

2. Set up the Hand Hold and Align the Joints

Take the receiver's upper arm into the palm of your hand and wrap your fingers around their bicep muscle. Take the end of their forearm farthest from their torso (distal end) into your other hand. The hand holding their upper arm becomes the anchor while the other hand pulses. See Figure 13-1.

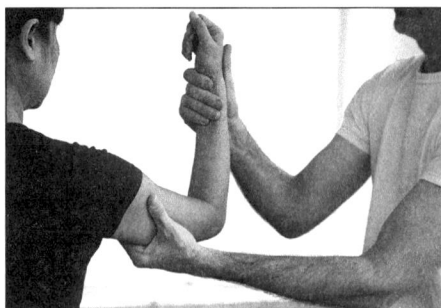

Neutral position

Figure 13-1:
Pulsing the Elbow   Hand Hold

During all pulsing processes, make sure the hand moves directly toward the shoulder on the flexion (bend) and directly away from the shoulder on the extension (stretch). The elbow tip always points directly downward. Make sure not to twist the joint at any point during the pulsing process.

3. Extend and Flex the Arm

From the neutral position (Figure 13-1):

- Extend and flex the receiver's elbow joint 100 percent in each direction, moving slowly and smoothly to feel the full range of the joint without going past the receiver's comfortable range (Figure 13-2a-b).
- Once you have a feeling for the full range of motion, back off to 70-percent extension/70-percent flexion (Figure 13-2c-d).

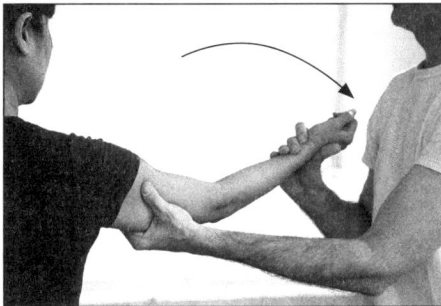

(a) 100-percent extension

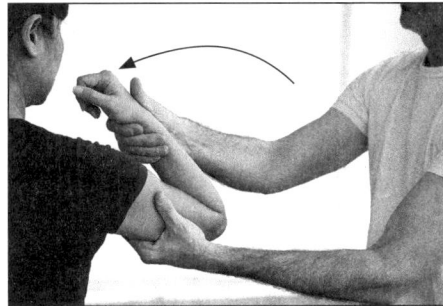

(b) 100-percent flexion

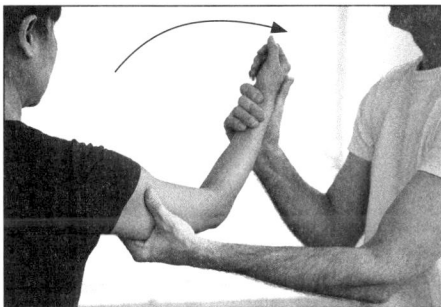

(c) 70-percent extension

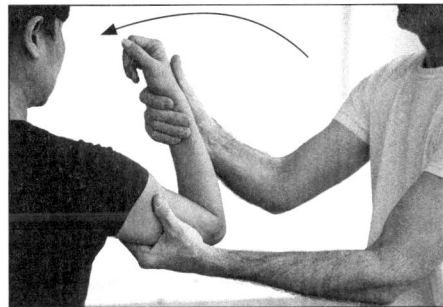

(d) 70-percent flexion

Figure 13-2: Pulsing the Elbow—Extend and Flex the Arm

When you are satisfied with this range, practice a few repetitions, moving smoothly and slowly to create a fluid and continuous operation. This action will give the receiver a clear experience of what it feels like when their elbow moves *without the pulse*. The receiver needs this feedback in order to know when the quality changes.

4. Activate the Two-Beat Cycle

From the 70-percent-flexed position:

- Draw the receiver's wrist and hand away from their shoulder (Figure 13-3a).
- As their forearm comes to the halfway point (50-percent flexed/50-percent extended), open the elbow angle to 70-percent extension, and use your little and ring fingers to start actively drawing the base of their forearm (i.e. the end closest to their elbow) away from their upper arm to internally open the joint. This action is all about leverage. You open the angle of the elbow and, at the same time, draw open the space within the joint by applying a downward-and-away-from-the-receiver pressure with your two fingers closest to their elbow, which will cause synovial fluid to be secreted in the joint capsule.
- After you open the joint, reduce your effort and allow the joint to return to neutral as you flex the elbow (Figure 13-3b).

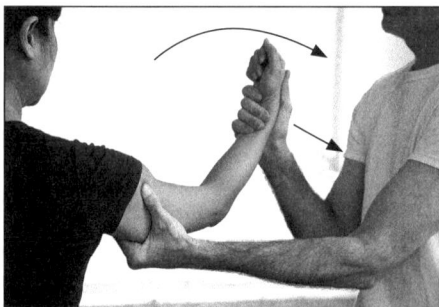

(a) 70-percent extension
while opening the joint 70 percent

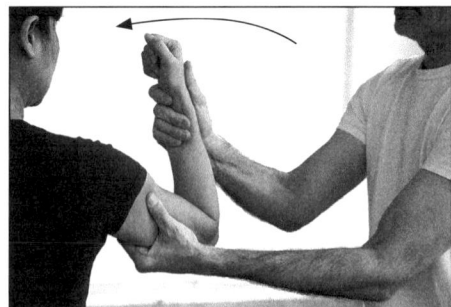

(b) Release to 70-percent flexion

Figure 13-3: Pulsing the Elbow—Two-Beat Cycle

Repeat this two-beat cycle half a dozen times or so to open up the joint. Check in with the receiver to make sure you do not overdo it, yet they feel a difference between when the elbow joint opens up and when it does not.

5. Close and Release the Joint

Now you will add the closing action:

- Begin with one more open and release (Figure 13-3).

- Then, as you pass the 50/50 position on the flex, have a sense of driving the inside of the elbow joint in toward itself to activate the synovial capsule (Figure 13-4a). You do not physically shut down the joint, but rather compress the fluid within the joint itself. If you just hinge the joint to the 70-percent-flexed position, there will not be any internal pressure. With your intent and the change of angle in the elbow, compress the fluid by gently driving the heel of your palm forward and toward your partner.

- Release the pressure in the joint to allow the recoil to open to neutral, that is 50-percent flexed/50-percent extended (Figure 13-4b).

Stay in communication with the receiver throughout this and all stages of the exercises.

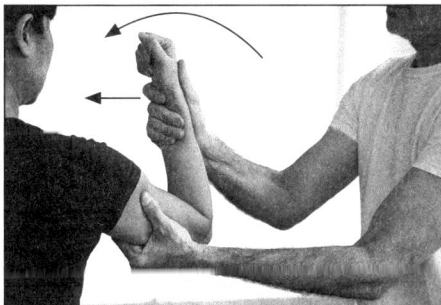

| (a) 70-percent flexion while closing the joint 70 percent | (b) Release to neutral position (50/50) |

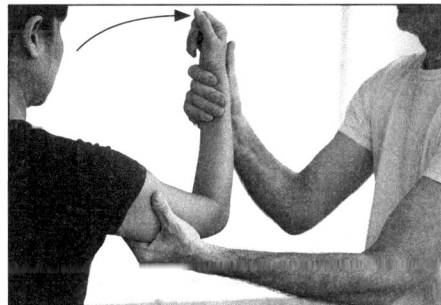

Figure 13-4:
Pulsing the Elbow—Close and Release the Joint

6. Activate the Four-Beat Cycle

Next you will activate the four-beat cycle, opening and closing the joint while extending and flexing the angle of the elbow, which should feel like you are operating a light water pump (Figure 13-5). There is a little resistance in the joint when the synovial fluid becomes engaged and the feeling should be markedly different to the simple hinging of the joint for both the pulser and the receiver.

- Shift into the four-beat cycle for a while—active open, passive release, active close, passive release—until the receiver has a tangible experience of the pulse and the compression-release cycle inside the elbow joint. Reflect on the "Five-Point Checklist for Pulsing a Partner" (see Chapter 11) as you pulse your partner's elbow.

- Once the internal pressure from activating the fluid in the joint is alive, apply your intent to draw qi from the receiver's elbow tip to their fingertips on the open, and drive the qi from their fingertips to their elbow tip on the close.

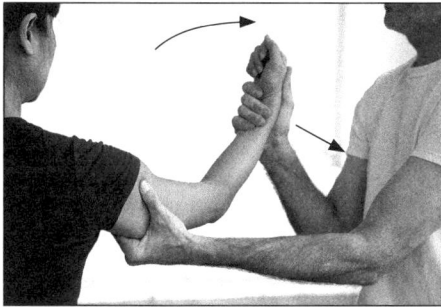

(a) 70-percent extension
while opening the joint 70 percent

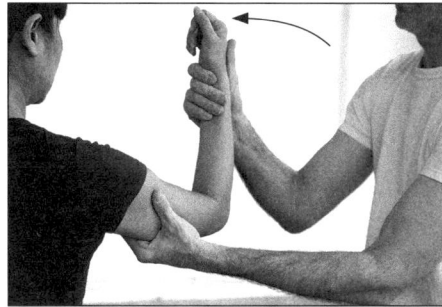

(b) Release to neutral position (50/50)

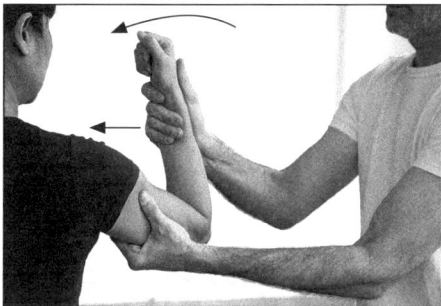

(c) 70-percent flexion
while closing the joint 70 percent

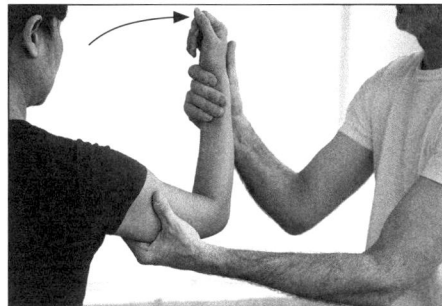

(d) Release to neutral (50/50)

**Figure 13-5:
Pulsing the Elbow—Four-Beat Cycle**

7. Hand off the Pulse

Once your partner feels the pulse come alive, shift into the handoff procedure (described in Chapter 11).

Repeat Stages 1-7 on the receiver's other elbow.

8. Practice the Self-Generated Pulse

Once the handoff is successful:

- The receiver stands and, with a very gentle elbow movement, pulses on their own. There is not any extension-flexion of the elbow while activating the qi flow from their elbows to fingertips and back again. The purpose is to consolidate their experiential knowledge while reflecting upon the "Four-Point Checklist for a Self-Generated Pulse" (see Chapter 11). When done well, there is a feeling of fluid and qi moving inside the arms between the fingertips and the elbows.

- Finally the receiver smoothly and fluidly transitions into the Heaven and Earth form while attempting to keep both the pulse and qi flows alive, opening during the opening phases and closing during the closing phases.

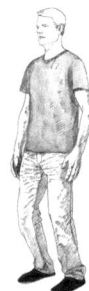

Change: Once all of the exercises in this chapter have been completed, the pulser and the receiver switch roles.

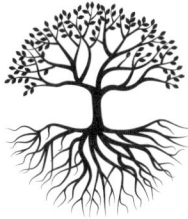

CHAPTER 14:

PULSING THE SHOULDERS

ANATOMY OF THE SHOULDER

The shoulder is comprised of several joints and a shoulder blade that slides across the rib cage, allowing the arm to perform a multitude of operations at various angles. In addition to opening and closing the shoulder blades, key joints, such as the AH (acromiohumeral) joint, GH (glenohumeral) joint and AC (acromioclavicular) joint, must also be activated in order to bring the shoulder fully alive. The shoulder pulse is therefore multilayered and is learned through a series of progressive exercises, which can also be used to deconstruct and rebuild the pulse in later stages of training to increase flexibility, range of motion and power. Initially, however, the focus is on releasing restrictions in the shoulder to restore healthy function.

The only direct bone-to-bone connection between the arm and the torso is where the shoulder blade (scapula) connects, via a bony protuberance on top of the blade (the acromion), to the collar bone (clavicle). The collar bone joins the arm-shoulder unit to the breast bone (sternum) via the sternoclavicular joint. This connection becomes really obvious when someone breaks their collar bone, as the shoulder droops and sits several inches lower than normal.

The upper arm bone (humerus) connects to the shoulder blade (scapular) at the GH joint and the shoulder blade is free to roam over the exterior surface of the back (posterior) of the rib cage. There are various muscles that connect the shoulder blade to the different parts of the torso, neck and spine, but no actual joints. This specific construction gives massive range of motion to the shoulder and the arm, unless of course they have become injured or remain dormant from lack of exercise and, thereby, stiff, tense and restricted.

THE AH, GH AND AC JOINTS

You will start by pulsing the three connecting joints of the shoulder blades—the AH (acromiohumeral) joint, the GH (glenohumeral) joint and the AC (acromioclavicular) joint—before activating the shoulder blades themselves, otherwise the motion in the shoulder blades can diminish the pulse in the shoulder joints.

The GH joint is the actual shoulder joint, where the head of the humerus bone sits into the glenoid cavity of the scapula, or where the upper arm bone joins to the shoulder blade. This joint is important to pulse as a means of supporting shoulder health and flexibility.

The AH joint, which is superficial to the GH joint, is a non-synovial joint that is connected through the deltoid muscle. It plays a major role in aiding qi flow from the spine, through the shoulders to the fingertips, and back again. When condensed, tense and tight, the AH joint shuts down or dramatically impedes qi flow into and out of the arm, thereby reducing the ability to pulse the GH joint. Conversely, when open and unrestricted, the qi of the shoulder can freely circulate and, by extension, fully engage the pulse in the shoulder joint.

The AC joint is a secondary joint, as you will see.

HOW TO PULSE THE GH AND THE AH JOINTS

1. Locate and Feel the Shoulder Bones

Locate your partner's shoulder blade on the back of their body above the height of their diaphragm on either side of their spine. Take a moment to familiarize yourself with the basic triangular shape and position of the shoulder blade before attempting to pulse the receiver's shoulder joints, including:

- The acromion - the top/outer aspect.
- The outer edge (lateral border) of the shoulder blade - i.e., the edge closest to the arm and farthest from the spine.
- The inner edge (medial border) of the shoulder blade - i.e., closest to the spine.

2. Set up the Hand Hold and Align the Joints

In order to pulse the GH and the AH joints, which are a matched pair that basically operate as one joint, the shoulder blade must be kept still in space. It is best for the receiver to sit in a chair, without making contact with the back of the chair, with their spine straight and their body and mind relaxed.

To find the beginning position, place one palm on the receiver's shoulder blade. With your other hand, take the receiver's upper arm, making sure their elbow remains bent and their forearm rests on your forearm, so that the receiver can fully relax. Using the hand holding and supporting their arm, draw their arm and shoulder blade away from their spine, so there is no slack in the soft tissues between their shoulder and their spine, and the receiver's posture is not distorted. See Figure 14-1a.

- As you draw out their arm, your hand that is holding their shoulder blade simply comes along for the ride (Figure 14-1b).
- Once the slack is out of their body, fix the hand connected to their shoulder blade in space with the heel of your palm up against the outside edge (lateral border) of their shoulder blade just below their armpit. Wrap your fingertips around the edge closest to their spine (medial border). When it feels like you have their shoulder blade in your grip and there is not any slack in their tissues between the blade and the spine, you have found the starting position and you are ready to begin pulsing (Figure 14-1c).

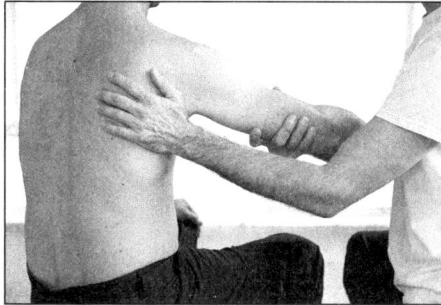

(a) Make contact with the shoulder blade

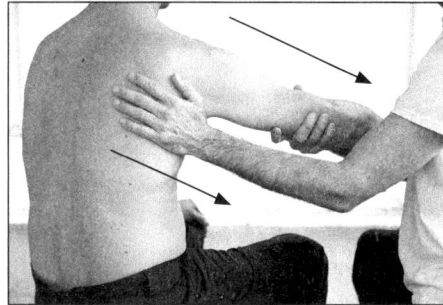

(b) Arm-and-shoulder-blade extension:
Draw the arm/shoulder away from the spine

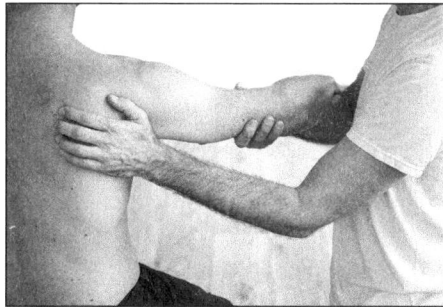

(c) Beginning position: The heel of the palm and fingertips contact
the outer and inner edges of the shoulder blade

Figure 14-1:
Pulsing the GH and AH Joints—Preparation

3. Activate the Two-Beat Cycle

Using the heel of your palm, hold the receiver's shoulder blade to prevent it from moving in space (Figure 14-1c) and:

- Draw their arm away from their shoulder blade to open up the GH and AH joints to 100 percent of their comfortable range, and slowly release to neutral (Figure 14-2a-b).
- Then back off to 70-percent open and release to initiate the two-beat cycle. Repeat a dozen times or so in order to free up the joints and begin releasing the localized tension. See Figure 14-2c-d.

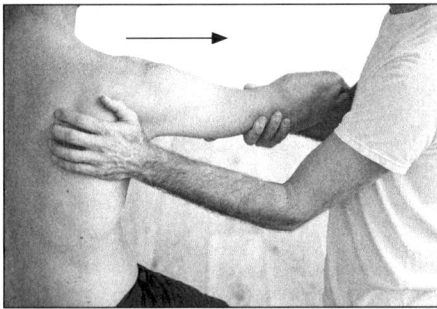

(a) Joints open 100 percent

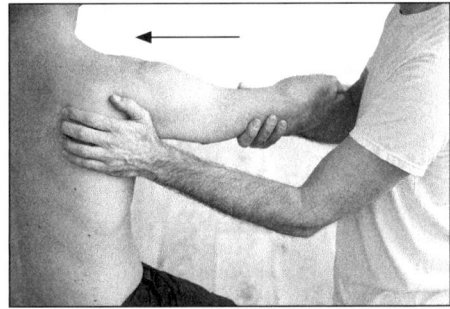

(b) Release to neutral

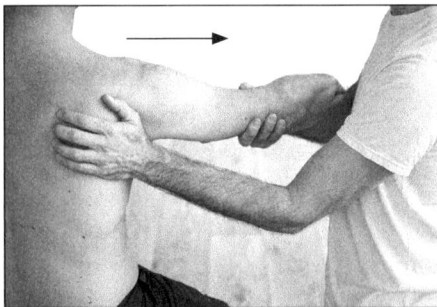

(c) Joints open 70 percent

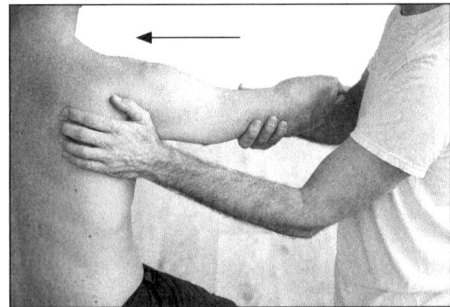

(d) Release to neutral

Figure 14-2:
Pulsing the GH and AH Joints—Two-Beat Cycle

4. Close and Release the Joints

After one more open-release:

- Smoothly close their joints 100 percent with the fingertips of your other hand supporting their blade to prevent their shoulder blade from moving toward their spine. During the close, do not allow their shoulder to rise. See Figure 14-3a.

- Then release to neutral (Figure 14-3b).

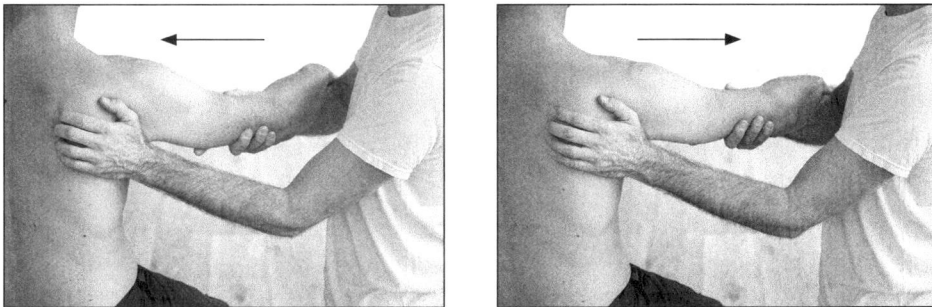

(a) Joints close 100 percent   *(b) Release to neutral*

Figure 14-3:
Pulsing the GH and AH Joints—Close and Release the Joints

5. Activate the Four-Beat Cycle

Initiate the four-beat cycle, 70-percent open/70-percent close (Figure 14-4).

- Adhere to the "Five-Point Checklist for a Pulsing a Partner" (see Chapter 11).

- The AC joint is close to the AH joint and, unless fused, will naturally come online (to some degree) once the pulse in the GH and the AH joints is strong enough. Over time and with more refined pulsing, the AC joint can become fully activated.

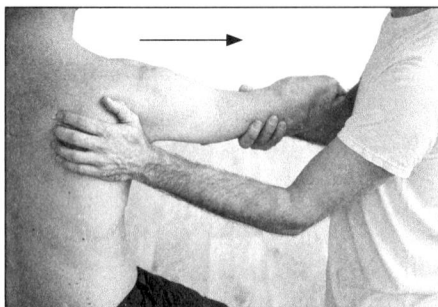

(a) Active open: 70 percent

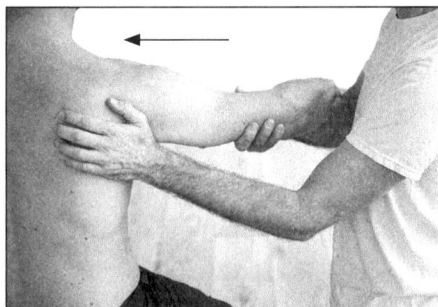

(b) Passive release to neutral

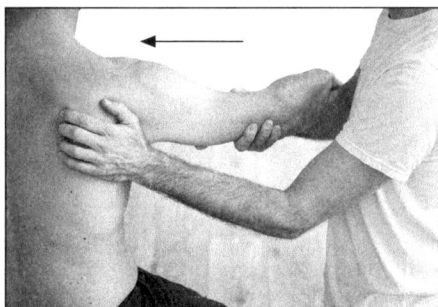

(c) Active close: 70 percent

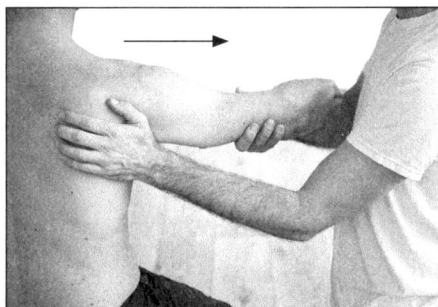

(d) Passive release to neutral

Figure 14-4:
Pulsing the GH and AH Joints—Four-Beat Cycle

6. Hand off the Pulse

Once the pulse is free and alive, follow the handoff procedure (described in Chapter 11).

Repeat Stages 1-6 on the receiver's other shoulder.

7. Practice the Self-Generated Pulse

Once the receiver has a connection to the pulse, they stand in the neutral posture (Figure 14-5a) and without any assistance:

- The receiver rounds their shoulders by extending their shoulder blades away from their spine (Figure 14-5b).

- Then the receiver pulses their shoulder joints in this position without allowing their shoulder blades to move back toward their spine.

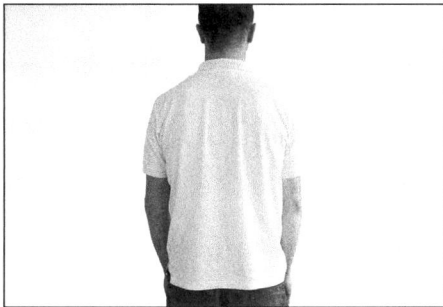

(a) Neutral position

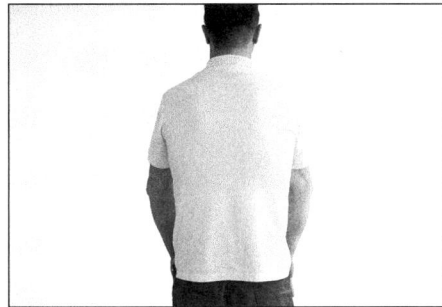

(b) Shoulders are spread open, the back is rounded, where pulsing begins

Figure 14-5:
Pulsing the Shoulder Joints

Once the pulse is alive in the shoulder joints, the receiver:

- Brings their arms up, out to the sides and forward with bent elbows in a very easy and comfortable position (Figure 14-6a).

- From this position and while maintaining a splay in their shoulder blades, the receiver initiates the four-beat pulse in their shoulder joints, elbows, wrists, hands and fingers—all in unison—while reflecting on the "Four-Point Checklist for a Self-Generated Pulse" (in Chapter 11). See Figure 14-6b-f.

- Once the pulse is alive, the receiver will fluidly shift into the Heaven and Earth form, opening the GH and AH joints as well as their elbows, wrists, hands and fingers during the opening phases and closing them during the closing phases.

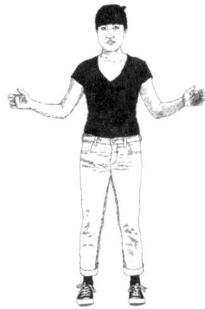 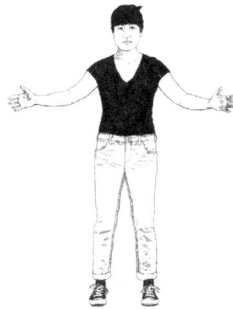

(a) Neutral position   (b) Open

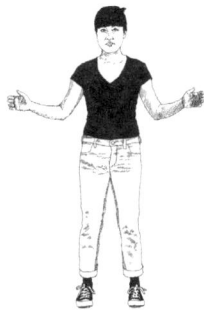 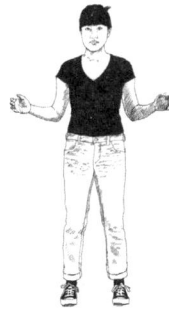

(c) Neutral   (d) Close

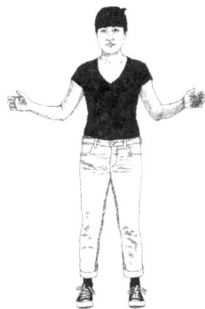 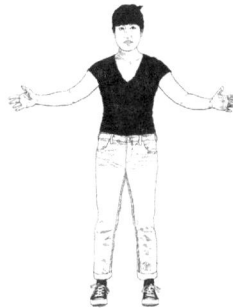

(e) Neutral position   (f) Open

Figure 14-6:
Pulsing the Shoulders, Elbows, Hands and Fingers

Always finish on an open before releasing to neutral

Change: Once the receiver has had a rest after solo practice, they will return the favor and pulse their partner's GH and AH joints.

PREPARATORY EXERCISES FOR PULSING THE SHOULDER BLADES

The shoulder blades move in three ways:

- Up and down.
- Sideways—away from the spine and toward the spine.
- Forward and backward.

LOOSENING THE SHOULDER BLADES

The following loosening exercises are initiated from the shoulder blades and, thereby, carry the arms and hands into motion. Because the shoulder blades initiate the motion of the upper limbs, there is no requirement for the arm and hand muscles to engage whatsoever. Such exercises are considered:

- **Warm-ups** - when the shoulder blades move to 100 percent of their range of motion, which is practiced to create more space.
- **Opening-and-closing techniques** - when the shoulder blades move within the space that has been created and remain within 70 percent of the practitioner's maximum range of motion.

Three warm-up exercises will help you connect to, identify any tension around and loosen up your shoulder blades. Eventually you can gain full control of your shoulder blades, which initiates all motion in the arms and connects the arms to the spine.

Warm-Up Exercise One: Raise and Sink the Shoulders

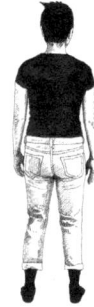

Start in the neutral standing position with your arms relaxed at your sides (Figure 14-7a).

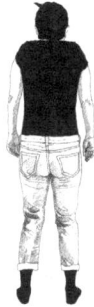

1. Raise your shoulder blades up to 100 percent of your comfortable range, while moving as smoothly and continuously as possible for you (see Figure 14-7b).

2. Lower your shoulder blades down to 100 percent of your comfortable range, while moving as smoothly and continuously as possible for you (see Figure 14-7c).

3. Repeat steps 1-2 a dozen times or so, gradually increasing the range of motion in your shoulder blades.

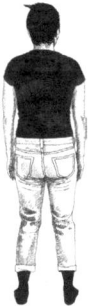

(a) Neutral position   (b) Raise the shoulders up   (c) Lower and
                                                                    sink the shoulders down

Figure 14-7:
Raise and Sink the Shoulders

Important Points

- Raising the shoulders unevenly or with tension can compress the muscles on either side of the neck, restrict blood flow in and out of the brain, disconnect the arms physically and energetically from the torso and the spine, and generate independent motion in the arms. Move slowly and remain present to create a balanced, smooth motion in the shoulder blades.

- To get the first action of up-and-down, relax your arms by your sides and make sure you do not use your arm muscles or hands. Many people bend their elbows during this exercise, which is a misunderstanding of the body mechanics required. It is the shoulder blade that moves the arm, not the other way around. When the shoulder blades move the arms, the arms feel empty and just hang down, and the hands will lightly contact the outer thighs. If the arms move the shoulder blades, the arms move away from the torso and the elbows will bend.

- While practicing this warm-up, note that although this exercise is good for loosening up the soft tissues that connect to and surround the shoulder blades, in qigong the shoulders always maintain a sense of sinking downward and are not meant to rise up.

Warm-Up Exercise Two:
Move the Shoulders Blades Away from and Toward the Spine

Start in the neutral standing position and bring your arms straight up and out to the sides to shoulder height with your elbows locked. This action is permissible in many warm-ups as the purpose is to stretch tight tissues around the shoulder blades, but is never practiced in internal arts as the elbows always remain bent (Figure 14-8a).

1. Simultaneously extend both of your shoulder blades and therefore your arms sideways away from your spine to 100 percent of your comfortable range of motion (Figure 14-8b).

2. Simultaneously move both of your shoulder blades sideways, back toward your spine to 100 percent of your comfortable range of motion (Figure 14-8c).

3. Repeat steps 1-2 a dozen times or so, gradually increasing the range of motion in your shoulder blades.

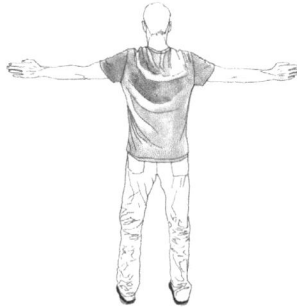

(a) Neutral position

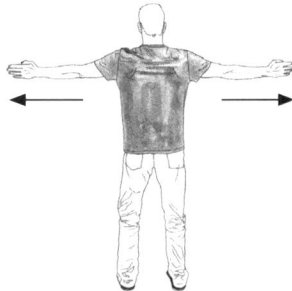

(b) Shoulder blades extend away from the spine

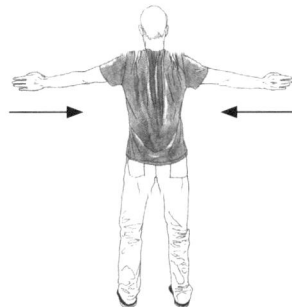

(c) Should blades draw back toward the spine

Figure 14-8: Move the Shoulder Blades Away from and Toward the Spine

Important Points

- As you move your shoulder blades side to side, relax and try not to let any tension build or the shoulder blades to rise up.

- Do not engage your arm muscles or move from your hands. The arms and hands only move because the shoulder blades move them, so they will not move independently.

- Do not bend your elbows. If you find yourself doing this, you know your arm muscles are trying to take over control of the action and you must reduce your effort. Focus on the shoulder blades becoming the source of the motion.

Warm-Up Exercise Three:
Move the Shoulder Blades Forward and Backward

Now you will attempt the forward-and-backward motion. This exercise is a lot smaller than the previous two movements since it requires the shoulder blades to press in toward the rib cage and then draw back out, away from the ribs. A small degree of sliding of the the shoulder blades around the rib cage prevents the buildup of internal pressure.

For this third exercise, stand in the neutral posture and put your arms straight out in front of you. Your arms should be parallel to each other at shoulder height with your elbows locked. Again, locking the elbows is permissible in warm-ups, but always maintain a bend in the limbs during qigong practice. See Figure 14-9a.

1. Move your shoulder blades forward to move your arms to 100 percent of your comfortable range—without any sideways motion in your arms or upward motion in your shoulder blades (Figure 14-9b).

2. Move your shoulder blades backward to move your arms to 100 percent of your comfortable range—without any sideways motion in your arms or upward motion in your shoulder blades (Figure 14-9c).

3. Repeat steps 1-2 a dozen times or so, gradually increasing the range of motion in your shoulder blades.

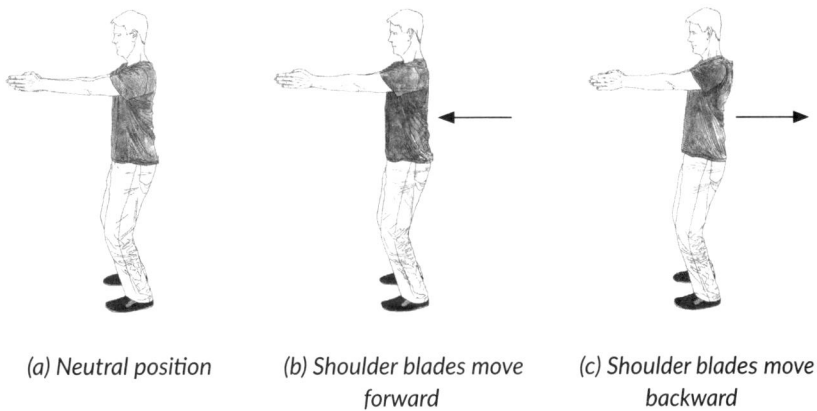

(a) Neutral position   (b) Shoulder blades move
                                    forward

(c) Shoulder blades move
        backward

Figure 14-9:
Move the Shoulder Blades Forward and Backward

HOW TO PULSE THE SHOULDER BLADES

Now you will apply the movements of the three warm-up exercises to initiate the pulse by backing off to 70 percent of your range of motion—except in the case of raising the shoulder blades, which always remain down in Heaven and Earth Qigong. Then you will learn how to integrate these motions in the Heaven and Earth form.

- When the shoulder blades open, they extend away from the spine—sideways or forward—or downward.

- When the shoulder blades close, they draw toward the spine—sideways or backward—or back up to their neutral position.

- When the shoulder blades open, the space in the armpits increases; when the shoulder blades close, the space in the armpits decreases.

- Do not engage your arm muscles or move from your hands. The arms and hands only move because the shoulder blades move them, so they will not move independently.

DEVELOP THE SIDEWAYS PULSING MOTION

1. Set up the Hand Hold and Align the Joints

First you will begin with the sideways motion, that is moving the shoulder blades away from and toward the spine. The receiver should sit upright with their back free from making contact with the back of the chair.

Take your partner's arm out to the side, just below their shoulder height. Place one hand on the back of their neck with your thumb on one side to adhere to their body's fascia and create a stability point from which to operate. Your other hand holds their upper arm. Their elbow remains bent and their forearm rests on your arm.

Initially give your partner's arm a gentle shake to help them relax. When their arm is relatively heavy, their nerves are letting go and their muscles are releasing tension. Check that this neutral position is comfortable for them (Figure 14-10).

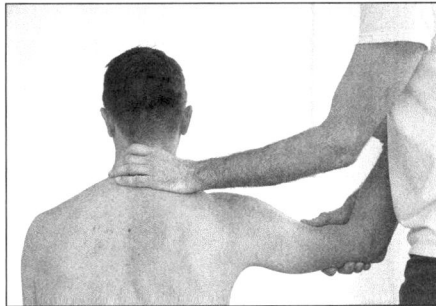

Neutral position

Figure 14-10:
Develop the Sideways Motion—Hand Hold

2. Activate the Four-Beat Cycle

Keeping your supporting hand at the base of their neck still in space:

1. Smoothly draw the receiver's shoulder blade 100 percent away from their spine and then 100 percent back toward their spine— without raising their shoulder (Figure 14-11a-b). The rising happens when the muscles are tight and tense, so only go as far as you can without causing their shoulder to scrunch up.

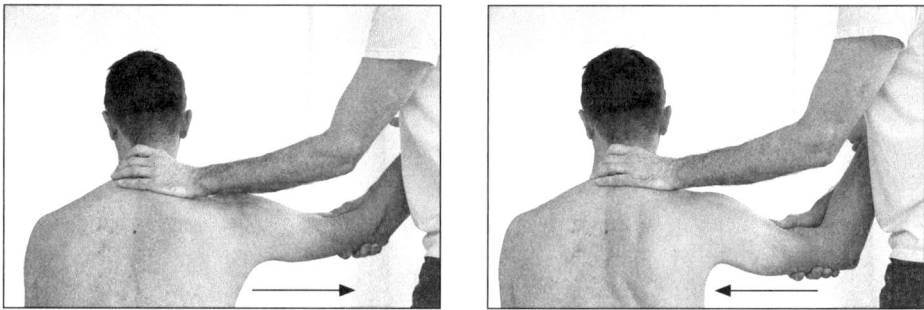

(a) 100-percent open   (b) 100-percent close

Figure 14-11:
Develop the Sideways Motion—
Find the Receiver's 100-Percent Range

2. There is not so much to be gained from the two-beat cycle as there is no local joint to pulse, unless there are a lot of restrictions in their shoulders. Simply back off and activate the four-beat cycle by staying within the receiver's comfortable 70-percent range, while letting the space in their armpit grow when you open and shrink when you close (Figure 14-12). As you pulse, adhere to the "Five-Point Checklist for Pulsing a Partner (see Chapter 11).

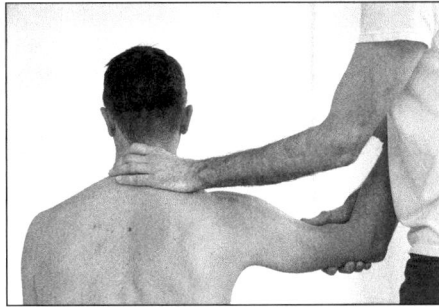

(a) Neutral position

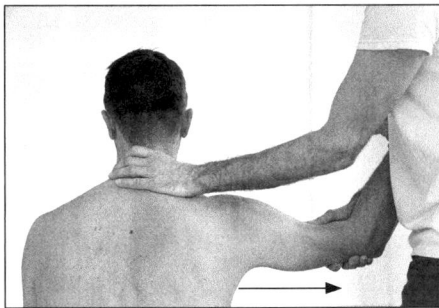

(b) Active open: 70 percent

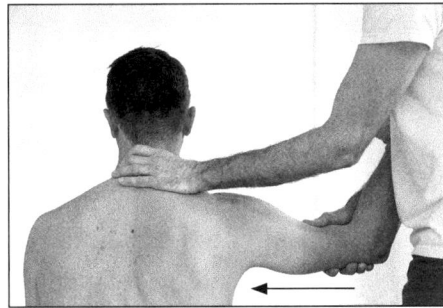

(c) Passive release to neutral

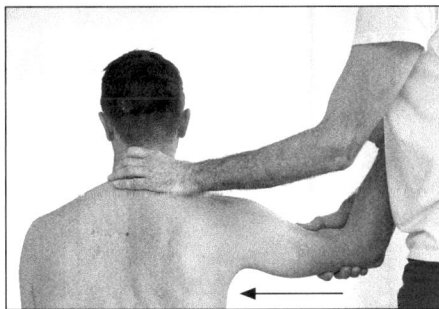

(d) Active close: 70 percent

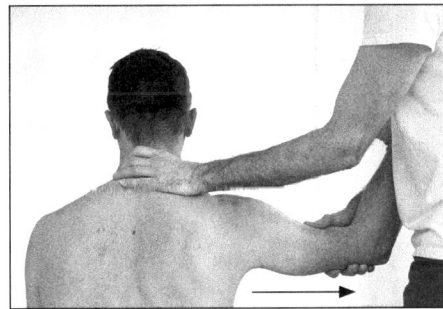

(e) Passive release to neutral

Figure 14-12:
Develop the Sideways Motion—Four-Beat Cycle

3. Hand off the Pulse

Follow the handoff procedure (from Chapter 11), so that the receiver gains full control over and smooth operation of their 70-percent range of motion in their shoulder blades.

Repeat Stages 1-3 on the receiver's other shoulder.

Change: Once both shoulders have been pulsed, switch roles, so the receiver returns the favor and pulses their partner's shoulder blades sideways.

DEVELOP THE FORWARD-AND-BACKWARD MOTION

1. Set up the Hand Hold and Align the Joints

This exercise may be done while standing or sitting.

Place one hand on the base of the side of the receiver's neck/top of their shoulder and adhere to their fascia for stability. Your other hand holds and supports their upper arm with their elbow bent and their forearm resting on yours. Bring their arm in front of their torso, just below their shoulder height and slightly outside their left or right channel in accordance with whether you are holding their left or right arm. See Figure 13-13.

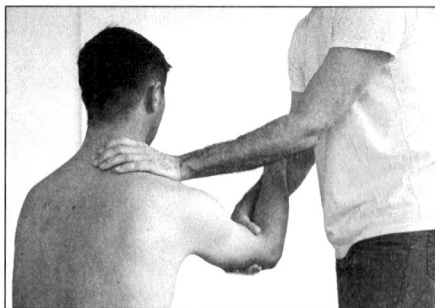

Neutral position

Figure 14-13:
Develop the Forward-and-Backward Motion—Hand Hold

2. Activate the Four-Beat Cycle

While keeping your supporting hand on the base of their neck still in space:

1. Smoothly draw their shoulder forward 100 percent and then backward 100 percent—without distorting their posture or raising their shoulder. The range will generally be much smaller than in the previous exercise. See Figure 14-14.

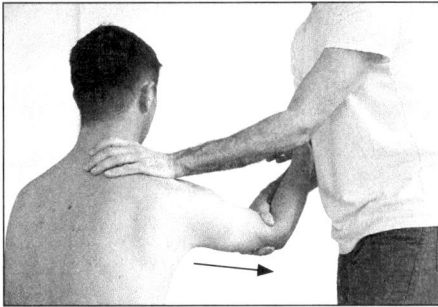

(a) 100-percent open   (b) 100-percent close

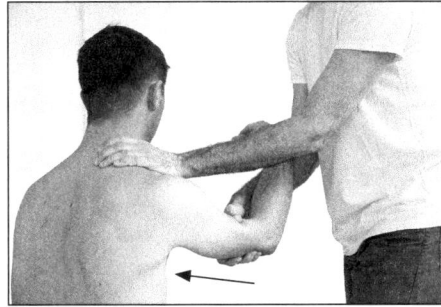

Figure 14-14:
Develop the Forward-and-Backward Motion—
Find the Receiver's 100-Percent Range

2. Back off to 70-percent forward/70-percent backward and adhere to the four-beat cycle, while letting the space in their armpit grow when you open and shrink when you close (Figure 14-15). Repeat until their tissues and shoulder blades move smoothly and easily while adhering to the "Five-Point Checklist for Pulsing a Partner" (see Chapter 11).

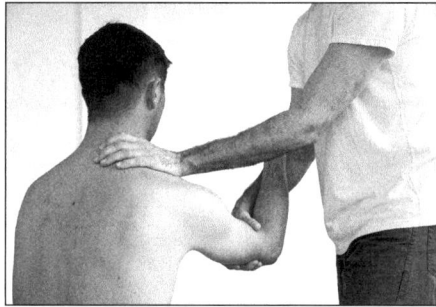

(a) Neutral position

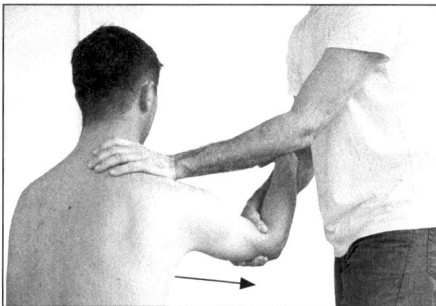

(b) Active open: 70 percent

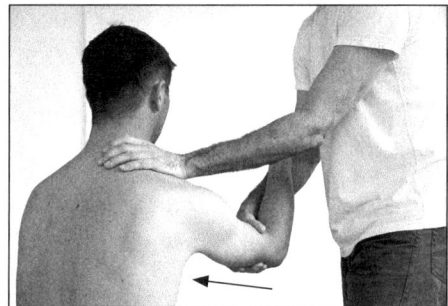

(c) Passive release to neutral

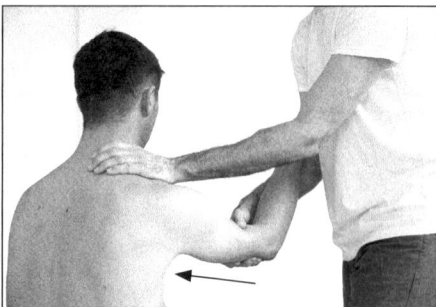

(d) Active close: 70 percent

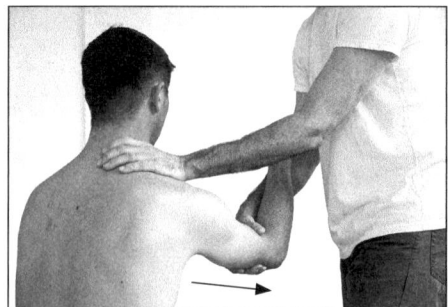

(e) Passive release to neutral

Figure 14-15:
Develop the Forward-and-Backward Motion—Four-Beat Cycle

3. Hand off the Pulse

Follow the handoff procedure (from Chapter 11), so that the receiver gains full control over and smooth operation of their 70-percent range of motion in their shoulder blades.

Repeat Stages 1-3 on the receiver's other shoulder.

Change: Once both shoulders have been pulsed, switch roles, so the receiver returns the favor and pulses their partner's shoulder blades using the forward-and-backward motion.

DEVELOP THE DOWNWARD-TO-NEUTRAL MOTION

1. Set up the Hand Hold and Align the Joints

This exercise is best done while standing.

With your partner standing in the neutral position, place one hand against the same side of their neck as the shoulder you will pulse and use the other hand to hold on and adhere to their corresponding upper arm (Figure 14-16).

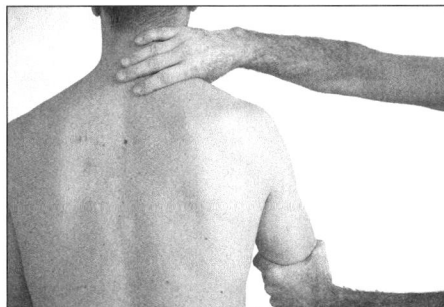

Neutral position

Figure 14-16:
Develop the Downward-to-Neutral Motion—Hand Hold

2. Activate the Two-Beat Cycle

Take the receiver's arm out to a minimum of one fist width from the side of their body to create space in their armpit and:

- Smoothly draw their arm and shoulder blade down toward the ground to 100-percent of their comfortable range of motion— without the receiver distorting their standing position. The space in their armpit will grow slightly. See Figure 14-17b.

- Then release and allow their shoulder to slowly return to neutral. The space in their armpit will shrink slightly. See Figure 14-17c.

- Back off to 70 percent and follow the two-beat cycle: 70-percent downward and then release to neutral (Figure 14-17d-e).

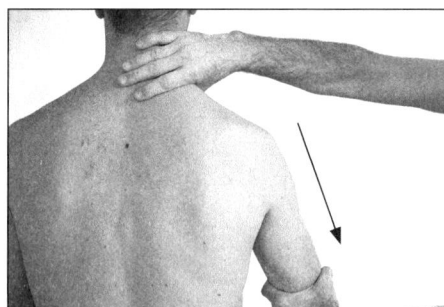

(a) 100-percent down

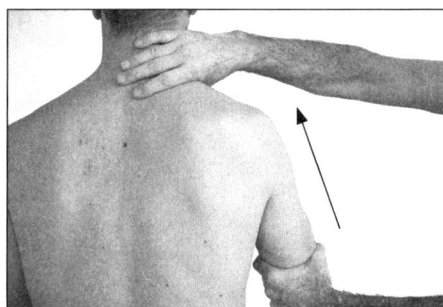

(b) Release to neutral

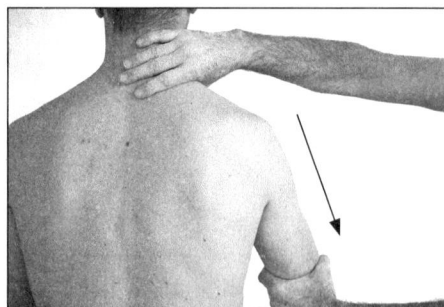

(c) 70-percent down

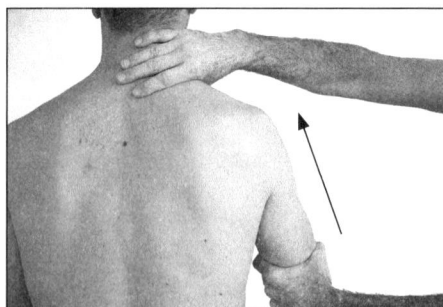

(d) Release to neutral

Figure 14-17:
Develop the Downward-to-Neutral Motion—Two-Beat Cycle

In the beginning, there will not be much movement. After the receiver has relaxed and their tissues have warmed up, the motion will likely increase in size, which is a sign that you are correctly amplifying the pulse.

3. Hand off the Pulse

Follow the handoff procedure (from Chapter 11), so that the receiver gains full control over and smooth operation of their 70-percent range of motion in their shoulder blades.

Repeat Stages 1-3 on the receiver's other shoulder.

Change: Once both shoulders have been pulsed, switch roles, so the receiver returns the favor and pulses their partner's shoulder blades using the downward-to-neutral motion.

JOINING THE SHOULDER BLADES TO THE PULSE OF THE JOINTS

Once you have control over pulsing your shoulder blades in the three directions, the next step is to join these motions with all of the previously covered joints in this section (i.e. shoulders, elbows, wrists, hands and fingers), as well as add bending and stretching the arms to mobilize and develop the qi of the upper limbs. Since the shoulder blades are the root of the arms, they initiate the motion, including bending-and-stretching and opening-and-closing techniques, as well as the flow of qi. The following three-stage exercise will help you integrate the various threads that you have already been practicing separately. This is the guiding Principle of Separate and Combine in action, which permeates all levels of training and allows you to continuously layer in more threads of neigong.

Stage One: Pulse the Arm Joints—Forward-and-Backward Motion

Stand in the neutral posture, bring your arms in front of you and parallel with each other. Your elbows remain bent while your forearms remain horizontal and parallel to the ground throughout the entirety of the exercise (Figure 14-18a).

1. Initiate the movement from your shoulder blades and:

   (a) Lightly stretch the soft tissues of your arms in sync with the open (Figure 14-18b).

   (b) Lightly bend the soft tissues of your arms in sync with the close (Figure 14-18c).

   You do not want the bending-and-stretching cycle to be so large or so strong that it inhibits your ability to go internal.

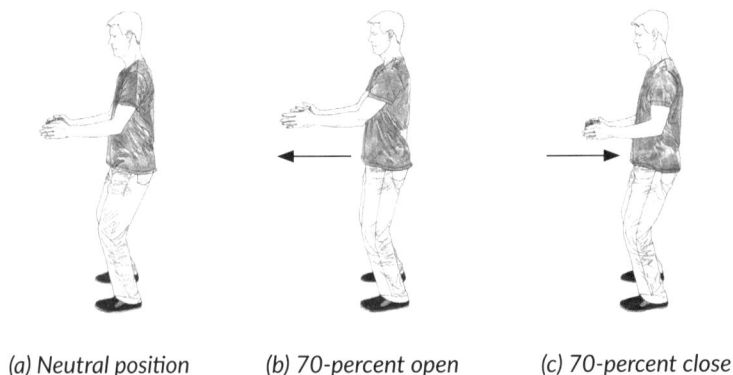

(a) Neutral position   (b) 70-percent open   (c) 70-percent close

Figure 14-18:
Pulse the Arm Joints—Forward-and-Backward Motion

2. Initiate opening and closing in your arms by:

(a) Moving your shoulder blades forward to open your arm joints (i.e., shoulders, elbows, wrists, hands and fingers). See Figure 14-18b.

(b) Moving your shoulder blades backward to close your joints (Figure 14-18c).

Establish a smooth, even and relaxed rhythm until all the joints of your arm are actively pulsing in sync with the motion of your shoulder blades, and the bending and stretching of your arm tissues. Only when all your arm joints are active should you move onto the next step.

3. Now use the motion of your shoulder blades to not only bend and stretch your soft tissues and open and close your arm joints, but also to mobilize your qi with your mind's intent as you:

(a) Drive qi to your fingertips on the open and move your shoulder blades forward (Figure 14-18b).

(b) Draw qi into your shoulder blades on the close and move your shoulder blades backward (Figure 14-18c).

Practice until the qi flows are smooth, fluid, complete and balanced in both arms. You want the motion of your shoulder blades to move in sync with your intent and direct the flow of qi.

4. The shoulder blades drive the flow of qi, so the next step is to connect the qi of the shoulder blades into and out of the spine. This is achieved by moving the shoulders:

(a) Backward to drive qi into the spine between the shoulder blades (Figure 14-18b).

(b) Forward to draw qi from the spine to the shoulder blades (Figure 14-18c).

Note: Suspend the qi flow from the shoulder blades to the fingers and back (step 3), as you amplify the qi flow into and out of your spine.

5. Once you can do steps 3 and 4 smoothly and independently, join the two flows together.

    (a) As you move your shoulder blades forward, extend your qi from your spine through your blades to your fingertips, while simultaneously stretching all your soft tissues and opening all the joints of your arms (Figure 14-18b).

    (b) As you move your shoulder blades backward, draw the qi back up your arms and through your shoulder blades into your spine from your fingertips, while simultaneously bending all your soft tissues and closing all the joints of your arms (Figure 14-18c).

Keep practicing until you integrate the three aspects—bend and stretch, pulsing and the qi flows—smoothly and continuously, at which point you will be ready to move on to Stage Two.

Relaxing your arms for a few moments before moving on to Stage Two will allow you to release any tension that has built up in your arms, shoulders and neck. Do not wait too long though, or you will lose momentum and interrupt qi flow.

Stage Two: Continue Pulsing the Arm Joints—Sideways Motion

6. Fluidly transition into bringing your arms out to the sides while maintaining a bend in both arms (Figure 14-19a).

7. Repeat steps 1-5 from Stage One. Only the position of the arms has changed and this time the shoulder blades pulse sideways—away from and toward the spine—to initiate the bending and stretching of the soft tissues, pulsing of the joints and the qi flows (Figure 14-19b-c).

8. Practice pulsing the shoulder blades sideways until they smoothly and easily control and integrate the three aspects in this position.

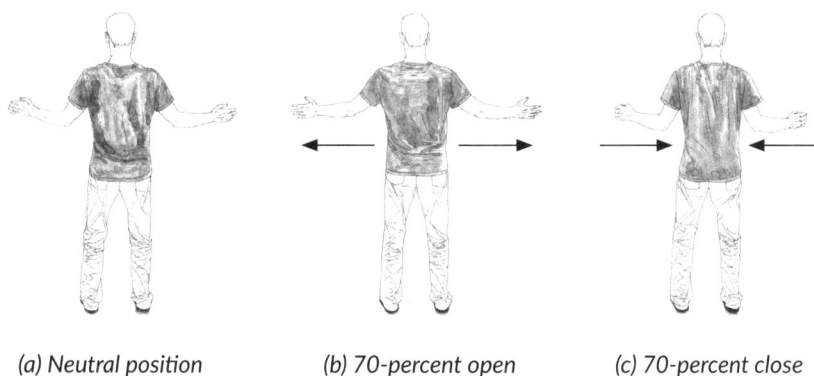

(a) Neutral position   (b) 70-percent open   (c) 70-percent close

Figure 14-19:

Pulse the Arm Joints—Sideways Motion

Once you have either achieved the goals of step 8 or you hit the point of diminishing returns, move on to Stage Three. A momentary pause, where you relax your arms down at your sides, can prevent tension from building up in your body.

Stage Three: Continue Pulsing the Arm Joints—Sink and Release

9. Bring your hands away from the sides of your body, maintaining one fist width distance between:

   (a) your upper arms and your torso; and

   (b) your hands and your hips/legs (Figure 14-20a).

10. Repeat steps 1-5 from Stage One with a shift of focus on the pulse. In this third position, the shoulder blades only sink and release to neutral, so you need to adjust the opening-and-closing action in the arm joints and the qi flow to fit the shoulder-blade motion.

    (a) As the shoulder blades descend, the joints open, the tissues stretch and qi travels from your spine to your fingertips (Figure 14-20b).

    (b) As the shoulder blades release to neutral, the joints close, the tissues bend and qi travels from your fingertips to your spine (Figure 14-20c).

11. Practice sinking and releasing your shoulder blades to bend and stretch your tissues and open and close your joints with the accompanying qi flows—until the three aspects integrate into one seamless whole.

Keep practicing until the qi flows and the pulse are smooth, fluid and continuous.

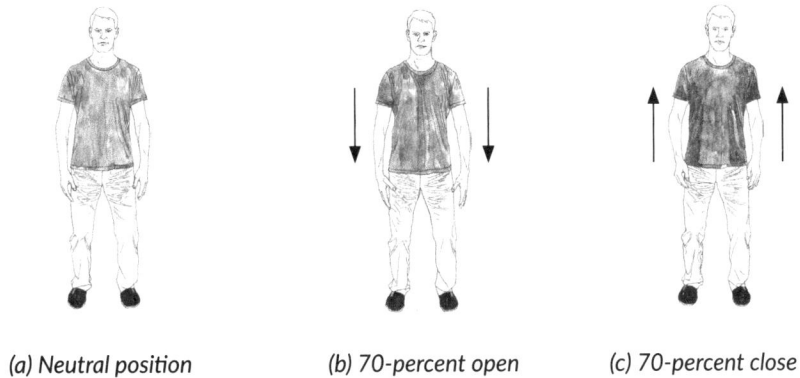

(a) Neutral position   (b) 70-percent open   (c) 70-percent close

Figure 14-20:
Pulse the Arm Joints—Sink and Release

ACTIVATING THE SHOULDER BLADES
IN HEAVEN AND EARTH QIGONG

When your shoulder blades move fluidly and smoothly, and control the physical motion of the pulse in the arms as well as the qi flows, you are ready to practice Heaven and Earth with all the material presented on the shoulders, arms and hands.

The opening and closing of the AH, GH and AC joints fits snuggly within the opening-and-closing phases of the form as do the previous joints of the elbows, wrists, hands and fingers. Simply open during the opening phases and close during the closing phases.

The shoulder blades, however, are different.

The main objective with the shoulder blades is to keep them moving smoothly, fluidly and continuously. Sometimes the blades will be in harmony with all of the other upper limb joints and sometimes they will not be. The reason the shoulder blades can do this is because they move in three dimensions so, from one perspective, they could be seen as closing and, from another, opening. Also, with the complexity of the arm movements required in Heaven and Earth, what actually happens is that the shoulder blades rotate a great deal, laying the foundation for deeper neigong downstream.

Follow the instructions on all of the material presented on the arms and, whatever you do, just keep your shoulder blades moving! For instance, on the first close, they extend away from the spine for all four steps—not just opening on the first step and remaining still for the next three.

As the movement of your joints becomes smoother, the fascia in your neck, back and around your shoulder blades will naturally begin to stretch. However, if you experience any sharp pains, this indicates you are pushing your body. Simply back off and adhere to the 70-Percent Rule, allowing your soft tissues to release and open up in their own time.

Take your time, go slowly and, if you feel you need assistance, seek out the support of a qualified Heaven and Earth Qigong Instructor to offer personal feedback to keep you from going off-track.

REVIEW: SIMPLIFIED INSTRUCTIONS

MACROCOSMIC ORBIT

First-Phase Open

Steps 1-2 - Open the shoulder blades forward (Figure 14-21a-c).

Step 3 - Open the shoulder blades sideways (Figure 14-21d-e).

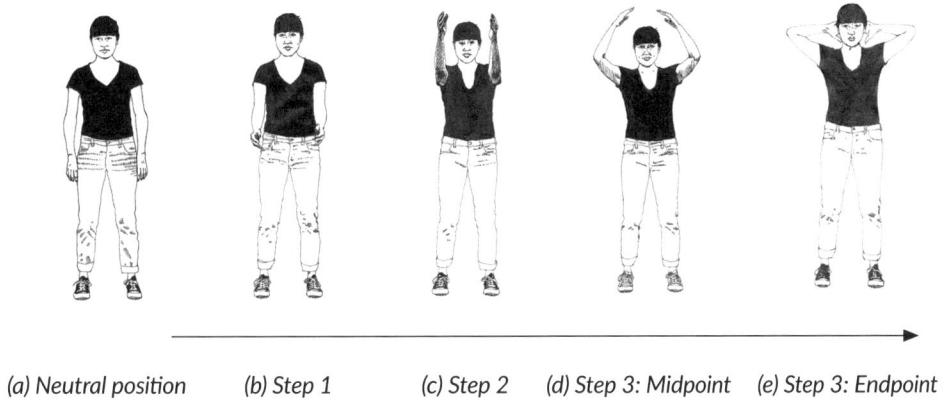

(a) Neutral position   (b) Step 1   (c) Step 2   (d) Step 3: Midpoint   (e) Step 3: Endpoint

Figure 14-21:
Open the Arm Joints—First-Phase Stretch

Second-Phase Close

Steps 4-7 - Extend and wrap the shoulder blades away from the spine and forward continuously (Figure 14-22).

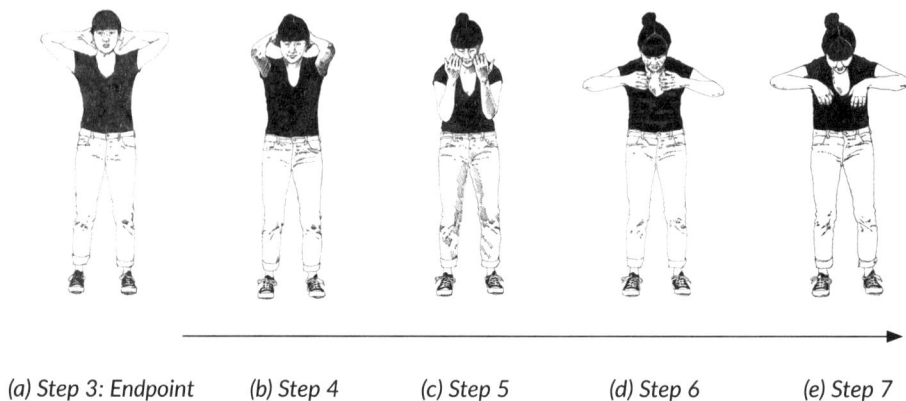

(a) Step 3: Endpoint   (b) Step 4   (c) Step 5   (d) Step 6   (e) Step 7

Figure 14-22: Close the Arm Joints—Second-Phase Bend

Third-Phase Open

Step 8 - Release the shoulder blades back to neutral and sink them down (Figure 14-23).

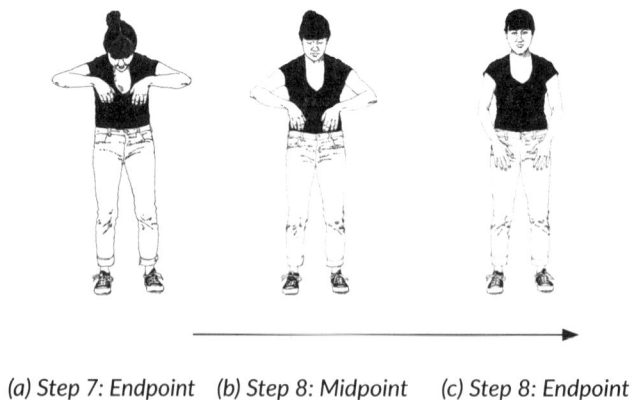

(a) Step 7: Endpoint   (b) Step 8: Midpoint   (c) Step 8: Endpoint

Figure 14-23:
Open the Arm Joints—Third-Phase Stretch

MICROCOSMIC ORBIT

Fourth-Phase Close

Steps 9-11 - Draw the shoulder blades back to the spine (Figure 14-24).

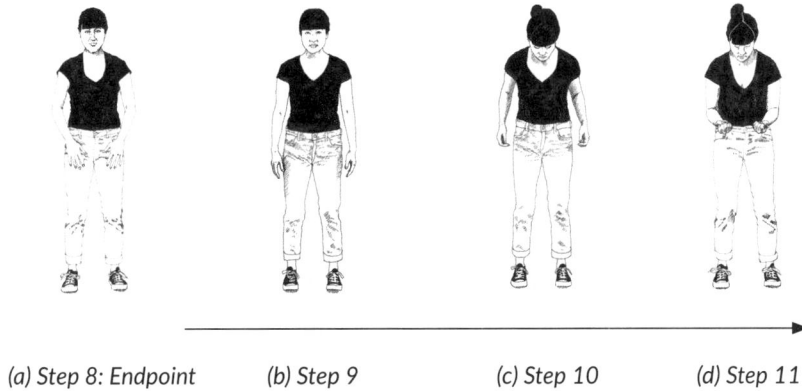

(a) Step 8: Endpoint   *(b) Step 9*   *(c) Step 10*   *(d) Step 11*

Figure 14-24: Close the Arm Joints—Fourth-Phase Bend

Fifth-Phase Open

Steps 12-13 - Open the shoulder blades forward (Figure 14-25).

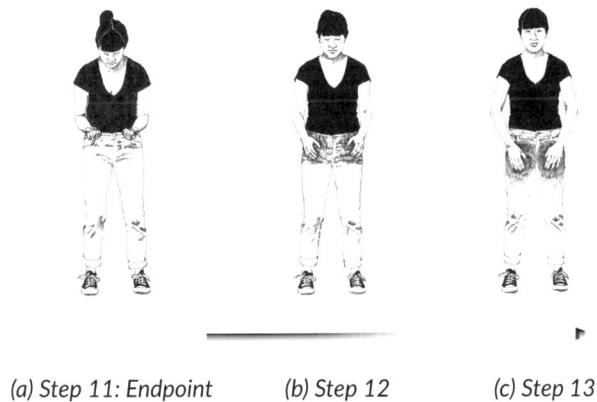

(a) Step 11: Endpoint   *(b) Step 12*   *(c) Step 13*

**Figure 14-25:
Open the Arm Joints—Fifth-Phase Stretch**

NEUTRAL

Sixth-Phase Release

Step 14 - Release the shoulder blades to neutral (Figure 14-26).

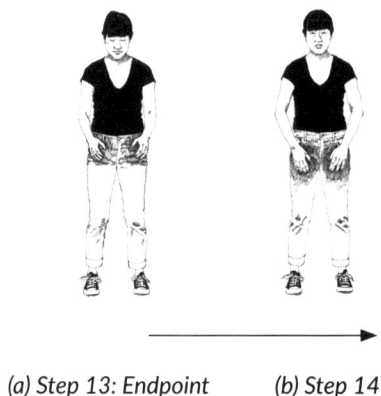

(a) Step 13: Endpoint   *(b) Step 14*

Figure 14-26:
Release the Arm Joints—Sixth-Phase Release

THE SHOULDER BLADES: INDICATORS OF HEART HEALTH

The influence of the military posture is widely apparent in Western culture. The shoulders are back, the chest is forward with the chin lifted; and the shoulder blades are locked into the spine and back of the rib cage (Figure 14-27). This causes undue pressure on various parts of the body—not the least of which is the heart. This posture reduces flexibility, blood and qi circulation, and generates a lot of tension. Over time all of this leads to imbalances that can degrade to serious health issues. Most people hardly feel and cannot directly move their shoulder blades at all. New students soon find that by learning qigong in general and Heaven and Earth specifically, they are embarking upon releasing a lifetime's worth of tension from this area.

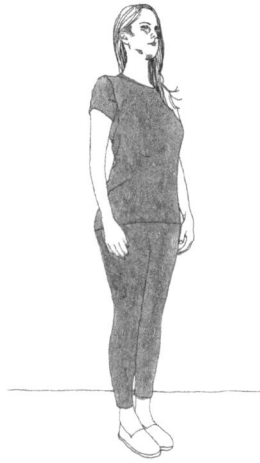

Figure 14-27:
Western Military Posture

If you observe a young child before they have been imprinted with Western cultural norms, you will notice a straight spine, open back, dropped shoulders and chest with a full belly. As we age, we pick up on the not-so-subtle yet widespread postural conditioning and subsequently begin to close down the area behind the heart, expand and lift the chest, and use the motion of the shoulder blades less and less frequently. When the blades move less, the connective tissues close down and become stuck. In time the back of the rib cage becomes rigid and the vertebrae between the shoulder blades contract, further restricting spinal movement. As this continues over decades, the internal organs—especially the diaphragm, heart and lungs—lose the space they need to function optimally. Eventually the shoulder blades move little and the rib cage and the spine lock down, which puts immense strain on the heart. Two words: cardiac arrest!

Additionally, the shoulder blades have a direct energetic connection to the heart and, when they do not move freely, the heart becomes restricted. The importance of freeing up the shoulder blades and the space behind the heart cannot be overstated—these exercises could literally become life-savers.

Together with the postural alignments and C-curve (presented in Chapters 1 and 4, respectively), the shoulder blades are critically important to reversing the contracting and shutting down process. As the body is exercised through the many stages of Heaven and Earth practice, the shoulder blades become freer and freer. When the shoulder blades move more, they open up the tissues on the surface of the torso, as explained earlier in this chapter. The more tension that is released from the tissues connected to the shoulder blades, the more the back of the ribs can move, which can eventually unlock the spine, back of the diaphragm, pericardium and heart.

One of the immediate benefits of engaging this level of practice with the shoulder blades is that circulation increases. Removing or even partially removing blockages behind the heart increases circulation of blood and qi quite dramatically. If left unaddressed, contractions in this area are likely to diminish the flow of blood away from the heart. Similarly tension in the chest and shoulders' nests reduces venous return.

Eventually and with sufficient practice, you can release a lifelong store of tension. As you penetrate your body deeper and deeper, you can release your ribs, spine, diaphragm, pericardium and even your heart muscle. Anybody who has progressively trained through this process will tell you it is like receiving a new lease of life, like a boa constrictor slowly and progressively releasing its grip. If you get nothing more from your Heaven and Earth practice, these benefits alone make training well worth the effort!

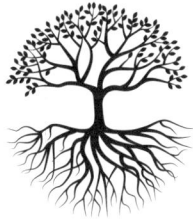

CHAPTER 15:

PULSING THE RIBS
AND THE STERNUM

Once the shoulder blades become free and loose, they release the tensions that prevent the ribs from moving well. The ribs themselves are moved via breathing and soft-tissue techniques, and can be pulsed by almost anyone who puts in the time and effort to develop the skill to do so.

THE STERNOCOSTAL AND INTERCOSTAL JOINTS

There are two primary ways to move the ribs:

- Extend them away from and back toward the breast bone (sternum).

- Increase and decrease the space in the intercostals—the space between each pair of ribs.

The ribs connect to each other via the intercostal muscles and into the sternum via the costal cartilages, which are long strips of thick, elastic ligamental material designed to generate flexibility in the chest (see Figure 15-1). The average Westerner breathes high into their chest cavity. As a result, the connections between the ribs and the sternum could remain flexible, but the connections between the ribs themselves become relatively inflexible. In order to open up the intercostal spaces, opening and closing the ribs-to-sternum (sternocostal) joints, along with the breathing material presented in Chapter 8, can be immensely useful.

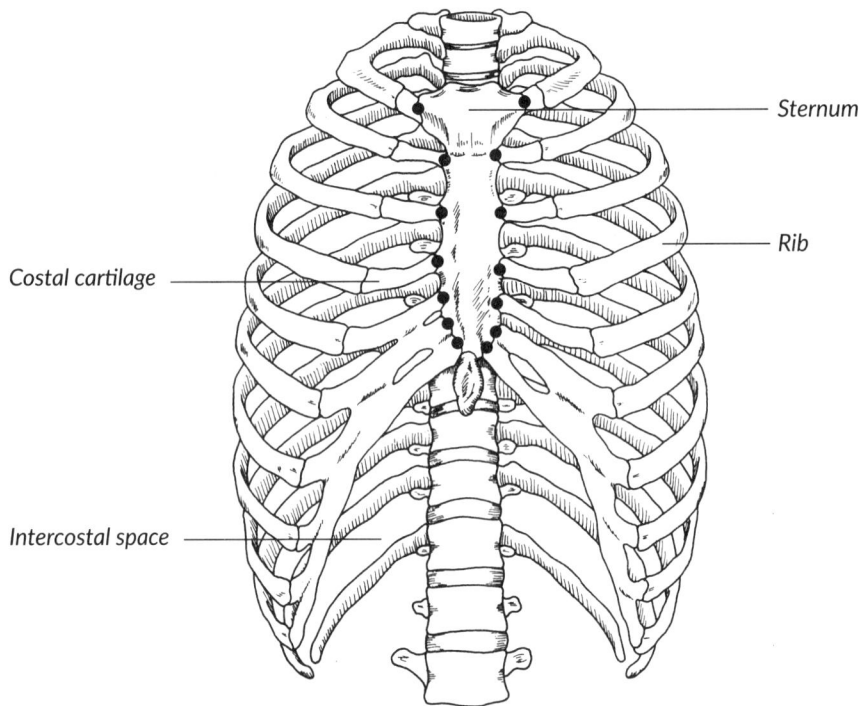

Figure 15-1:
The Ribs and the Sternum

HOW TO PULSE
THE RIBS-TO-STERNUM CONNECTIONS

The technique that follows is radically different from all previous pulsing exercises for the simple fact that a rib cannot be held by a hand. Be sure to familiarize yourself with the ribs, the sternum and the connections between the two before moving ahead.

LOCATE THE RIBS-TO-STERNUM CONNECTIONS

1. At the front of your chest, a couple of inches either side of your centerline, place your fingertips on a vertical line. Feel around this area and you will find that the ribs protrude and the spaces between the ribs (intercostal spaces) dip in.

2. Once you have found the spaces between your ribs, follow the depressions toward your centerline. These depressions will disappear when you reach your sternum bone.

3. Now that you have found the junction of the ribs and sternum, keep your fingers there and follow the edge of the sternum upward and downward, so you can identify the connections from the ribs to the sternum.

4. Repeat this exercise on your partner.

PULSING THE RIBS-TO-STERNUM CONNECTIONS

1. Prepare to Pulse

In order to pulse these connections on a partner, you will need to use a certain quality of pressure and adhesion between your fingers and the receiver's chest. Too much pressure leads to the receiver recoiling and/or contracting; too little pressure and your fingers will slide or you will only move their skin—both scenarios prevent rather than support amplification of the pulse.

The best method for activating the pulse in the ribs is to ask the receiver to stand with their back against a wall. As you sink your finger pads into their chest, this position will prevent them from losing their balance or pushing back against your pressure and tightening up.

Place the pads of your fingers on their ribs, which are located on either side of the sternum (Figure 15-2).

- Slowly and gently, yet firmly, sink your finger pads into the soft tissues covering their ribs until you feel like you "stick" to their ribs.

- Separate your hands, left and right, without losing your grip or sinking in deeper.

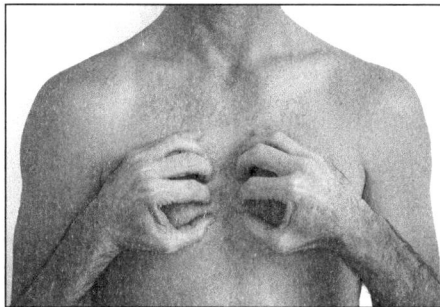

Neutral position

Figure 15-2:
Pulsing the Ribs-to-Sternum Connections—Hand Position

Because you are dealing with thick cartilage rather than synovial joints containing fluid, there is no need to work through the normal procedure, so you can skip the two-beat cycle.

2. Activate the Four-Beat Cycle

Use your intuition developed via all of the previous pulsing techniques and start directly with the four-beat cycle of 70-percent open/70-percent close (Figure 15-3).

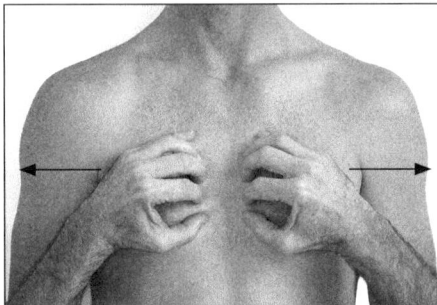

(a) Active open: 70 percent

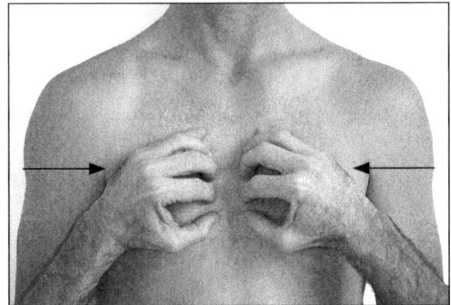

(b) Release to neutral

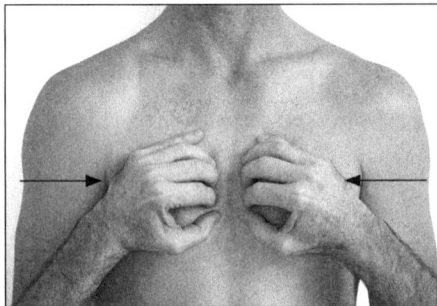

(c) Active close: 70 percent

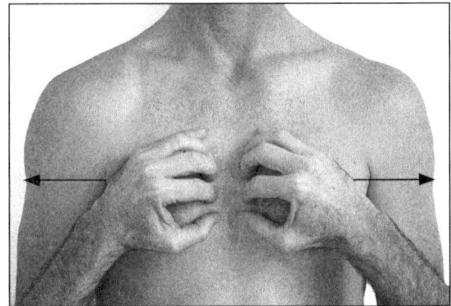

(d) Release to neutral

Figure 15-3:
Pulsing the Ribs-to-Sternum Connections—Four-Beat Cycle

If the receiver's tissues are tight, there will be little or almost no motion initially, but after a number of repetitions, you will normally notice the motion build. Repeat a dozen times or so while staying in verbal communication with your partner to make sure you do not overdo it or only move their skin.

There is little chance that the receiver will be able to pick up the pulse from a single experience, so skip the handoff procedure too, at least for a while. Activating the pulse in the sternocostal joints initially relies on the correct physical form of Heaven and Earth, and unifying the pulse in all of the previous joints to jumpstart the motion.

3. Practice the Self-Generated Pulse

Once the receiver has experienced their ribs being pulsed, they should stand and pulse on their own.

- Repeat the exercise on pulsing their whole arm via their shoulder blades in the sideways position (from Chapter 14).

- Then, after focusing on bringing their whole shoulder, arm and hand alive on both sides of their body, the receiver uses that pulse to link to and affect their ribs and sternum while reflecting upon the "Four-Point Checklist for a Self-Generated Pulse" (see Chapter 11). A strong pulse in the arms, shoulders and ribs is required before moving on.

- Once the ribs are moving well, the receiver releases into neutral and transitions into the Heaven and Earth form, opening their ribs and sternum during the opening phases and closing them during the closing phases.

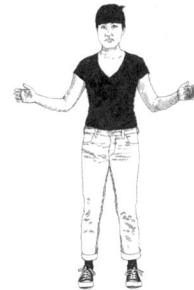

PULSING THE RIBS-TO-STERNUM CONNECTIONS IN HEAVEN AND EARTH QIGONG

Important Points

- The sternocostal joints will open during the opening phases and close during the closing phases; however the strongest opening of the chest joints will be in the first phase, step 3, as the elbows go out to the sides (Figure 15-4).

- The focus is on using the sideways spreading of the elbows and shoulder blades to grab the rib cage and draw it out from the sternum—one rack of ribs in either direction!

- Extending the fingertips back in to the occiput will increase the opening, if the elbows are stretching out from the spine.

- Both closing phases are equally as strong when closing the sternocostal joints.

- The other two opening phases (i.e., the third and fifth phases) will induce some degree of opening in the beginning and, once the pulse is initiated, will grow over time.

Change: Once all the exercises in this chapter have been completed, the pulser and the receiver will switch roles.

Figure 15-4: The Marriage of Heaven and Earth Qigong—Pulsing the Sternum

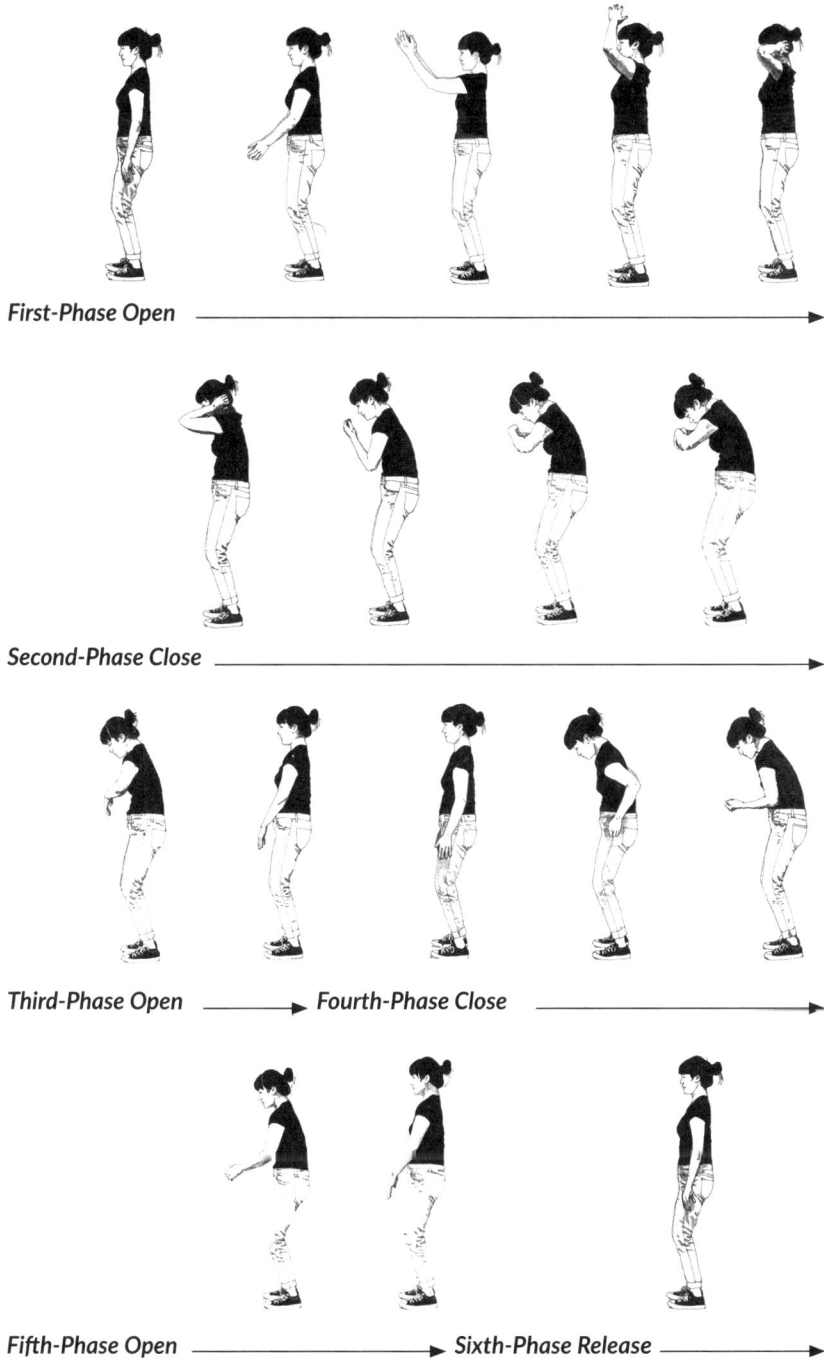

First-Phase Open ────────────────────────────▶

Second-Phase Close ────────────────────────────▶

Third-Phase Open ──────▶ *Fourth-Phase Close* ──────────────▶

Fifth-Phase Open ──────────────▶ *Sixth-Phase Release* ──────▶

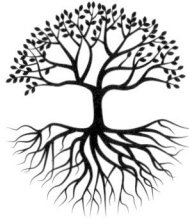

CHAPTER 16:

PULSING THE FEET
AND THE ANKLES

ABOUT OPENING AND CLOSING THE LOWER BODY

When moving on to pulsing the lower body, a few more considerations are necessary. Pulsing the lower body is more difficult for both the pulser and the receiver. This is due to the weight of the lower limbs being much heavier, as well as the tissues being much denser and thicker than those of the upper limbs. Most people also have a stronger connection to and so can perform more intricate movements with their arms. As a result, the lower body requires more time and effort to bring alive. Of course you have the added issue of the torso's weight going through the legs during standing and moving practices too. This causes the joints to compress, which at least initially, will restrict the motion of the pulse. If you practice, these hurdles will be temporary and you will become more familiar with and develop the skill to pulse your lower body. The effort is well worth your time as pulsing the lower body develops qi faster and more strongly than is possible in the upper body.

THE SIX CONNECTIONS

The six connections are:

- The hands, wrists and fingers to the feet, ankles and toes.
- The elbows to the knees.
- The shoulders to the hips.

These three pairings are on both the left and right sides of the body, and thereby form the six connections.

This energetic connection between pairs of upper- and lower-body joints can be observed in any four-legged animal, such as a dog or cat—in both anatomy and physiology. Their spine is horizontal: the roots of their limbs are their shoulders and hips, which connect to their spine; these are followed by the elbows and knees; followed by the wrists and ankles; and complete at their paws (the equivalent to human fingers and toes). When they walk, they move their left-rear leg with their front-right leg and, in opposite, their right-rear leg with their front-left leg. This alternating action allows them to maintain their balance as they would fall over by moving both right limbs or both left limbs at the same time. Like animals, human beings are created from a similar design, which can be observed when a baby crawls or an adult walks and swings their arms in the opposite direction to their step. All of these actions are instinctual because of the underlying energetic connections and framework with which we are all born.

For this reason, we will work through the lower body in a similar pattern to the upper body, using similar pulsing exercises for each correlated pair of joints.

HOW TO PULSE THE FOOT

Feet do not move much in the modern age of restrictive footwear and the lack of proper exercise. However, your feet can become loose and open and, if you put in sufficient effort, can perform intricate motions. As proof, some people who lose their upper limbs develop incredible skills with their feet, such as carving, painting or playing musical instruments.

The feet pulses are the same as the hands with one small difference—toe pulses are almost impossible to achieve joint by joint, especially in the small toes. So you will pulse each toe as one whole, doing your best not to bend or buckle the toes, and keeping the integrity of the alignment through the toe-to-foot during the entirety of the pulsing exercises.

PULSING THE TOES

In the following instructions, you will pulse all ten of your partner's toes individually before moving onto the lengthwise and widthwise pulses for the whole foot.

1. Locate and Feel the Foot Bones

Familiarize yourself with the joints and the structure of the foot and toes, then make contact with the receiver's foot with a gentle intent.

2. Set up the Hand Hold and Align the Joint

Hold the receiver's foot in one hand with your fingers on the top of their foot and your thumb on their arch (Figure 16-1). Keep you partner's toes in alignment with their foot such that:

- From the side, their toe, ball of their foot and their heel are in a straight line.
- From the top, their toe and their foot bone (metatarsal) to which it is attached is in a straight line.

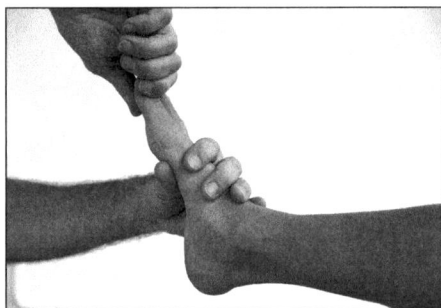

Neutral position

Figure 16-1:
Pulsing the Toes—Hand Hold

3. Activate the Two-Beat Cycle

Working with one toe at a time, starting with the big toe:

- Open up the receiver's toe joints to 100 percent of their comfortable range, then release smoothly and slowly (Figure 16-2a-b).

- Reduce your effort and open their toe joints to 70 percent of their comfortable range of motion, then release to neutral (Figure 16-2c-d).

- Continue with the two-beat cycle a dozen times or so, until you feel their toe joints loosen up and their tissues elongate.

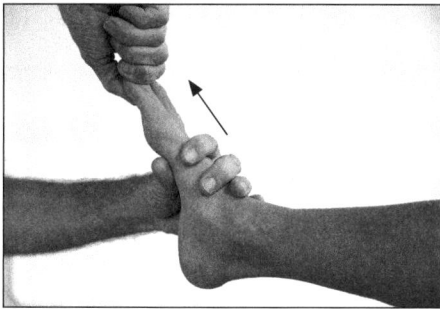

(a) 100-percent open

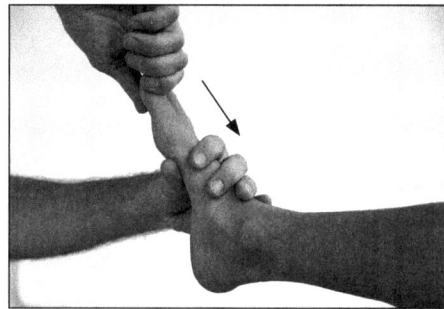

(b) Release to neutral

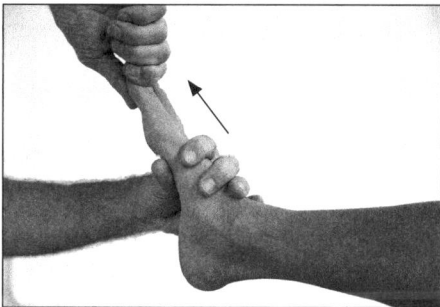

(c) 70-percent open

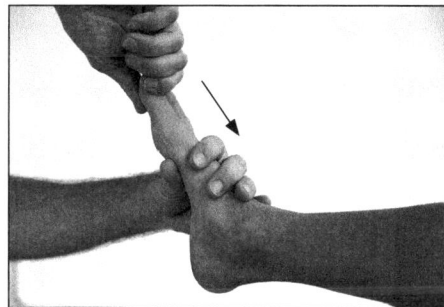

(d) Release to neutral

Figure 16-2:
Pulsing the Toes—Two-Beat Cycle

4. Close and Release the Joints

Repeat one more open-release, before:

- Shifting into the 100-percent close (Figure 16-3a).
- Releasing to the neutral position (Figure 16-3b).

Be careful as you close: it is here that you could bend and buckle the toes if your alignment is out or the pressure of your push is uneven or too fast.

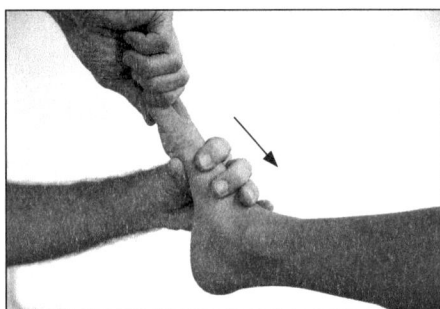

(a) 100-percent close   (b) Release to neutral

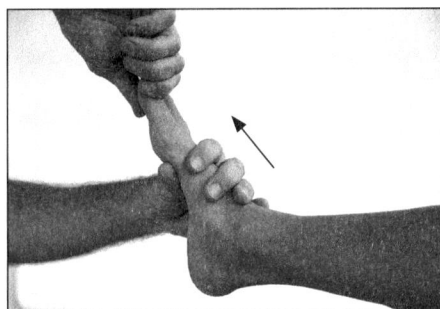

Figure 16-3:
Pulsing the Toes—Close and Release the Joints

5. Activate the Four-Beat Cycle

Shift into the four-beat cycle, 70-percent open/70-precent close (Figure 16-4), while reflecting on the "Five-Point Checklist for Pulsing a Partner" (see Chapter 11).

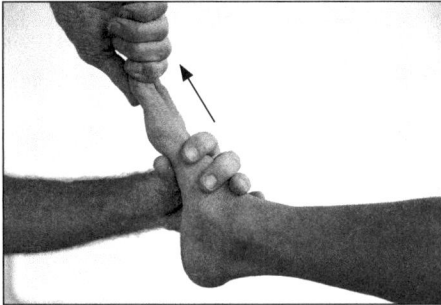

(a) Active open: 70-percent

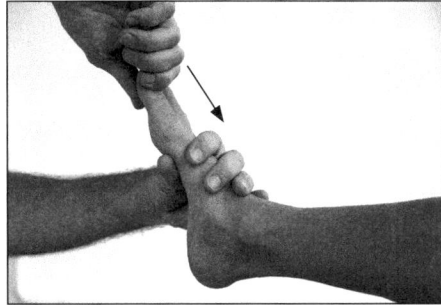

(b) Passive release to neutral

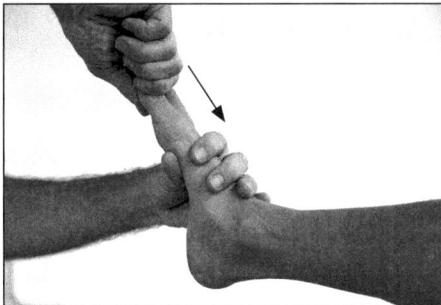

(c) Active close: 70-percent

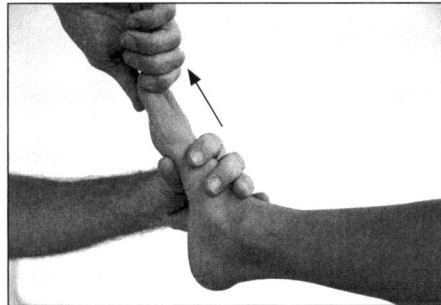

(d) Release to neutral

Figure 16-4:
Pulsing the Toes—Four-Beat Cycle

Note: Skip the handoff procedure until all the toes of both feet have been pulsed and you have also pulsed both feet lengthwise.

Repeat Stages 1-5 on the receiver's other foot.

PULSING THE FOOT LENGTHWISE

All of the following pulsing techniques can help to relieve the compressions commonly found in the feet. Normally, due to these compressions and the tightness of the ligaments within the foot, more effort is required to pulse a foot than a hand. First you will pulse along the length of the foot and then you will add the toes.

1. Set up the Hand Hold and Align the Foot Bones

With one hand, grab the heel of your partner's foot by wrapping your thumb, index finger and middle finger around their heel. Your ring and little fingers will cradle the bottom of their heel. Take your other hand and hold the ball of their foot. See Figure 16-5.

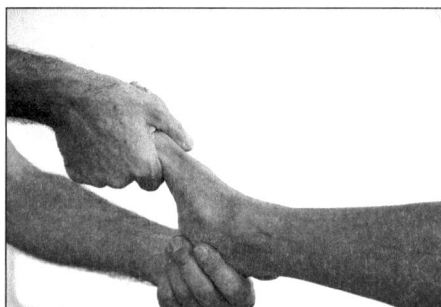

Neutral position

Figure 16-5:
Pulsing the Foot Lengthwise—Hand Hold

2. Activate the Two-Beat Cycle

From the neutral position:

- Draw the ball of their foot in one direction and their heel in the opposite direction to open up the foot to 100 percent of the receiver's comfortable capacity, then release (Figure 16-6a-b).

- Use the two-beat cycle to open-release the foot to 70 percent of the receiver's comfortable range a dozen times or so in order to open up the foot and begin releasing any tension (Figure 16-6c-d).

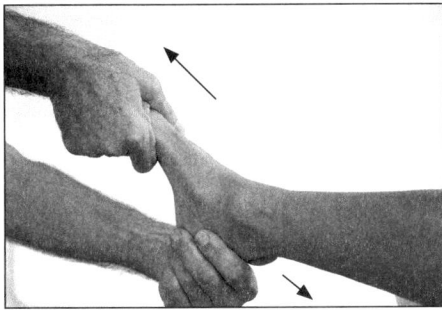

(a) 100-percent open

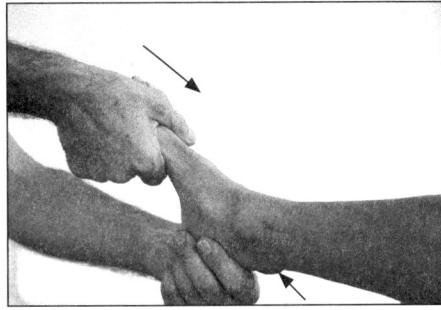

(b) Release to neutral

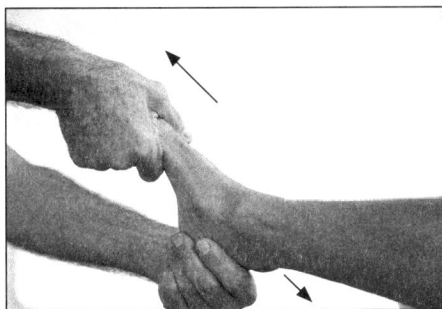

(c) 70-percent open

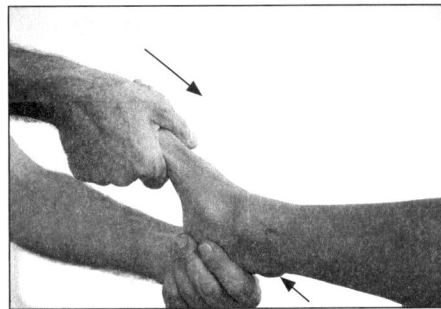

(d) Release to neutral

Figure 16-6:
Pulsing the Foot Lengthwise—Two-Beat Cycle

3. Close and Release the Foot Joints

Repeat one more open-release, before:

- Closing the foot 100 percent (Figure 16-7a).
- Releasing to the neutral position (Figure 16-7b).

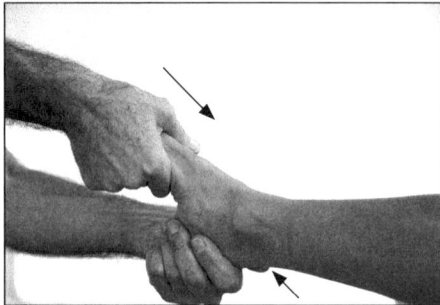

(a) 100-percent close   (b) Release to neutral

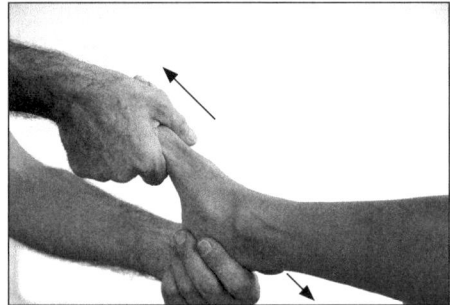

Figure 16-7:
Pulsing the Foot Lengthwise—Close and Release the Joints

4. Activate the Four-Beat Cycle

Shift into the four-beat cycle, 70-percent open/70-percent close, to pulse the foot lengthwise (Figure 16-8a-d).

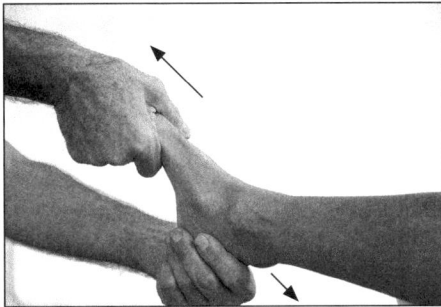

(a) Active open: 70 percent

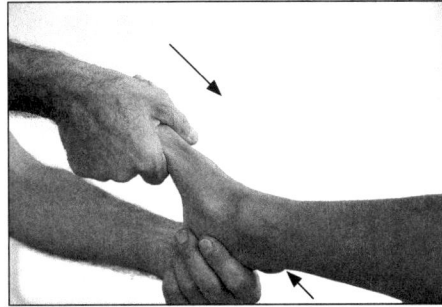

(b) Passive release to neutral

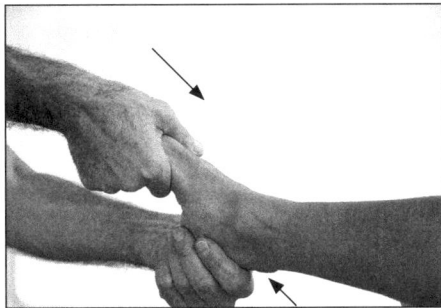

(c) Active close: 70 percent

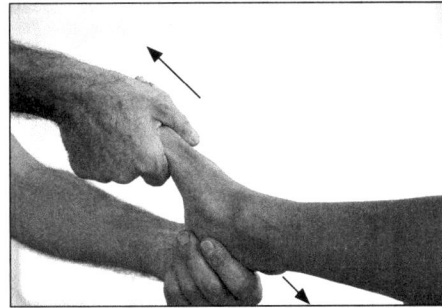

(d) Passive release to neutral

Figure 16-8:
Pulsing the Foot Lengthwise—Four-Beat Cycle

Note: Skip the handoff procedure until the toes have been connected lengthways to the pulse of the foot.

Repeat Stages 1-4 on the other foot.

JOINING THE TOE AND LENGTHWISE FOOT PULSES

Once the foot and all ten toes have been opened up individually from the previous two exercises, you are ready to move on to joining the pulses into one.

1. Set up the Hand Hold and Align the Joints

Use one hand to hold the receiver's heel, as done in the previous exercise. Use the pads of your fingers to the heel of your other palm to grab and "sandwich" all their toes in a comfortable way for your partner (Figure 16-9).

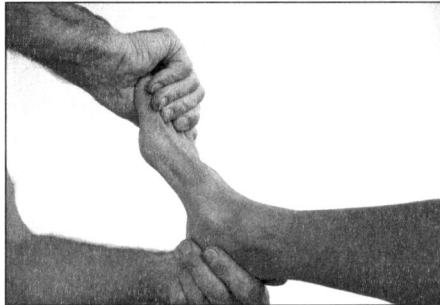

Neutral position

Figure 16-9:
Join the Foot and Toe Pulses Lengthways—Hand Hold

2. Activate the Four-Beat Cycle

Since the individual pulses have already brought the toe and foot joints alive, shift directly into the four-beat cycle and pulse all the toes and the whole foot lengthwise (Figure 16-10). Be sure to maintain the alignment between the toes and the foot, especially on the close, so that you do not bend or buckle the toes.

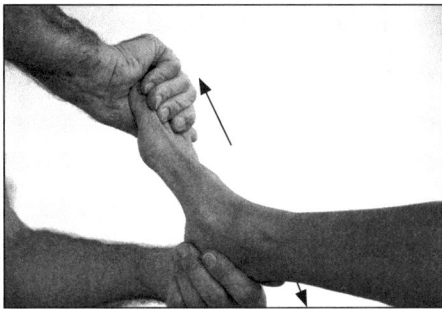

(a) Active open: 70 percent

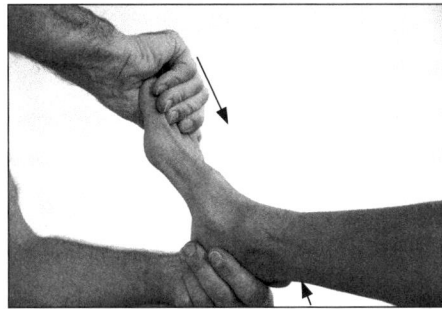

(b) Passive release to neutral

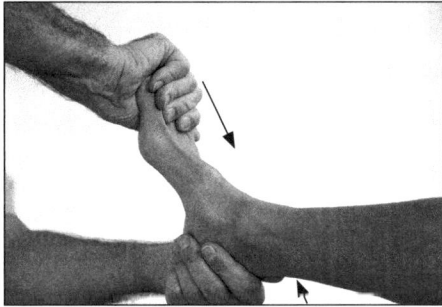

(d) Active close: 70 percent

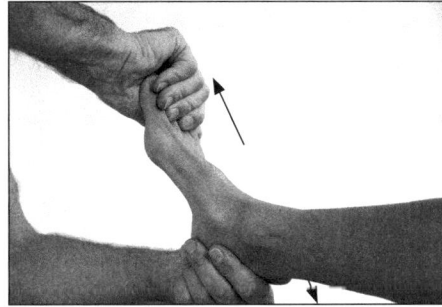

(e) Passive release to neutral

Figure 16-10:
Join the Foot and Toe Pulses Lengthwise—Four-Beat Cycle

3. Hand off the Pulse

Follow the handoff procedure (see Chapter 11) once their foot is fully activated by the pulse, so that the receiver takes over the pulse of their foot and toes on their own.

Repeat Stages 1-3 on the other foot.

4. Practice the Self-Generated Pulse

Once the handoff procedure is complete on both feet, the receiver:

- Sits in a comfortable position with their back supported, their feet stretched out in front of them and their knees bent. In this position, they will pulse without assistance for a few minutes to solidify the pulse on their own.

- Stands with their feet parallel and firmly on the ground while continuing to pulse on their own. The sensation of pulsing while sitting is different to standing with the body's weight evenly distributed between both feet.

- Seamlessly shifts into the Heaven and Earth form, opening the feet and toe joints during the opening phases and closing the feet and toe joints on the closing phases.

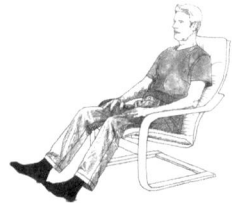

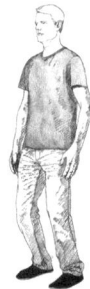

Change: Once the receiver has had a rest after solo practice, they will return the favor and pulse their partner's feet and toes, following all of the instructions in this chapter so far.

PULSING THE FOOT WIDTHWISE

Once both partners feel they have assimilated the lengthwise pulse in their feet, they move on to pulsing their feet widthwise.

1. Set up the Hand Hold and Align the Joints

The hand hold is similar to the one used for pulsing the hands: with one hand you grab the bone of their big toe (first metatarsal) and your other hand grabs the bone of their little toe (fifth metatarsal) between your finger pads and the heel of your palm/thumb (Figure 16-11).

Again, pulsing a foot widthwise takes more effort than pulsing a hand widthwise.

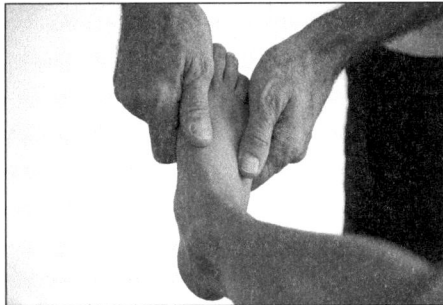

Neutral position

Figure 16-11:
Pulsing the Foot Widthwise—Hand Hold

2. Activate the Two-Beat Cycle

Without letting the bones of the receiver's foot slip through your fingers:

- Fix one hand in space and use your other hand to spread the bones of their feet sideways to 100 percent of their comfortable capacity, then release (Figure 16-12a-b).

- Maintaining your grip, move into the two-beat cycle, 70-percent open, then release (Figure 16-12c-d). Repeat half a dozen times or so, until their foot begins to open up.

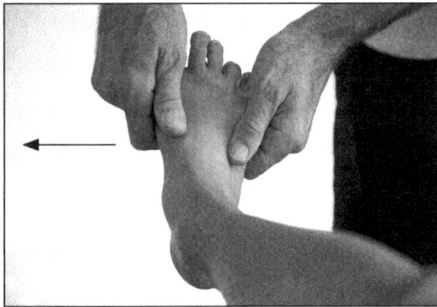

(a) 100-percent open

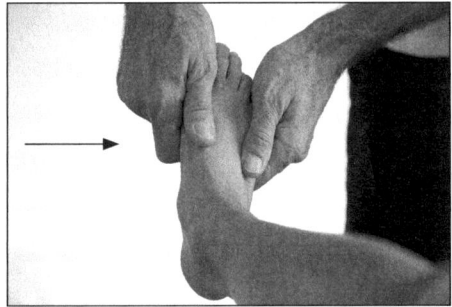

(b) Release to neutral

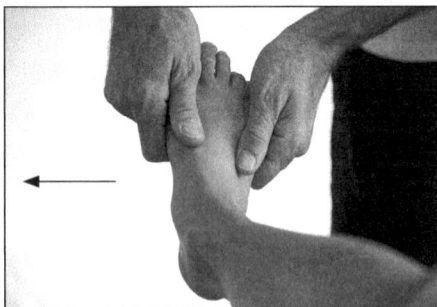

(c) 70-percent open

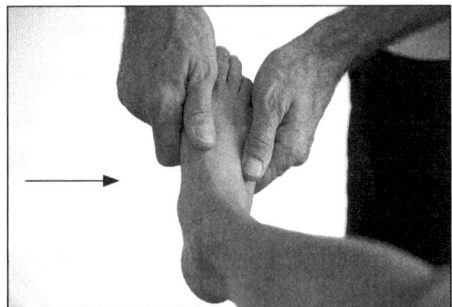

(d) Release to neutral

Figure 16-12:
Pulsing the Foot Widthwise—Two-Beat Cycle

3. *Close and Release the Foot Joints*

Repeat one more open-release, before:

- Closing the receiver's foot widthwise 100 percent (Figure 16-13a).
- Releasing to the neutral position (Figure 16-13b).

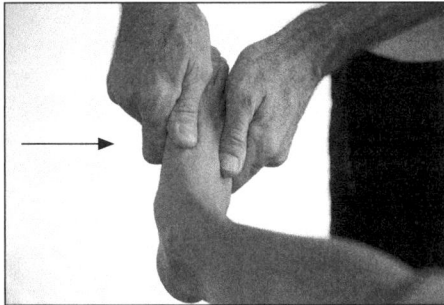

(a) 100-percent close   (b) Release to neutral

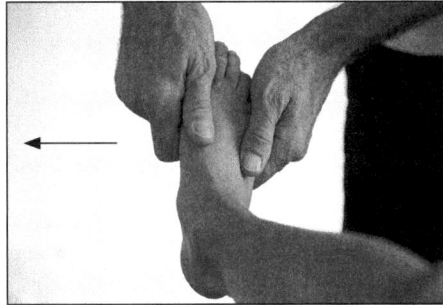

Figure 16-13:
Pulsing the Foot Widthwise: Close and Release the Joints

4. Activate the Four-Beat Cycle

Shift into the four-beat cycle, 70-percent open/70-precent close (Figure 16-14) while adhering to the "Five-Point Checklist for Pulsing a Partner" (see Chapter 11). Repeat until there is some fluidity in their foot or the hand-off will not be successful.

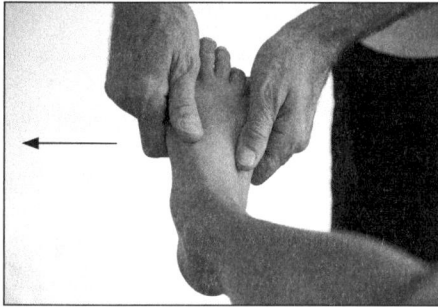

(a) Active open: 70 percent

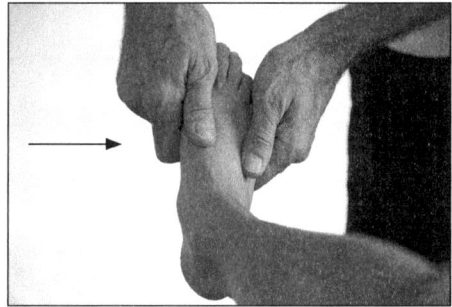

(b) Passive release to neutral

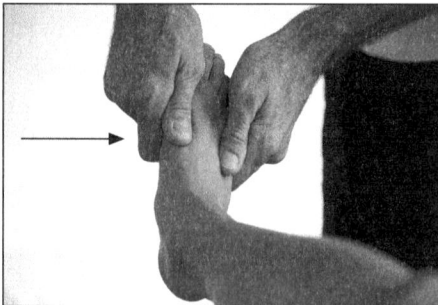

(c) Active close: 70 percent

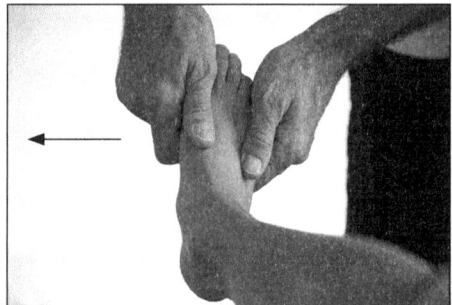

(d) Passive release to neutral

Figure 16-14:
Pulsing the Foot Widthwise—Four-Beat Cycle

5. Hand off the Pulse

Shift into the handoff procedure (see Chapter 11), where the receiver takes over both pulses along the length and across the width of their foot.

Repeat Stages 1-5 on the other foot.

6. Practice the Self-Generated Pulse

Once the handoff procedure is complete and both feet have been pulsed, the receiver sits in a chair and pulses both of their feet in unison without any assistance for a few minutes while adhering to the "Four-Point Checklist for a Self-Generated Pulse" (see Chapter 11). It is easier to pulse the feet without the bodyweight on them, so the pulse must be strong before standing.

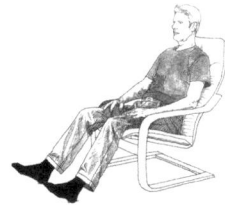

Change: Once the receiver has had a rest after solo practice, they will return the favor and pulse their partner's feet widthwise.

SOLO PRACTICE:
UNIFY THE FOOT PULSES AND QI FLOWS

1. While sitting in a chair, pulse your feet to once again activate the lengthwise and widthwise pulses, including all your toes, until the two pulses become balanced and integrated.

2. Focus on moving qi from the bubbling-well points to the periphery (toe tips and edges of your feet) on the open and back to the bubbling-well points on the close. Keep going until this qi flow is alive and strong.

3. Let go of the previous flow of qi and next focus on applying your mind's intent to running qi from your heels to the tips of your toes on the open, and back from the tips of your toes to your heels on the close.

4. When the flow along the length of the foot is strong, add the previous qi flow (bubbling-well points to periphery and back again). Try to balance and integrate the two qi flows as much as possible.

5. Once you have solidified the pulse and the two qi flows in your feet, stand and pulse using the weight shift (see Chapter 3, Figure 3-1) to aid the pulse while reflecting on the "Four-Point Checklist for a Self-Generated Pulse" (see Chapter 11).

   (a) On the open - shift forward onto the balls of your feet and run qi from your heels to the tips of your toes and, simultaneously, from your bubbling-well points out to your extremities (the edges of the feet and toes).

   (b) On the close - shift back to the heels of your feet and run qi back from the toes to your heels and, simultaneously, from the extremities of your feet back to your bubbling-well points.

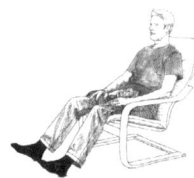

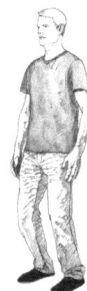

6. When the pulse is as good as it can be standing, fluidly shift into the Heaven and Earth form, following the usual pattern of opening the feet in the opening phases and closing the feet in the closing phases.

ANKLES

Many people walk with poor leg alignments, which closes down their ankle joints. When the alignments are out on either side of the midline of the leg, the ankle collapses and the nerves tighten to prevent potential damage, which generates a lot of tension. This, combined with the fact that the whole weight of the body goes through the ankle during standing and walking, can lead to a very tight ankle.

Even though the ankle joint is complex, the pulsing technique is straightforward, similar to the wrists. In this case, the foot moves away from the shin and calf, and back toward them. The difficulty is in finding the correct grip and using the correct amount of effort. Some of the lower-body pulses can be particularly demanding on the pulser.

HOW TO PULSE THE ANKLE

1. Prepare to Pulse the Ankle and Align the Joint

This exercise is best done with both the pulser and the receiver in a seated position. The receiver should sit in a comfortable chair in a reclined position, so they can relax and let go. This enables a deep, internal pulse to come alive.

Start by placing the receiver's lower leg on your thighs and familiarizing yourself with their ankle joint. Then grip the area of their leg just above the ankle, and wrap your fingers and thumb as far around their leg as possible to give you maximum contact and stability. Your other hand holds their foot in such a way that your palm is in contact with the heel of their foot, and your fingers and thumb wrap around the sides of their foot.

Align their foot and ankle correctly, so that when viewed from above there is a straight line that runs through the center of the foot, ankle and knee. This ensures that, during the pulse, the receiver feels an even pressure around their whole ankle joint. See Figure 16-15.

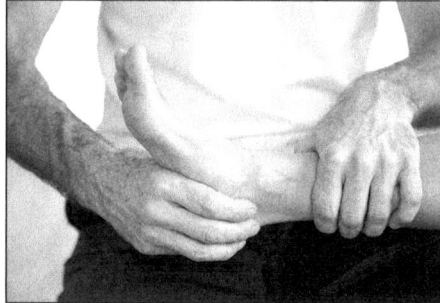

Neutral position

**Figure 16-15:
Pulsing the Ankle—Hand Hold**

2. Activate the Two-Beat Pulse

From the neutral position:

- Draw their foot away from their leg to 100 percent of their comfortable capacity and release (Figure 16-16a-b).

- Shift into the two-beat cycle, 70-percent open, then release (Figure 16-16c-d). Repeat until their ankle begins to open up.

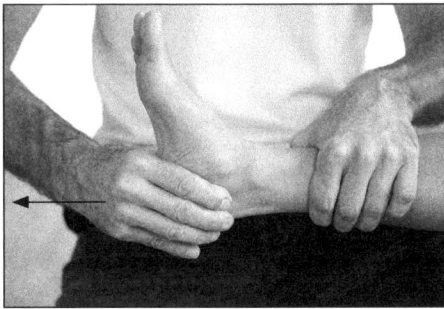

(a) 100-percent open

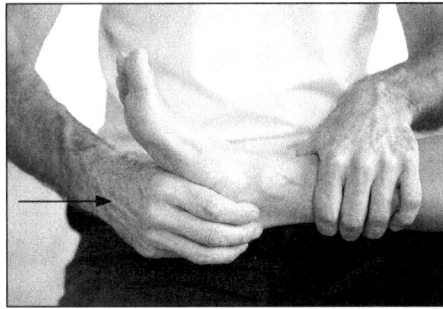

(b) Release to neutral

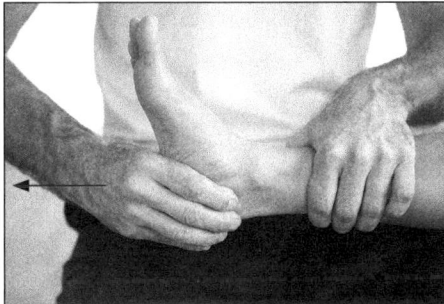

(c) 70-percent open

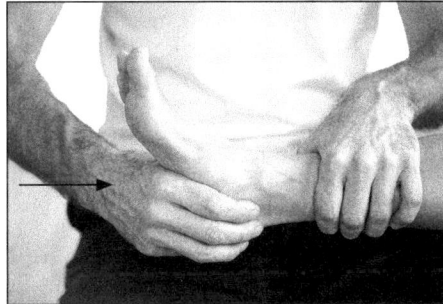

(d) Release to neutral

Figure 16-16:
Pulsing the Ankle—Two-Beat Cycle

3. Close and Release the Ankle

Repeat one more open-release, before:

- Closing their ankle to 100 percent of their comfortable capacity (Figure 16-17a).
- Releasing to the neutral position (Figure 16-17b).

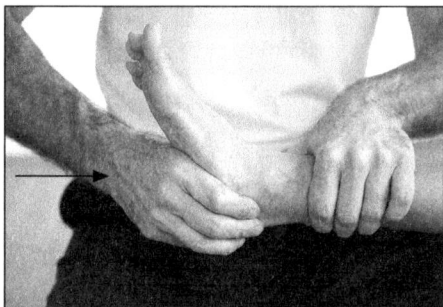

(a) 100-percent close   *(b) Release to neutral*

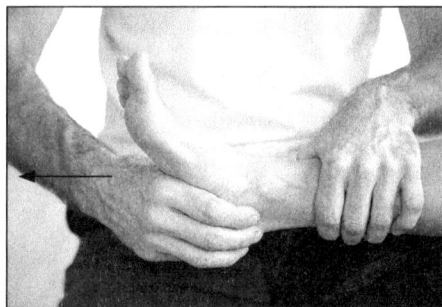

Figure 16-17:
Pulsing the Ankle—Close and Release the Joint

4. Activate the Four-Beat Pulse

Shift into the four-beat cycle, 70-percent open/70-percent close, until the pulse is alive and the ankle moves freely (Figure 16-18). Adhere to the "Five-Point Checklist for Pulsing a Partner" (see Chapter 11).

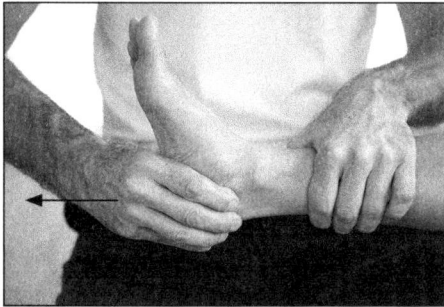

(a) Active open: 70 percent

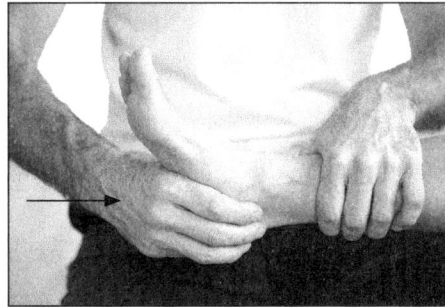

(b) Passive release to neutral

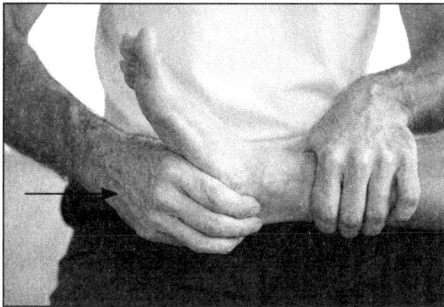

(c) Active close: 70 percent

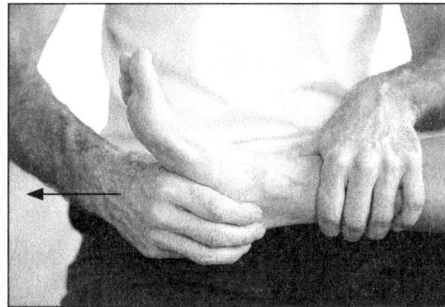

(d) Passive release to neutral

Figure 16-18:
Pulsing the Ankle—Four-Beat Cycle

5. Hand off the Pulse

Complete the handoff procedure (see Chapter 11) until the receiver pulses on their own without any assistance.

Repeat Stages 1-5 on the other foot.

6. Practice the Self-Generated Pulse

The receiver then sits and pulses on their own to activate their ankles, feet and toes, combining the lower-body techniques covered so far while reflecting on
the "Four-Point Checklist for a Self-Generated Pulse"
(see Chapter 11).

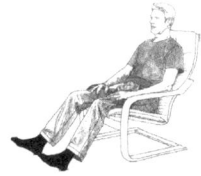

- To close - draw qi into the ankle.
- To open - extend qi to the heel and tips of the
  toes and the whole foot.

Next the receiver stands and continues to pulse on
their own without any assistance, this time without the
weight shift.

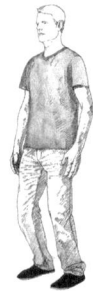

Finally, the receiver fluidly transitions into the Heaven
and Earth form, following their natural opening-and-
closing rhythm.

Change: Once the receiver has had a rest after solo practice, they will return the favor and pulse their partner's
ankles.

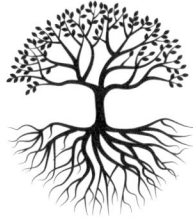

CHAPTER 17:

PULSING THE KNEES

Every step you take in a day involves bending your knees, not to mention each time you sit down, stand up, lie down and move your legs. Rarely do you move a leg without some kind of flexion or extension in the knee joint.

A WEIGHT-TRANSFERRING JOINT

The knee is a weight-transferring joint, not a weight-bearing joint. The knee transfers weight from the upper body and pelvis through the ankle and onto the foot. Its construction is relatively weak when compared to the two load-bearing joints on either side, namely the hip and the ankle. For this reason, caution should always be exercised when pulsing someone else's knee as they may have old injuries or structural weaknesses of which you and/or your partner may not be aware.

PROTECTING THE KNEES

In qigong, the knees are never bent as much as the elbows because it would cause disconnection from the synovial fluid inside the joints, plus there is the potential to overstretch the front of the knees. Likewise, the knees are never hyperextended, whereby the knee joints become locked. This action is common in Western sports (and bad tai chi), and creates many knee and lower-back problems.

Whenever standing or moving, always make sure a weighted knee does not project forward beyond your toes to ensure you do not overstretch the front of your knee, or allow your knee to collapse in or splay out. Maintaining these alignments will reduce how low you can squat down, reduces the range of flexing in the knees and takes the motion deeper into the body. The farthest even the most flexible and advanced internal arts practitioners will go down in long stances is to the point that their thigh is horizontal or parallel to the ground. Going lower simply downgrades the motion to external movement, which lacks the fundamental internal connections that define Taoist arts training.

HOW TO PULSE THE KNEE

THE WATER-PUMP METHOD

The knee is the middle joint in the leg, just as the elbow is in the arm, so you will once again use the water-pump method of pulsing for the knee joint.

1. Set up the Hand Hold and Align the Knee Joint

The receiver should either lie down on a mat or be seated quite high up relative to the pulser. For the seated position, when the pulser pumps the knee, the foot should not make contact with the ground toward the end of the closing half of the cycle. This can be achieved by the receiver sitting in a chair and resting the underside of their thigh on top of your thigh.

In the exercise that follows, you will learn how to pulse the receiver's knee while the receiver lies down on a mat. You will kneel down on one leg using a cushion or mat to support your own knee with the weight of your other leg on your foot. Lift the receiver's leg and rest their thigh on your own, leaving a good gap between your thigh and your partner's knee. If your partner is too close, you will not be able to pump properly, which prevents the pulse from coming alive or overstretches the front of the knee.

Place the hand closest to the receiver's torso on the top of their thigh while your other hand holds their lower leg, just above their ankle. Grip their leg where it is thin, so you can control the pumping action smoothly and evenly. This should give you the leverage to generate the pump within the knee joint itself. See Figure 17-1.

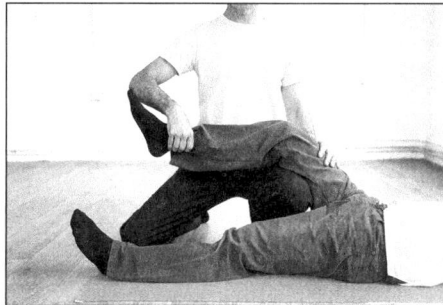

Neutral position

Figure 17-1:
Pulsing the Knee—Hand Hold

Be sure to keep the receiver's leg properly aligned throughout the entirety of the pulsing exercise, which requires that the foot, ankle, knee and hip remain in line with either the left or right channel, as it corresponds to the side of the body on which you are pulsing. The leg joints will be on a straight line with the shoulder when viewed from above.

2. Extend and Flex the Knee

Become comfortable with the posture and the grips before beginning.

- Extend and flex the knee 100 percent—or just under, that is nearly straight to a 90-degree bend (Figure 17-2a-b).

- Once you have found the 100-percent range of motion, back off to 70-percent extension-flexion.

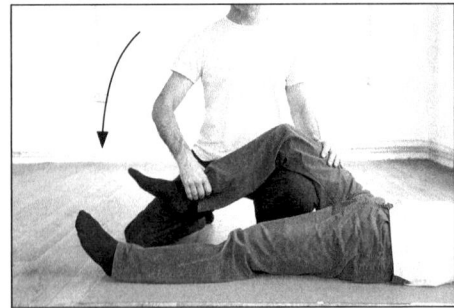

When you are satisfied you have found the 70-percent range, practice a few repetitions smoothly and slowly to create a smooth motion to give the receiver a clear experience of the feeling *without the pulse* (Figure 17-2c-d).

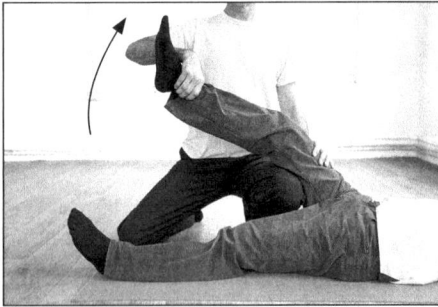

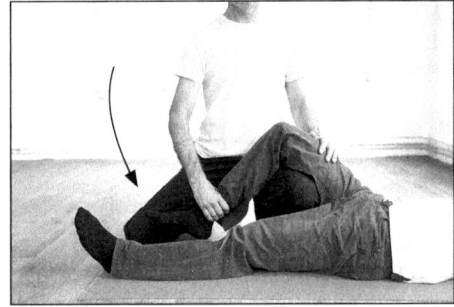

(a) 100-percent extension (or slightly less) *(b) 100-percent flexion (or less)*

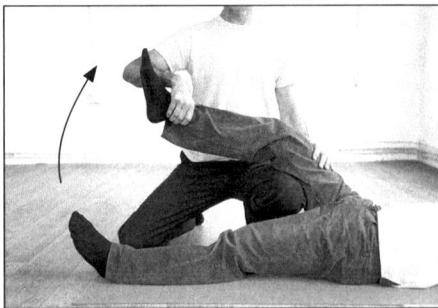

(c) 70-percent extension *(d) 70-percent flexion*

Figure 17-2:
Pulsing the Knee—Extend and Flex the Knee

3. Activate the Two-Beat Cycle

From the 70-percent flexed position:

- Raise the receiver's foot and open the angle of their knee joint to 70-percent extension, while drawing the receiver's ankle away from their knee to create more internal space inside the knee joint itself. Make sure to hold their thigh still in space between your own thigh and hand, or the joint will not open and you will simply displace the leg. See Figure 17-3a.

- After opening both the angle of the knee (extension) and the internal space of the knee joint to 70 percent, reduce your effort and allow the joint to return to the original, neutral position as you flex their knee to 70 percent of their comfortable capacity (Figure 17-3b).

Repeat this two-beat cycle half a dozen times or so while staying in communication with your partner to prevent overdoing it or reverting to the simple extension-flexion action.

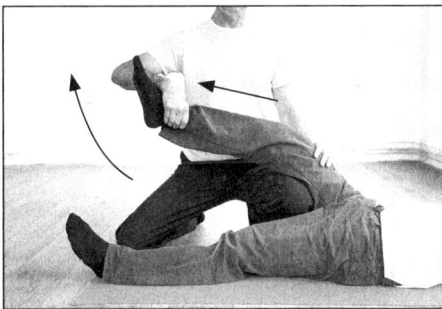

(a) 70-percent extension while opening the joint 70 percent

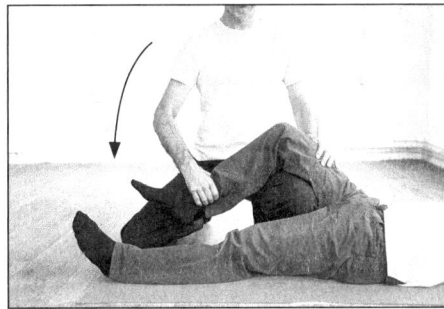

(b) Release to 70 percent flexion

Figure 17-3:
Pulsing the Knee—Two-Beat Cycle

4. Close and Release the Knee Joint

Next add the closing action.

- Begin with one more open-release (Figure 17-3).

- Then, as you pass the 50/50 position on the flex, use your intent to further close the internal space inside their knee joint to 70 percent of their comfortable capacity as you flex their knee. Rather than trying to physically push their knee closed, use gravity to assist with the compression of the fluid inside the joint. See Figure 17-4a.

- After compressing the joint, release to neutral while extending the leg to the 50/50 position (Figure 17-4b).

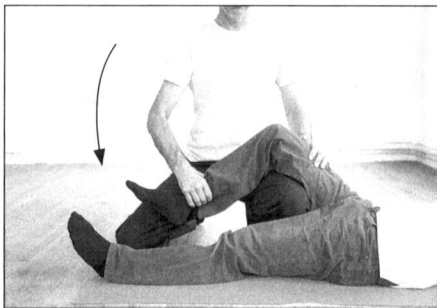

(a) 70-percent flexion while closing the joint 70 percent

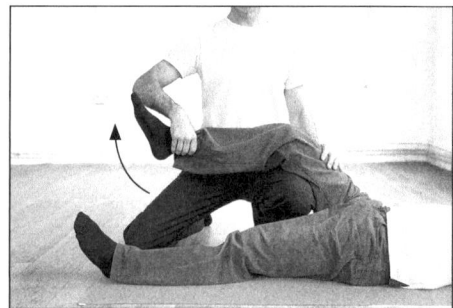

(b) Release to neutral 50/50

Figure 17-4:
Pulsing the Knee—Close and Release the Joint

5. Activate the Four-Beat Cycle

Shift into the four-beat cycle, 70-percent opening/70-percent closing of their joint, while extending and flexing the angle of their knee (Figure 17-5).

- The operation should feel like a light water pump and markedly different to simply hinging the joint to both the pulser and the receiver.

- Make sure you feel and remain conscious of the receiver's subtle feedback signals and cues as you continue the four-beat cycle and reflect upon the "Five-Point Checklist for Pulsing a Partner" (see Chapter 11).

- On the open, apply your intent to draw qi from the receiver's knee to their toes and, on the close, from their toes to their knee.

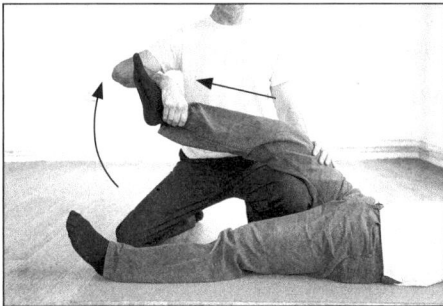

(a) Active open: 70 percent

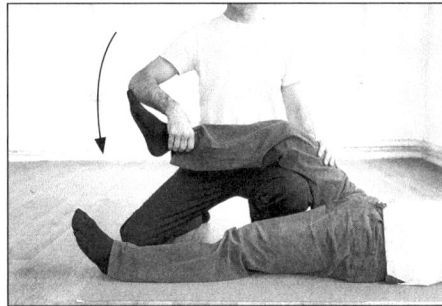

(b) Passive release to neutral

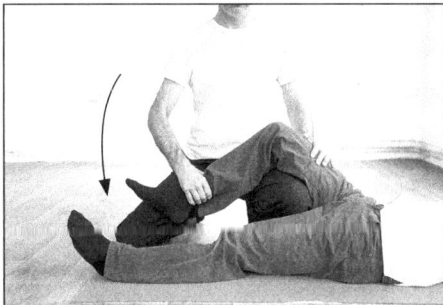

(c) Active close: 70 percent

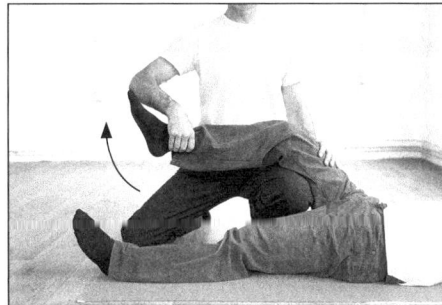

(d) Passive release to neutral

Figure 17-5:
Pulsing the Knee—Four-Beat Cycle

It is better to achieve half a dozen to a dozen well-connected pumps of the knee joint and rest than to keep going to the point of diminishing returns, where the quality of the motion becomes a simple flexion-extension. Pulsing the knee is much more demanding than its upper-body counterpart, the elbow, and the pulser can tire quickly.

6. Hand off the Pulse

Once your partner feels the pulse come alive, shift into the handoff procedure (see Chapter 11) until they can pulse on their own.

Repeat Stages 1-6 on the other knee.

7. Practice the Self-Generated Pulse

To consolidate their experiential knowledge:

- The receiver sits in a chair and tries to initiate the pulse inside their knee joint (without any extension or flexion), ankles, feet and toes on their own, while simultaneously projecting their qi from their knees to their toes on the open and back to their knees on the close.

- Once the pulse and qi flows are unified, the receiver stands with their feet parallel and repeats the same procedure done previously while sitting.

- Finally, the receiver smoothly transitions into the Heaven and Earth form while keeping both the pulse and qi flows alive—opening all of the lower-body joints covered so far on the opening phases and closing them on the closing phases.

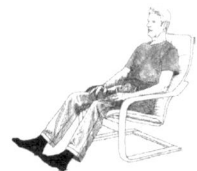

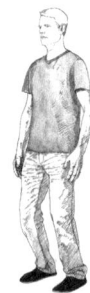

Change: Once the receiver has had a rest after solo practice, they will return the favor and pulse their partner's knees.

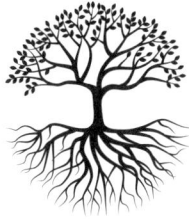

CHAPTER 18:

PULSING THE HIPS

A BALL-AND-SOCKET JOINT

The hip joints are simple yet deep ball-and-socket joints that can bear weight at various angles and hold the potential to perform a large range of motions. Repetitively sitting in chairs for prolonged periods has a particularly negative effect on the hips as the soft tissues that surround and connect to them can become compressed, dormant, stiff and inflexible, which dramatically reduces range of motion.

The hips are internally connected to the kwa (covered in Chapter 4) via the psoas muscles and, if the hips do not move well, nor does the kwa. The kwa is partially responsible for the health of the lower organs, including the kidneys and the bowels. For these reasons, we will revisit the pelvic roll exercises from the C-curve (i.e. bowing and straightening the spine, also from Chapter 4) with a change in emphasis.

HOW TO PULSE THE HIP

PREPARATORY EXERCISE: THE PELVIC ROLL

Stand in the neutral posture with your knees aligned and slightly bent. Your tailbone is dropped and your spine is straight.

1. Place the palm of one hand on your lower belly and the back of your other hand on your sacrum/tailbone area.

2. Roll your pelvis so that your tailbone moves downward, forward and slightly upward.

   (a) Your front hand will rise and move back slightly.

   (b) Your back hand will drop and move forward slightly.

3. To return, gently drive your tailbone downward. If it descends, the return is guaranteed; if you simply move it back, you will arch your spine and disconnect your tailbone from your legs. Use the back of your hand to monitor the back of your pelvis. Your spine becomes straight—or at least as straight as it is in the beginning, neutral posture.

4. Repeat the pelvic roll and the return a dozen times or so while focusing on creating a smooth and continuous motion in your hip sockets.

   Remember: When practicing the pelvic roll, the inguinal grooves will go flat as you roll your tailbone under and forward.

When the pelvis rolls and the thigh bones remain still in space, the hip socket (acetabulum) rotates on the head of the thigh bone (femur), which loosens the hip socket and the associated connective tissues. With regular practice this exercise will prepare the hips for pulsing as well as improve your kwa squat and your spinal C-curve.

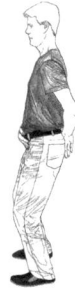

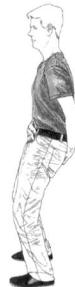

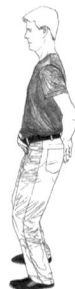

PULSING THE HIP

1. Prepare to Pulse

The receiver will lie on the floor on a carpet or mat to be comfortable and warm. The pulser uses a similar stance as with the knee-pump-pulsing exercise—one foot and one knee in contact with the ground or a cushion placed on the ground.

The receiver completely relaxes and the pulser lifts their leg, making sure the ankle, foot, knee and hip remain in alignment with the associated left or right channel—without twists or kinks. When viewed from above, a straight line could be drawn through the receiver's foot, ankle, knee, hip and shoulder. Your back hand-forearm holds their calf muscle and supports the weight of their leg from below, while your other hand cups their knee. This hand can then assist in both the open and the close. Keep a good bend in their knee at all times. See Figure 18-1.

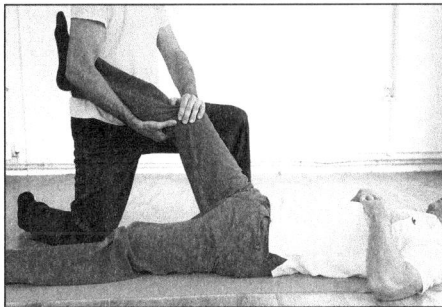

Neutral position

Figure 18-1
Pulsing the Hip—Hand Hold

2. Activate the Two-Beat Cycle

From the neutral position, smoothly and slowly open the receiver's hip socket 100 percent by drawing their leg away from their torso and then allow the hip to return to the neutral position (Figure 18-2a-b).

- The hips are made of thick, fibrous muscle and strong tendons and ligaments, so the opening must be done slowly and gradually.

- Make sure you do not lift the receiver's pelvis off the floor. If this happens, you know you are moving too fast and the joint has not opened, or you have gone too far.

- The opening of the joint can be achieved simply by fixing your arms to your body and leaning back slightly, moving slowly and smoothly with your torso. When you lean back, your arms come with you, as does your partner's leg—neither are left behind.

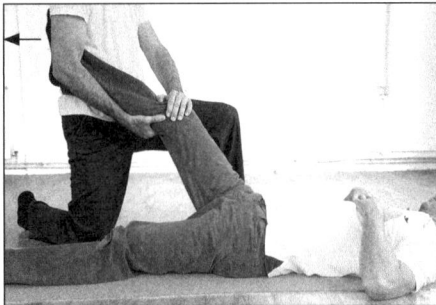

(a) 100-percent open

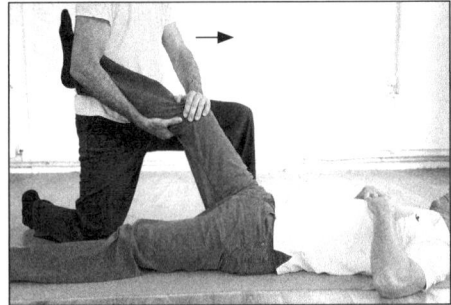

(b) Release to neutral

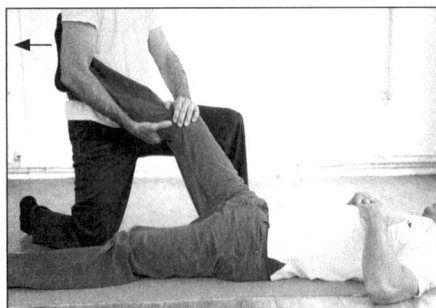

(c) 70-percent open

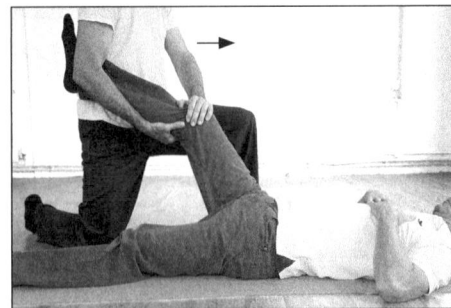

(d) Release to neutral

Figure 18-2 Pulsing the Hip—Two-Beat Cycle

Shift into the two-beat cycle, opening 70 percent and releasing back to neutral a dozen times or so, until the hip loosens up (Figure 18-2c-b).

- This can be achieved by simply rocking your body back and forth, slowly and smoothly, while observing the hip fold (inguinal groove) and pelvis of the receiver.

- If the space in the hip fold increases slightly as you lean back and decreases as you release and return, you are on the right track.

- If the receiver tenses up or their pelvis lifts, you know you have moved too far, too fast and/or too suddenly.

3. Close and Release the Hip Joint

Repeat one more open-release, then:

- Using the hand covering their knee, lean in slightly toward the receiver and close the joint 100 percent (Figure 18-3a). When you lean in, you must not rely on the receiver for balance. Instead, balance on your front foot and rear knee, as well as the ball of your back foot in contact with the ground. The lean is simply to apply pressure through your front hand in contact with the receiver's knee, that is, downward through their thigh and into their hip joint.

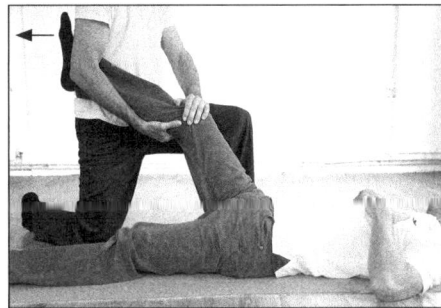

- Release back to the neutral position (Figure 18-3b).

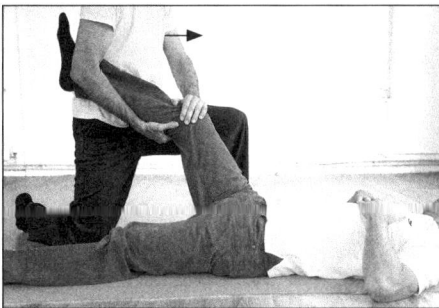

(a) 100-percent close   (b) Release to neutral

Figure 18-3 Pulsing the Hip—Close and Release the Joint

4. Activate the Four-Beat Cycle

Shift into the four-beat cycle, 70-percent open/70-percent close, via your torso leaning backward and forward—move smoothly, slowly and gently (Figure 18-4). Stay in communication with your partner and follow the "Five-Point Checklist for Generating the Pulse in a Partner" (see Chapter 11).

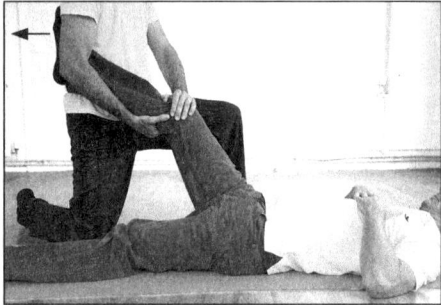

(a) Active open: 70 percent

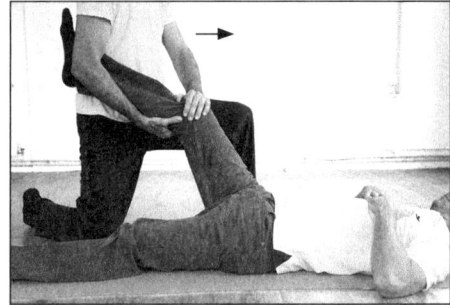

(b) Passive release to neutral

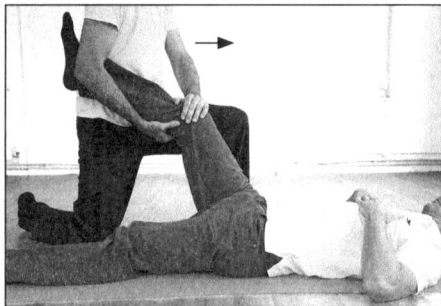

(c) Active close: 70 percent

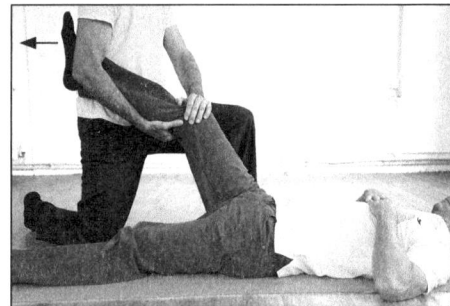

(d) Passive release to neutral

Figure 18-4 Pulsing the Hip—Four-Beat Cycle

5. Hand off the Pulse

After a dozen repetitions or so, shift into the handoff procedure (see Chapter 11) until the receiver pulses on their own purely with their mind and without any assistance.

Repeat Stages 1-5 on the other hip.

6. Practice the Self-Generated Pulse

Once both hips have been pulsed, the receiver should assume the sitting position.

- First they pulse their hips.

- Once the pulse in their hips is active, they add their knees, ankles and feet.

- When all the joints in their legs are active, they move qi from their hips to their toes, and back to their hips—until both the pulse and the qi flows are smooth and continuous.

- When all of the joints in their legs are active, the receiver stands and pulses their legs for a few minutes. Refrain from transitioning into the Heaven and Earth form until after the pulses have been unified in the lower body.

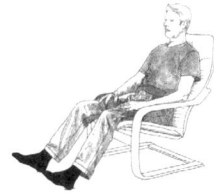

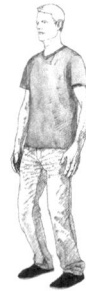

Change: Once the receiver has had a rest after solo practice (and the pulser has practiced the pelvic roll), they will return the favor and pulse their partner's hips.

UNIFYING THE LOWER BODY

The next process is to unify the pulse and qi flows in the lower body, which uses the pelvic roll and kwa squat. Once you have activated the pelvic roll and kwa squat, the pulse and qi flows in your legs, you will integrate these internal techniques into the Heaven and Earth form.

JOINING THE PULSES AND QI FLOWS OF THE LOWER BODY

If you had a break after practicing the last section on the hips, repeat the pulsing-while-sitting exercise to bring alive the pulse before standing. If you are directly following on, simply stand and pulse your hip, knee, ankle and foot joints.

1. Activate the Pelvic Roll

To begin, roll under your pelvis and tailbone to close your joints and gently drive your tailbone downward to open your joints.

- As the tailbone rolls under and slightly upward, it initiates the flow of qi up the legs, from the toes to the hips.

- As the tailbone drives downward, it initiates the flow of qi down the legs, from the hips to the toes.

Repeat this exercise until you integrate the pulse and qi flows with the pelvic roll while moving smoothly, evenly and continuously—without any sinking or rising in the kwa.

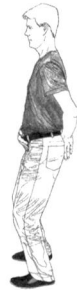

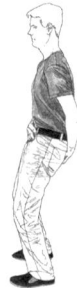

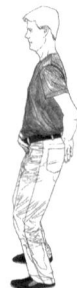

2. Activate the Kwa

Now you will add the opening and closing of your kwa to the pelvic roll. When you do, the rolling of your pelvis will diminish somewhat. You do not want to allow your inguinal grooves to go flat as that would cause you to internally disconnect. However, the kwa, which is the engine of the pulse and the whole physical motion, can now take its rightful position and amplify the flow of qi, bringing that qi flow all the way to your lower spine. This is the equivalent of the shoulder blades bringing qi into the upper spine in the pulsing exercises for the upper body.

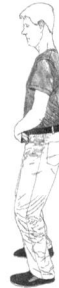

The kwa generates the power to supercharge the qi flows while the movement of the pelvis/tailbone governs the direction of that flow. Qi moves up the legs as the tailbone rolls under, and qi moves down the legs as the tailbone drives downward.

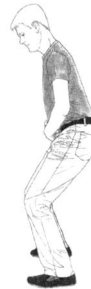

- Close your kwa by rolling your tailbone under, while simultaneously folding in the inguinal grooves and sitting in your heels to close the joints of your legs.
- Open your kwa by gently driving your tailbone forward and downward onto the bubbling-well points of your feet, while simultaneously shifting your weight onto the balls of your feet to open the joints of your legs.

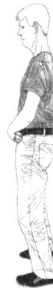

Direct qi in accordance with the kwa closing and opening.

- On the close - draw qi from your toes up your legs, through your hips and into your lower spine via your tailbone
- On the open - send qi from your lower spine, through your tailbone and hips, down your legs to your toes.

Continue until you can move smoothly and fluidly throughout the entirety of the exercise, both physically and energetically.

3. Practice the Self-Generated Pulse in Heaven and Earth Qigong

Fluidly transition into the Heaven and Earth form while keeping both the pulse and all the qi flows of the lower body alive. Be sure to follow the correct weight-shift pattern (balls-arches-heels-balls-heels-arches) as covered in Chapter 3, Figure 3-1.

UNIFYING THE UPPER AND LOWER BODY

With the pelvic roll and the kwa active, balanced and integrated, they can fully engage the pulse of all the joints and qi flows of the lower body as one unified whole. The next step is to activate the entire upper body pulse, including the qi flows from the spine to the fingertips, and back to the spine. Once both the upper and lower body pulses are alive—with their associated qi flows—join both together and begin trying to balance your whole system so that:

- A center-to-periphery and periphery-to-center qi flow is generated from your spine to your extremities (fingertips and tips of your toes) and back from your extremities to your spine.
- Both the pulse and the qi flow are equal in your upper and lower body with the feeling that each is mutually activating the other.
- Both the pulse and the qi flow are equal in the right and left sides of your body.

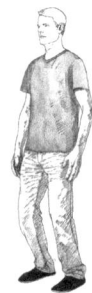

First practice while standing and pulsing your whole body, then fluidly transition into the Heaven and Earth form.

Remember: Pulsing techniques might be in sync with other neigong threads and qi flows, but sometimes they are not. This is true for all forms of qigong, tai chi and other internal arts.

HOW THE PULSE HARMONIZES BODY, MIND AND QI

Consider that a healthy baby is made up of about 75-78 percent water, whereas an elderly person is on average only 45-50 percent water. We literally dry out if we do not do something to counter the aging process.

As with all Water tradition neigong, pulsing is designed to open up the body, release unnecessary tensions and allow the body to function optimally. Pulsing specifically and directly affects the body's ability to remain well hydrated—not just in the joints, but systemically. This is because pulsing the joints is only the beginning of a cascade of fluid production throughout the body. Eventually the pulse can permeate the entirety of the physical body and its subtle energy anatomy.

Resonance Between Joints

Once you achieve a pulse in one joint it resonates at a particular frequency, which can help kick off the next joint in the chain. The effect is similar to plucking one guitar string, which causes others to resonate with it. Therefore, when you pulse the wrist, the hand joints get a little boost. When you pulse the hand joints, the finger joints get a boost. When the whole hand, wrist and fingers pulse, the elbow joint receives a boost.

Once you work through your body and can pulse all your joints, they each boost the capacity of neighboring joints, which is precisely how joints that are stiff or restricted open up without the use of excessive force. When this happens, the whole pulse is integrated throughout your entire skeletal frame, which once again amplifies the pulse and creates a jump in energy. This is one example of how neigong training yields an overall effect that is far greater than the sum of its parts.

When the pulse goes beyond two (or more) bones of a joint moving apart and back again, and engages the fluids and qi of that joint, a spherical expansion occurs. Each joint also becomes the microcosm of the whole body's macrocosm, where all joints pulse in unison, from center-to-periphery and periphery-to-center. In this scenario, the kwa becomes the center and origination point of the motion, which kicks off all other joints in concentric rings out to the periphery on the open and draws in or closes all joints back into the kwa on the close.

When this level of the pulse emerges, the effect on the flesh, nerves, qi and mind is profound. Normal mental functioning is suspended and a timeless, harmonious mental state temporarily opens up, where the physical body synchronizes and becomes balanced as one whole. The need to achieve, know or get something simply drops away and the contentment "to be" takes over, leaving the practitioner at peace ... even if only for a fleeting moment or two.

ABOUT THE SPINE

At this level of practice, the spine is not involved in the pulse. Pulsing the spine is a more advanced technique, which is generally taught in Bend the Bow Spinal Qigong. Preparatory practices must be honed before adding spinal expansion-compression cycles, which start with methods for contacting, controlling, opening, releasing and loosening the spine to a great degree. This is done using the C-curve techniques presented in Chapter 4 and activating the longitudinal ligaments of the spine in more advanced stages of Heaven and Earth practice. When you gain access to and control over these ligaments, the whole spine can move as one unit, deepening the connection and integration of the upper and lower body.

THE JAW: OMITTED FOR SAFETY REASONS

Instructions for pulsing the jaw have been intentionally left out due to its delicate nature and the potential risk of causing harm by misinterpreting or not correctly following instructions. If you wish to learn how to pulse the jaw, which can be tremendously beneficial for people suffering from temporomandibular joint (TMJ) disorders, seek out the instruction of a well-qualified neigong instructor or a *qigong tui na* specialist.

> *Qigong tui na* is an energy-based bodywork system that incorporates all aspects of qigong and is applied to healing another person. Traditionally in China a practitioner would have to clearly demonstrate that they could activate any specific neigong thread in their own body before being allowed to work with that specific on another person.

A Word to the Wise: If you have steadily worked your way through the instructions of this book up to this point, the authors highly recommend resisting the urge to continue on to Section Four immediately. Spend a few weeks solidifying your current level of practice, so that you do not lose any important components by layering in too many neigong techniques too quickly.

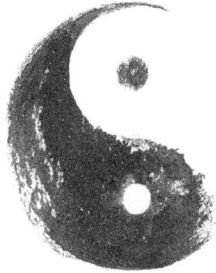

SECTION FOUR:

EMBEDDING DEEPER NEIGONG IN THE HEAVEN AND EARTH FORM

Neigong and component practices covered in this section:

- Lengthening the soft tissues of the body

- Wrapping the soft tissues of the body

- Activating indirect and direct qi flows

- Cleansing the brain

- Circulating qi through the macrocosmic and microcosmic orbits of energy

- Banking qi.

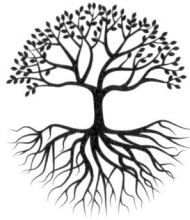

CHAPTER 19:

LENGTHENING THE SOFT TISSUES OF THE BODY

Lengthening techniques call for moving the body's soft tissues in ways that are far from the norm, so first the conceptual framework must be established. This neigong component is very different from bending-and-stretching and radically different from the Western reciprocal-inhibition model (as covered in Chapter 6). Lengthening is in a realm of its own and, as a quality of opening and closing, is sometimes referred to as "opening and closing the body's soft tissues." One of the main operating principles is to separate the yang and yin tissues (see Figure 19-1 on the next page), so that one surface of the body is exercised while the other rests. These tissue stretches are done at the level of the fascia just below the skin, where wei qi flows through the acupuncture meridian lines. This is why lengthening is so closely tied to the macrocosmic and microcosmic orbits (to be discussed in Chapter 22).

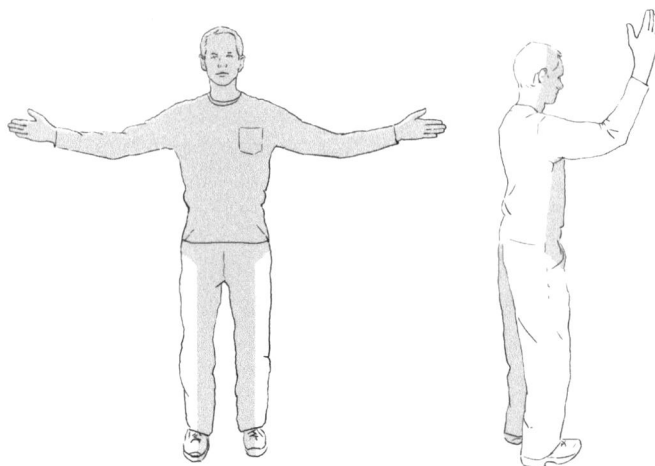

Figure 19-1:
Yin and Yang Surfaces of the Body

The shaded areas are the yin surfaces and the white areas are the yang surfaces

NINE EXERCISES TO ACTIVATE LENGTHENING THROUGHOUT THE FASCIA OF THE BODY

Whether activating the yin or the yang soft tissues of the body, generally the guiding principles are the same. The beginning method requires lengthening in the following way:

- From bottom to top through the yang tissues—since yang energy naturally rises up.
- From top to bottom, through the yin tissues—since yin energy naturally sinks down.

This is the easiest, simplest and most direct lengthening process for beginners, which must be *fully* embodied before attempting more advanced techniques that are beyond the scope of this text. If you jump ahead too quickly, you will simply limit your longer-term development.

Additionally, lengthening can only occur with a soft, open and relaxed body and intent. Similar to practicing the pulsing techniques described in Section Three, tension, excess effort or strength of any kind tightens the nerves and shuts down the process. However, with lengthening, the aim is not just to relax the nerves, but actually stretch them along with the soft tissues they inhabit. This is what dramatically empties the bound tension within the nerves and supercharges qi flows within the meridian lines themselves.

First you will learn methods for initiating lengthening in the yang tissues since the Heaven and Earth form begins and ends with a yang stretch. Also, most people find yin stretching techniques more difficult, so you will develop your skill with that which is easy before moving on to that which is more challenging.

ACTIVATING THE YANG TISSUES: BEGINNING METHOD

In bending-and-stretching techniques, you used the extension of your arms to engage the soft tissues of your back: that is, you extended your elbows away from your spine during the stretching half of the cycle. Now the operation begins at the spine and runs down the arms to the fingers. This motion requires the back tissues to move a microsecond before the elbows *and not the other way around*. What follows is the beginning soft-tissue lengthening process that sets the arms into motion.

Exercise One: Initiating the Yang Stretch

Begin in the neutral standing posture. Bring your arms parallel to each other with your forearms horizontal to the ground and in front of you. This is approximately the halfway point of the first-phase stretch, step 2, in the Heaven and Earth form (Figure 19-2).

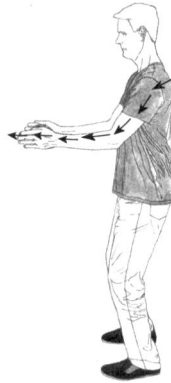

Figure 19-2: Exercise One

Initiate the yang stretch from the spine to the fingertips

1. Sink your mind into the soft tissues between your shoulder blades, the area from which you initiate the yang stretch in your arms.

2. Once your mind has fully contacted this area:

   (a) Spread open the yang fascia on your back left-right across your shoulder blades, out to your upper arm muscles (deltoids) and down the outside of your upper arms.

   (b) Continue down the outside of your forearms, back of your hands and fingers to your fingertips.

3. Then relax and let your tissues return to neutral. As you lengthen the yang tissues, the shoulder blades and arm bones will move to some degree with a small extension of the elbow joint, all of which will return to neutral when you let go.

4. Repeat steps 1-3 while trying to physically move the fascia from your spine sideways and down your arms in a smooth, soft and continuous wave—without using any excess force, tension or strength and without distorting your posture. This is only achievable if you have sufficiently released tension from your body via bending-and-stretching and opening-and-closing techniques, and refined your ability to feel and move your flesh—all while operating within 70 percent of your comfortable range of motion.

Play with this exercise for some time before moving on or you will miss the many subtleties it has to offer as well as the refinements to come downstream.

Exercise Two: Activating the Yang Tissues of the Upper Body

Start in the neutral standing posture with your hands resting on the outside of your thighs (Figure 19-3).

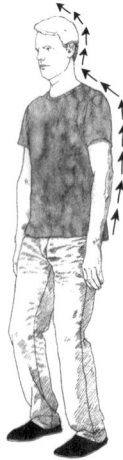

Figure 19-3: Exercise Two

Activate the yang tissues of the upper body from the pelvis to the crown of the head

1. Sink your mind into the area around your sacrum (back of the pelvis), from where the yang stretch in the torso is initiated.

2. Once your mind has fully contacted this area, begin lifting your body's fascia:

   (a) From the back of your pelvis

   (b) Up your back

   (c) Through the space between your shoulder blades

   (d) Up your neck

   (e) To the crown of your head.

3. Relax and let your tissues return to neutral. Although there will not necessarily be a visible change in the torso, neck and head during this exercise (as the fascia moves over the bones of the spine, ribs and skull), the experience will be radically different from normal muscular motion.

4. Repeat steps 1-3 while focusing on creating one smooth wave, from bottom to top, without distorting your posture or raising your shoulders at any time.

Play with this exercise for some time before moving on.

Exercise Three: Combining Exercises One and Two

Now you will combine the flows of the first two exercises into one seamless motion, simultaneously arriving at your fingertips and the crown of your head. This coordinated stretch will require you to move much faster down your arms, and comparatively slower up your neck and head. This is because of the bifurcation that happens at the space between the shoulder blades, as you will see.

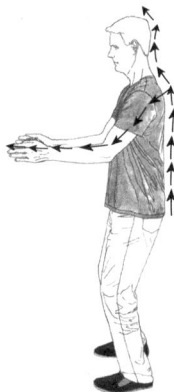

Figure 19-4:
Exercise Three

Combine the two yang flows in the upper body, from the back of the pelvis and simultaneously arriving at the fingertips and the crown of the head

Begin in the neutral standing posture with your hands out in front of you and relax (Figure 19-4).

1. Put your mind into the back of your pelvis/sacrum area and let it rest there for a minute.

2. Start lifting the fascia upward along your back to the space between your shoulder blades.

3. At this point, the yang movement of fascia splits into three branches—out to each arm and up your neck.

4. Continue until you reach the back of your hands and all your fingertips, and the crown of your head—ideally at the same moment in time.

5. Relax everything back to neutral.

A Word to the Wise: Copious practice is required to perform this exercise well and it can always be refined by even the most competent and gifted practitioners. If lengthening is fairly new to you, remain at this stage for at minimum of three to six months of daily practice before attempting to lengthen the yang tissues of your lower body and skip to Exercise Five for initiating the yin stretch.

Exercise Four:
Activating the Lower Body for Intermediate Practitioners

Important: If you can perform the exercises presented so far with relative ease, then you are ready for lengthening through your legs. If you have any ambiguity or a training partner cannot tangibly feel and verify that your tissues are moving, you know you have not yet fully activated the tissues of your upper body and you should save the leg techniques for another day. Neigong processes done with the legs are usually much more challenging than those for the arms as the mind is generally less accustomed to deeply connecting to the lower body—unless something hurts!

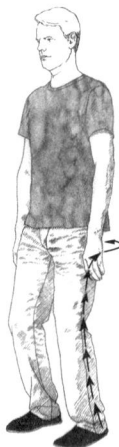

Figure 19-5:
Exercise Four (Intermediate Practitioners)

Activate the yang tissues of the lower body
from the outside edges of the feet to the back of the pelvis

Begin in the neutral standing posture and take a moment to relax (Figure 19-5).

1. Start by sinking your mind into the outside edges of both of your ankles and feet.
2. From there, stretch up the outside of your legs and thighs to your buttocks (gluteal muscles) on the back of your pelvis.
3. Relax and let your tissues return to neutral. Let go of all your muscles, fascia, nerves and mind to allow everything in your system to rest.
4. Continue practicing steps 1-3 with the aim of running through the fascia in a smooth, soft and continuous wave, from your feet to your buttocks—without igniting any sense of strain, force or strength.

This exercise is excellent for developing body awareness and patience as it requires a lot of practice even for the most gifted students.

ACTIVATING THE YIN TISSUES: BEGINNING METHOD

The yin stretch is almost the same as the yang stretch, only it runs in the opposite direction and on the opposite surface of the body (see Figure 19-1). Many people struggle with this technique because they are not used to stretching inward. Stretching outward is normal, but the concept of refined inward stretching is generally nonexistent in Western exercise paradigms.

Exercise Five: Initiating the Yin Stretch

Start in the neutral standing posture with your arms parallel, horizontal to the ground and in front of you, as before (Figure 19-6).

1. From the pads of your fingertips, without moving your physical frame, stretch the fascia inward:

    (a) Into your palms

    (b) Down the inside of your forearms, upper arms and shoulders' nests

    (c) Into your chest.

2. Aim for a tangible feeling of movement from your fingertips moving down your arms and into your chest.

3. Relax and let your tissues return to neutral.

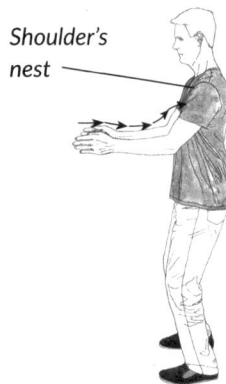

Figure 19-6:
Exercise Five

Initiate the yin stretch from the fingertips to the chest

Exercise Five: Initiating the Yin Stretch—the Fudge

In the beginning, the yin stretch described in Exercise Five is very difficult to achieve. In order to get the tissues to move, you can use a fudge for a temporary period of time. The aim is to learn how to kick-start your system and gain control over your body's soft tissues without ongoing use of the crutch.

Start in the neutral standing position as before (Figure 19-7). Then sink your chest physically down into your belly, which initiates a drawing of the yin tissues from your upper arms to your shoulders and chest—*if* your arms remain still in space, that is. Eventually you can use this technique to draw out all the yin tissues in your arms and hands. Once your tissues move, you can shift the action to start at your fingertips and run down your arms to your chest.

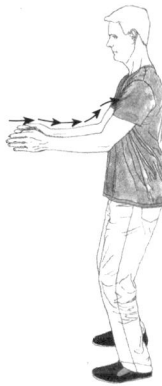

Figure 19-7:
Exercise Five—the Fudge

Gently sink your chest down into your belly
to draw the yin tissues inward

Exercise Six: Activating the Yin Tissues of the Upper Body

Begin in the neutral standing posture with your hands resting on your outer thighs (Figure 19-8).

1. Sink your mind into the tissues on your forehead and face.

2. Lengthen/drop:

   (a) From your forehead down your face, neck, chest and belly

   (b) Down to your pubic region/inguinal grooves—without distorting your torso and spine.

3. Relax and let your tissues return to neutral.

4. Repeat steps 1-3 until you experience a tangible feeling of this yin stretch or you hit the point of diminishing returns.

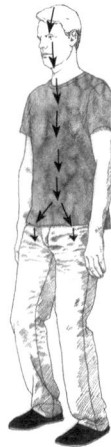

Figure 19-8:
Exercise Six

Activate the yin tissues of the upper body
from the forehead to the inguinal grooves

Exercise Seven: Combine Exercises Five and Six

Start in the neutral standing posture with your arms parallel, horizontal to the ground and in front of you, as before (Figure 19-9).

1. Simultaneously lengthen:

    (a) Down your face, from your forehead

    (b) Down the inside of your arms from your fingertips.

    Run the two pathways so that they meet and join in the chest— ideally at the same moment.

2. Continue down your belly to the pubic area/inguinal grooves.

3. Relax and let your tissues return to neutral.

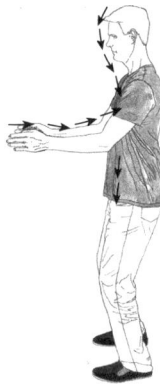

Figure 19-9: Exercise Seven

Combine the two yin flows in the upper body from the crown of the head and fingertips, to the chest and down to the inguinal grooves

As previously stated, this yin stretching method is more difficult to achieve than the yang stretching method and, therefore, may take more time to develop than the yang. Playing with these exercises on a daily basis will give you the best chance of embedding them in your system.

A Word to the Wise: Do not move on to the intermediate section until you have grasped physical control over your upper body or you will simply impede your longer-term development.

Exercise Eight:
Activating the Lower Body for Intermediate Practitioners

Start in the neutral standing posture with your hands on the outside of your thighs (Figure 19-10).

1. Sink your mind into the uppermost part of the inside of your thighs.

2. From there, stretch the fascia down the inside of your thighs, calves, ankles and feet.

3. Relax and let your tissues return to neutral.

4. Continue practicing while focusing on creating a smooth, uninterrupted flow—without using strength, tension or force.

After each attempt, make sure you rest until your nerves have fully released and your mind is calm before repeating the next repetition.

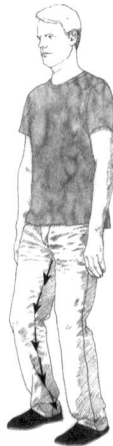

Figure 19-10:
Exercise Eight (Intermediate Practitioners)

Activate the yin tissues of the lower body
from the inguinal grooves to the inside of the feet

PUTTING IT ALL TOGETHER

Exercise Nine: Linking the Yin-Yang Flows

The aim here is to link together all of the previously covered lengthening processes in order to create one, continuous flow. What follows is the "ideal method" at this beginning stage of development. If you have not moved on to the legwork yet, simply skip it and engage only your torso, head and arms. Later you can add the legs and complete the circuit. This process underpins and supports the generation of the macrocosmic and microcosmic orbits of energy, so its importance cannot be overstated.

Start in the neutral standing posture. Bring your arms up until they become parallel with each other, horizontal to the ground and in front of you, as before (Figure 19-11). Put your mind in the outside edges of your ankles and feet.

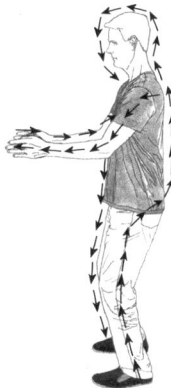

Figure 19-11:
Exercise Nine

Link the yin-yang flows

1. Stretch the fascia of the outside of your legs and thighs, upward and backward to the buttocks and up your back to the height of your heart.

2. Next the stretch goes in three directions:

    (a) Out to and down the outside of each arm to the fingertips of each hand

    (b) Up the back of your neck to the crown of your head.

3. From your fingertips and crown, stretch the fascia down the inside of your hands and arms and your face and neck to join the three flows in your chest.

4. Continue down your belly to your inguinal grooves, then down the inside of your thighs to the inside of your calves and ankles and to the arches of your feet.

5. Relax and rest for a minute before repeating steps 1-4. Each time you cycle around the circuit, *feel* more deeply what happens inside your body and try not to only visualize or simply create a mental map. Look for the gaps and, over time, develop the skill to move your fascia as one continuum—up and down your body.

The aim in Taoist qigong is to move your flesh. Moving flesh means you should physically feel a change and, if somebody were to put their hands on your body, that person too would be able to feel the motion with absolute clarity. Use your kinesthetic "feeling" sense to give you feedback on what is and, equally, that which is not moving. Asking a training partner to put their hands on an area of your body on which you wish to focus can help you develop your awareness of that area and maintain contact with it. Of course you would only do this for static practices and not while practicing a form.

Use each round to find the glitches and holes in your skill set, bringing awareness to and fixing them to create wholeness and unity. When there are no gaps, no glitches, no stuck places, the effect in your soft tissues, nerves and qi will be profound.

LENGTHENING IN HEAVEN AND EARTH QIGONG

If you have practiced and embodied the previous nine exercises to a good degree, the unification of yin and yang lengthening techniques in your form will be relatively easy. In fact this is your rule of measure: if you find the integration points come together well, you know you have embodied the layers and you are ready to move on. Conversely, if you find that your form or any piece becomes hard, sticky, bitty or nonexistent, then you know you have skipped ahead too early. Go back and practice the nine component exercises for some time and try again later. Rushing ahead yields less for your effort because lengthening as a preliminary exercise alone yields more than the choreography of the Heaven and Earth form without it.

MACROCOSMIC ORBIT

First-Phase Open

From the neutral standing posture, lengthen up the yang tissues of your body, from your feet to the crown of your head and fingertips (Figure 19-12).

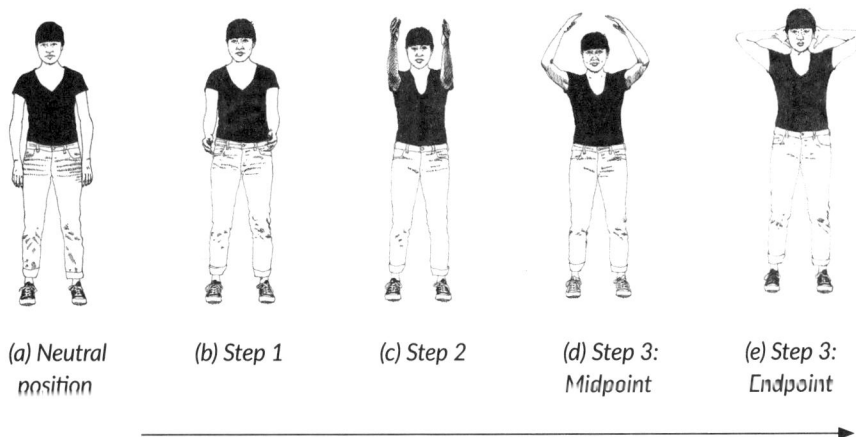

| (a) Neutral position | (b) Step 1 | (c) Step 2 | (d) Step 3: Midpoint | (e) Step 3: Endpoint |

Simultaneously lengthen upward to the crown of the head and the fingertips

Figure 19-12: First Phase—Lengthen Upward

Second-Phase Close

During the second-phase close, lengthen downward and inward, from the crown of your head and fingertips along the yin tissues to your chest (Figure 19-13).

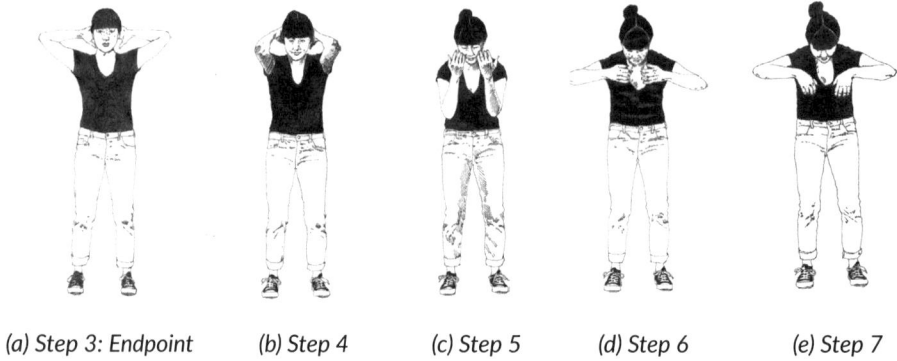

(a) Step 3: Endpoint   (b) Step 4   (c) Step 5   (d) Step 6   (e) Step 7

Lengthen downward and inward to the chest

Figure 19-13:
Second Phase—Lengthen Downward and Inward

Third-Phase Open

During the third-phase open (Figure 19-14), simultaneously lengthen:

- Down your chest, belly and front of your pelvis to the inside of your legs and the soles of your feet.
- From your spine down the yang tissues of your arms to your fingertips.

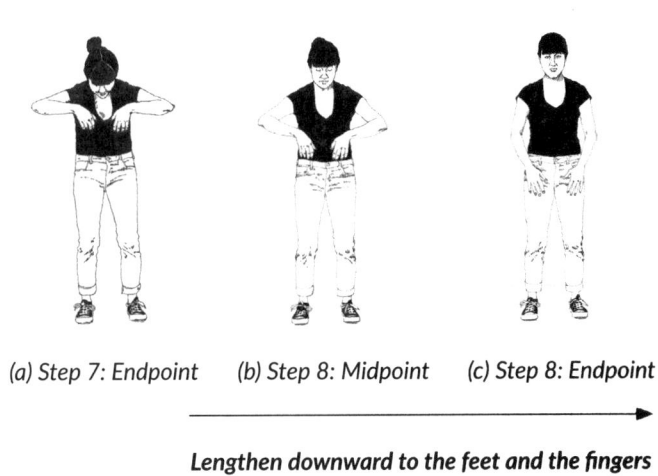

(a) Step 7: Endpoint   (b) Step 8: Midpoint   (c) Step 8: Endpoint

Lengthen downward to the feet and the fingers

Figure 19-14:
Third Phase—Lengthen Downward

MICROCOSMIC ORBIT

Some of the movement of fascia is different in the microcosmic orbit, as you will see, so pay close attention to the details that follow.

Fourth-Phase Close

While closing and moving into the C-curve in the fourth phase:

- Lengthen upward from your feet along your yang tissues of your legs and back, all the way up to the crown of your head.
- Simultaneously lengthen inward from your fingertips along the yin tissues of your arms to your chest (Figure 19-15).

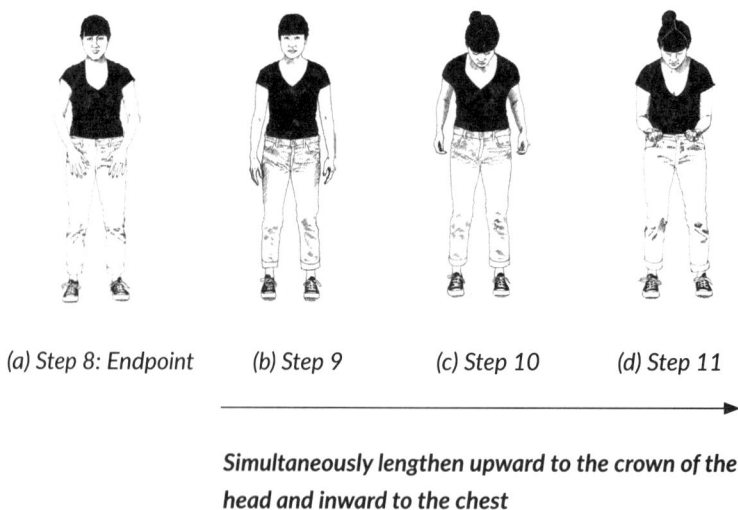

(a) Step 8: Endpoint   (b) Step 9   (c) Step 10   (d) Step 11

Simultaneously lengthen upward to the crown of the head and inward to the chest

**Figure 19-15:
Fourth Phase—Lengthen Upward and Inward**

Fifth-Phase Open

While opening in the fifth phase:

- Lengthen from the crown of your head down to your feet along the yin tissues of your torso and legs.

- Simultaneously lengthen down your arms along the yang tissues, from your spine to your fingertips (Figure 19-16).

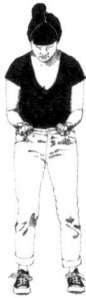 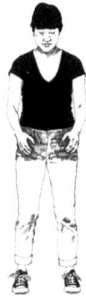 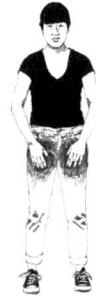

(a) Step 11: Endpoint   *(b) Step 12*   *(c) Step 13*

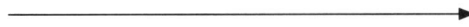

Lengthen downward to the feet and the fingers

Figure 19-16:
Fifth Phase—Lengthen Downward

NEUTRAL

Sixth-Phase Release

Release into the neutral position, softening your nerves, fascia, qi and mind (see Figure 19-17).

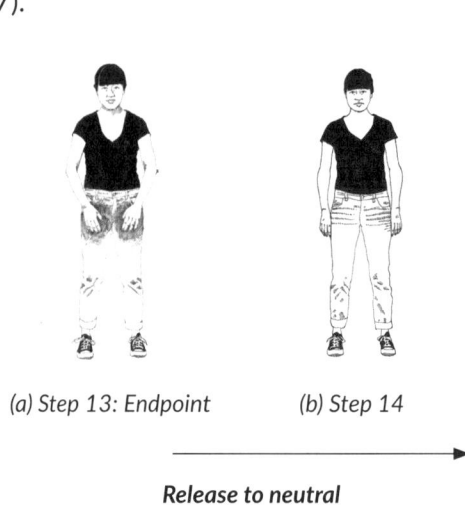

(a) Step 13: Endpoint   (b) Step 14

Release to neutral

**Figure 19-17:
Sixth Phase—Release**

TO ADVANCE, FIRST RETREAT

All of the material presented in this chapter comprises the beginning method for lengthening the body's soft tissues to help students engage and develop this essential neigong thread. If you experience any difficulties attempting to embody these lengthening processes, it indicates that your tissues house too much tension and are most likely being activated via reciprocal inhibition—instead of via relaxation. You must go back and practice bending-and-stretching techniques (from Chapter 6) for a period of time before returning to lengthening. In order to embody lengthening—or any other complex and multi-layered neigong thread for that matter—you cannot only practice the technique within the form itself, in this case Heaven and Earth. Each day, run through the nine component exercises presented in this chapter before practicing lengthening within Heaven and Earth and, when you do, observe what integrates well and if anything does not. Then, in your next practice session, focus on the dormant areas as a stand-alone exercise before recombining the technique back into your form.

Later, once these beginning-level lengthening techniques are fully embodied, there are more advanced methods to deepen and advance lengthening in your practice. These include exercises for lengthening up and down each of the yin and yang surfaces, and generating a figure-eight loop through lengthening up the yin tissues and down the yang tissues of the legs. These processes, when practiced with precision, can and will increase the quantity of qi running through your meridians—if you have successfully embodied the material presented so far. Therefore, whether or not you have been taught intermediate methods of lengthening, the authors recommend spending some months practicing the beginning methods. Then, if and when you move on to the next step in the process, you will have created a solid foundation that can support an exponential jump in qi development.

> *"To advance, first retreat."*
> —Lao Tzu

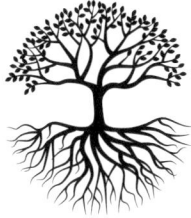

CHAPTER 20:

WRAPPING THE SOFT TISSUES OF THE TORSO

Wrapping is the horizontal equivalent to lengthening and activates the collateral (or horizontal) acupuncture meridians, which connect and integrate the body's vertical qi pathways.

Whereas lengthening is vertical in nature, either up or down the body, wrapping techniques activate the soft tissues of the torso horizontally, from the spine to the front centerline and back to the spine. Later, wrapping can be done in other areas of the body, but this usually can only be achieved after you have embodied the wrapping of your torso tissues.

- The motion of **wrapping forward** - originates at the spine and the torso tissues extend sideways (simultaneously left and right) from the spine, forward and around to the front centerline of the torso.
- The motion of **wrapping backward** - originates at the front centerline of the torso and again the tissues extend sideways in both directions, backward and around to the spine.

Wrapping, as in lengthening, is done at the level of the fascia below the skin and influences movement of qi in the horizontal/collateral (acupuncture) meridians. These link to and provide more qi for the yang and yin meridians, which are contacted and engaged through lengthening practices. Wrapping and lengthening are a matched pair, a yin and yang that supercharge the flows of each other and complete aspects of the macrocosmic and micro-cosmic orbits to be presented in Chapter 22.

HOW TO INITIATE WRAPPING

The first stage of wrapping is initiated by moving the shoulder blades. The arms and hands move, but only as a result of the movement in the shoulder blades. The shoulder blades are directly and indirectly connected to various tissues active in wrapping, such as the *latissimus dorsi* muscles (commonly known as the "lats") that run down the sides of the rib cage. Therefore, when the shoulder blades move correctly, the tissues to which they are connected become activated, which begins the process of moving qi in the collateral meridians. It is like a fishing rod: the hook catches the fish via a fishing line, but the reel pulls in the fish. In this case, the shoulder blades are the fishing reel, which move the tissues (line and hook) to catch the fish (your qi).

PRELIMINARY EXERCISE: MOVE THE TISSUES OF THE TORSO

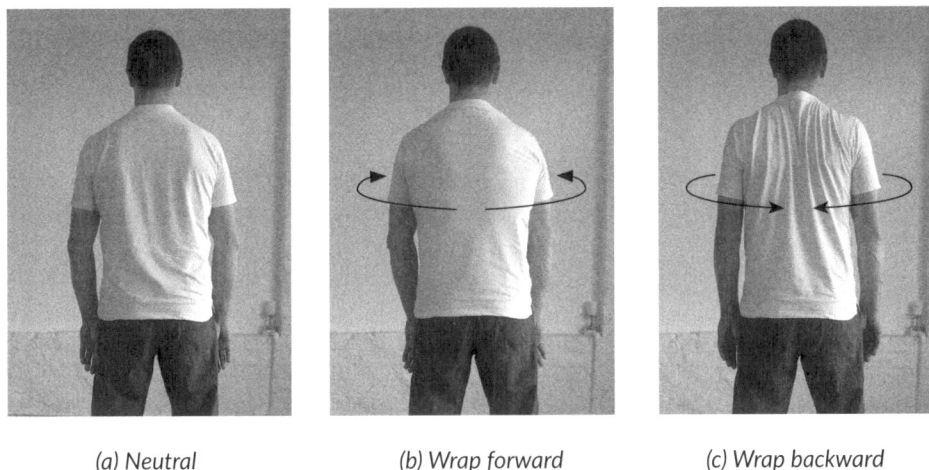

(a) Neutral   (b) Wrap forward   (c) Wrap backward

Figure 20-1:
Move the Torso Tissues

Begin in the neutral standing position with your hands resting on your thighs and put your mind into your shoulder blades.

1. Without independently moving your hands or arms, wrap your shoulder blades sideways, away from your spine and forward.

2. Next wrap your shoulder blades backward and toward your spine. If your arms and hands move as a result of the shoulder blades moving, that is correct, but do not deliberately engage your arm or hand muscles, or let them take over control of the movement.

3. As you continue to move your shoulder blades forward and backward, just feel and notice what moves and that which does not, while making sure your spine, neck and head remain upright and still in space.

4. With the intent of making the movement smooth, continuous, fluid and deliberate, begin to increase the range of motion in your shoulder blades. This will also further engage the depth and range of soft tissues activated in the region of and throughout your torso.

5. Make adjustments to induce a stretch in your back and a gathering in your chest—without allowing your chest to tense or puff up—as your shoulder blades extend forward. Look for a stretch in your chest and a gathering in your back as your shoulder blades wrap backward—without any distortions in your spine, neck or head.

Note: If you experience any difficulty performing this exercises, go back and practice the shoulder exercises presented in Chapter 14 for a period of time before attempting this exercise again.

Eventually the idea is to wrap the fascia from your spine to your front centerline, and from your front centerline back toward your spine. Over the practice sessions that follow, gradually increase your range of motion, giving your soft tissues the time needed to open and release their bindings. In time you will naturally connect to all the surrounding tissues, including everything from C7 (the base of the neck) down to the bottom of your rib cage.

Intermediate Considerations

When the tissues from C7 to the bottom of your rib cage are active, fluid and free from surface-level tension, begin moving both farther up and down your spine in incremental stages, stabilizing each gain before moving on to the next. The nervous system prevents the body from being forced into submission, so allow your body to open of its own accord.

The three major stability zones for wrapping the soft tissues are from:

- C7 down to the lowest ribs.
- The occiput down to the L5 vertebrae (just above the sacrum).
- The crown of the head down to the perineum (the soft space between your legs, anus and genitals).

Important: Until you can smoothly wrap the soft tissues between C7 and your lowest ribs—especially your fascia—forward and backward, and without strain, there is no point in attempting to wrap the tissues above and below these points. When wrapping is strong in this zone, it will naturally begin to transfer to the neighboring tissues since they are connected. Conversely, weak wrapping in this zone will prevent your ability to wrap at all in the neighboring tissues. As you practice and develop skill with this essential neigong component, you will naturally and incrementally progress to wrapping all of your tissues in the adjacent zone. When you reach the second stage of wrapping (between the occiput and L5), again practice within this zone until the final stage begins to come online of its own accord. Once you have integrated this level of wrapping, your entire torso, neck and head get involved in the action and the whole sheet of fascia will move as one—forward to the front centerline and backward to the spine.

WRAPPING IN HEAVEN AND EARTH QIGONG: BEGINNING METHOD

The Heaven and Earth form has both beginning and intermediate methods of wrapping, initially directed by the motion of the shoulder blades, which must be trained progressively. Focus on training only the beginning method until you stabilize your skill set sufficiently to provide a sound foundation for the intermediate method. Refinements are offered in the sections on intermediate considerations that follow.

The beginning method is:

- From the first-phase open, the start of step 3, to the end of the second-phase close, step 7 (Figure 20-2a-f)
- From the start of the fourth-phase close, step 9, to the fifth-phase open, step 13 (Figure 20-2g-l).

Figure 20-2: Wrapping in Heaven and Earth—Beginning Method

SECOND-PHASE CLOSE

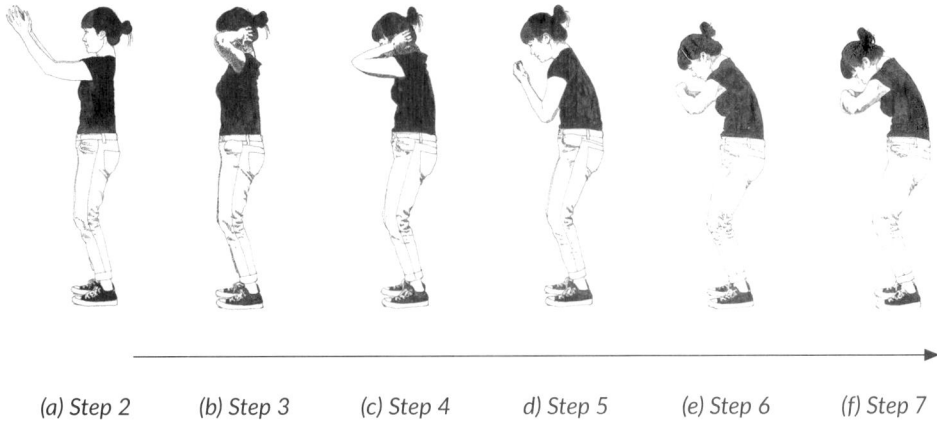

(a) Step 2 (b) Step 3 (c) Step 4 d) Step 5 (e) Step 6 (f) Step 7

FOURTH-PHASE CLOSE AND FIFTH-PHASE OPEN

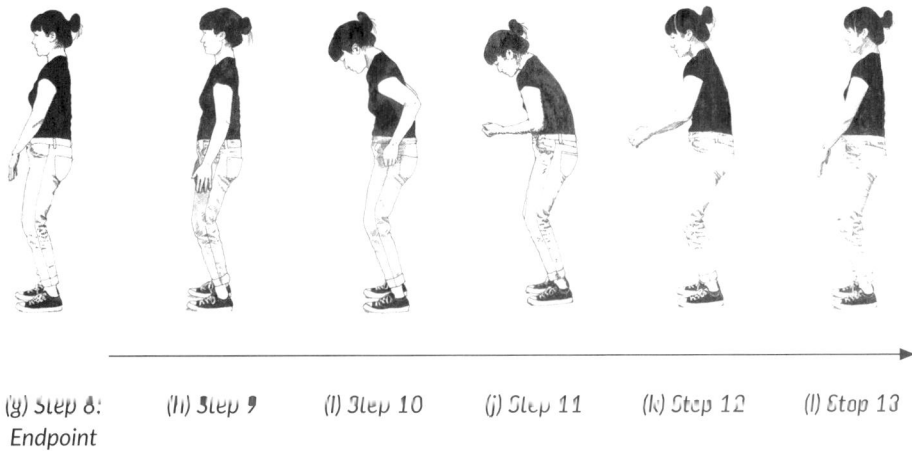

(g) Step 8:   (h) Step 9   (i) Step 10   (j) Step 11   (k) Step 12   (l) Step 13
Endpoint

*The beginning method is from step 3 to the end of step 7,
and step 9 to the end of step 13*

MACROCOSMIC ORBIT

First-Phase Open

Steps 1 and 2 - Focus on lengthening up your body.

Step 3 - As your hands come over your head, use your mind to contact the tissues at the front of your torso to whatever degree you can. Wrap these tissues back toward your spine without closing your shoulder blades toward your spine.

Be sure not to stick out or raise your chest, or bring your elbows too far back (Figure 20-3).

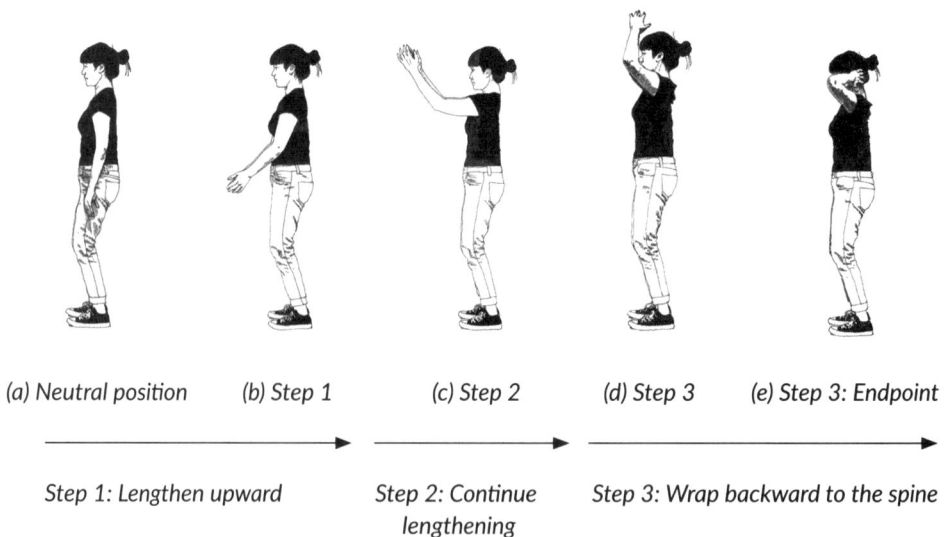

(a) Neutral position   (b) Step 1   (c) Step 2   (d) Step 3   (e) Step 3: Endpoint

Step 1: Lengthen upward   Step 2: Continue lengthening   Step 3: Wrap backward to the spine

Figure 20-3:
First-Phase Open—Lengthen Upward and Wrap Backward

Second-Phase Close

Steps 4-7 - Throughout the four steps of the first close, wrap forward from your spine to your front centerline (Figure 20-4). Try not to use all of your wrapping capacity at the beginning of the close (step 4) when bringing your elbows forward. Continuously wrap until your fingers drop at the end of the close in preparation for the second open (step 7).

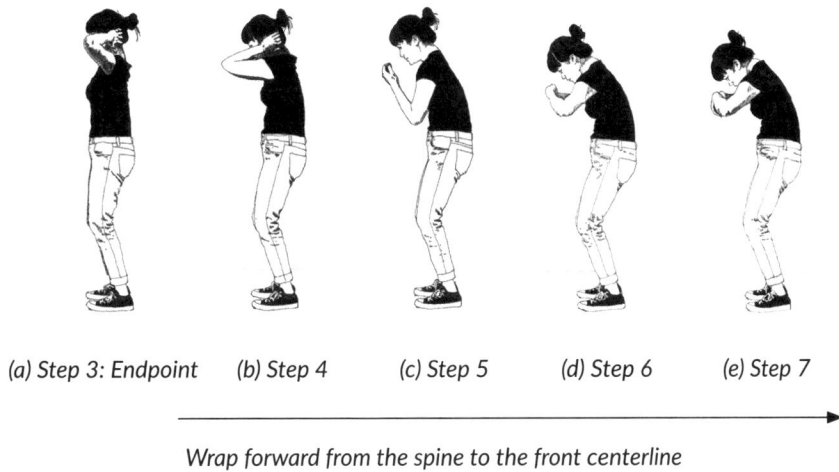

(a) Step 3: Endpoint   (b) Step 4   (c) Step 5   (d) Step 6   (e) Step 7

Wrap forward from the spine to the front centerline

Figure 20-4:
Second-Phase Close—Wrap Forward

Third-Phase Open

Step 8 - Focus on lengthening down the front of your body as your spine straightens (Figure 20-5).

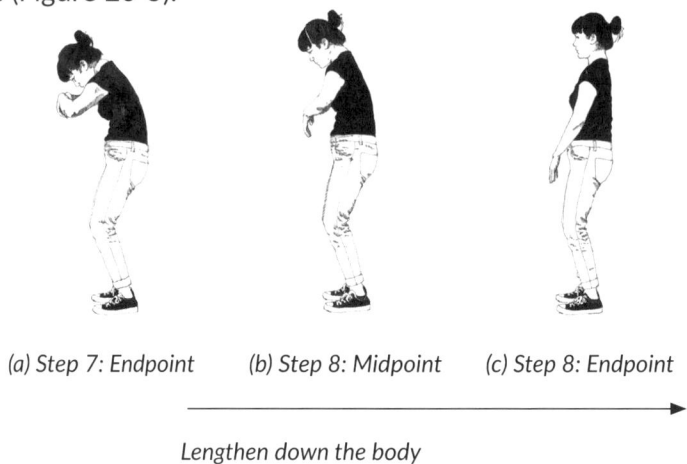

(a) Step 7: Endpoint   *(b) Step 8: Midpoint*   *(c) Step 8: Endpoint*

Lengthen down the body

Figure 20-5: Third-Phase Open—Lengthen Down the Body

MICROCOSMIC ORBIT

Fourth-Phase Close

Steps 9-11 - As your spine bows and your hands and elbows circle backward, upward and forward, wrap the tissues back toward your spine (Figure 20-6).

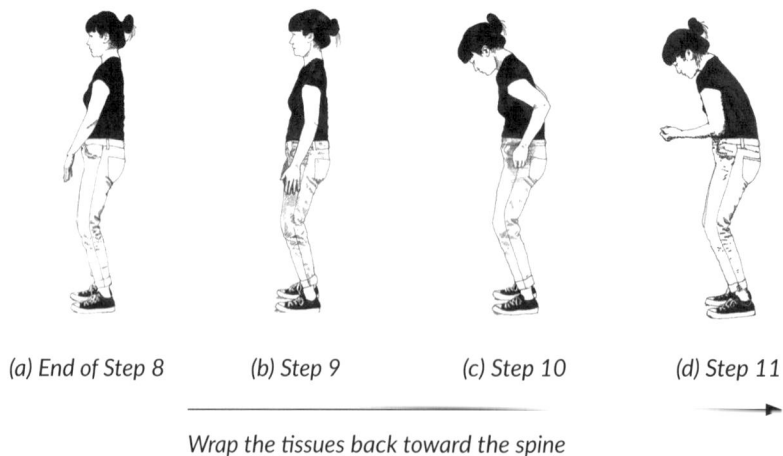

(a) End of Step 8   *(b) Step 9*   *(c) Step 10*   *(d) Step 11*

Wrap the tissues back toward the spine

Figure 20-6: Fourth-Phase Close—Wrap Backward

Fifth-Phase Open

Steps 12-13 - As your spine and hands stretch open and your elbows and hands circle forward, downward and backward, wrap the tissues forward to your front centerline (Figure 20-7).

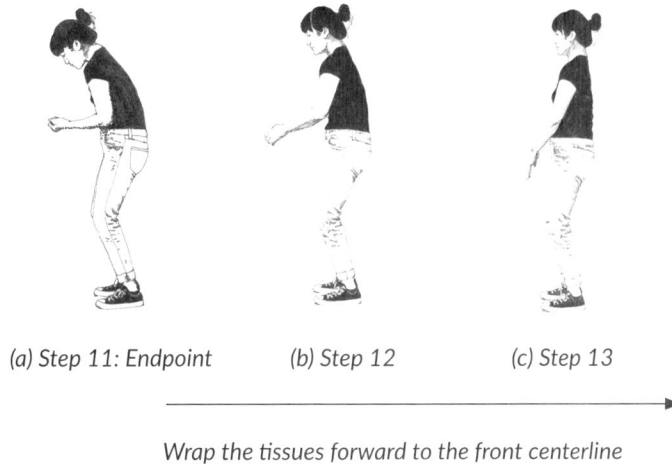

(a) Step 11: Endpoint   *(b) Step 12*   *(c) Step 13*

Wrap the tissues forward to the front centerline

Figure 20-7:
Fifth-Phase Open—Wrap Forward

NEUTRAL

Sixth-Phase Release

Step 14 - As always, release into neutral and completely let go to allow your tissues to relax and regain slack in preparation for the next round (Figure 20-8).

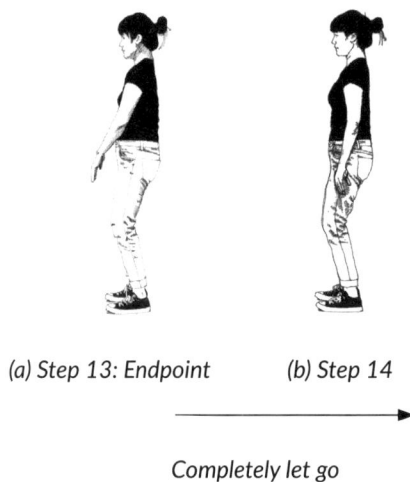

(a) Step 13: Endpoint   (b) Step 14

Completely let go

**Figure 20-8:
Sixth-Phase Release**

INTERMEDIATE CONSIDERATIONS

Moving the shoulder blades to activate the soft tissues is a very indirect method as you are using one body part (i.e. the shoulder blades) to move another (i.e. the fascia). Now there is another point to consider: Are you moving your shoulder blades to activate your tissues, or can you shift the origin of the motion to the fascia of your torso, so that it moves your shoulder blades?

Repeat the previous component exercises from the beginning of this chapter, only this time initiate from the fascia of your torso to move your shoulder blades away from and toward your spine.

The Shoulder Blades and Wrapping

In the internal arts of qigong, tai chi, bagua and hsing-i the shoulder blades do not always move in the same direction as the wrapping of the torso tissues: sometimes they are in sync with each other and other times they move in opposite to each other, so you must be able to operate these two techniques independently in order to bring them fully alive. Eventually you want to be able to stand and wrap the fascia of your torso while keeping your shoulder blades absolutely still in space.

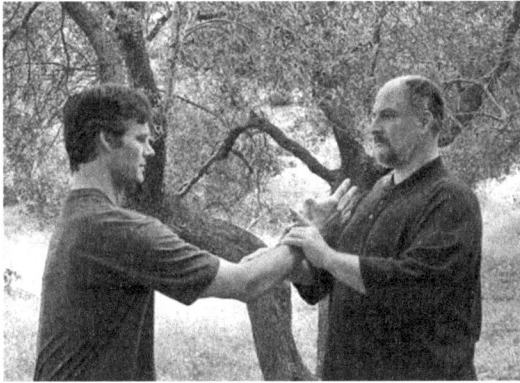

Master Frantzis helps Senior Student Paul Cavel
activate the tissues of his upper body

WRAPPING IN HEAVEN AND EARTH QIGONG: INTERMEDIATE METHOD

The instructions that follow are the intermediate method for continuously wrapping the soft tissues of the torso.

MACROCOSMIC ORBIT

First-Phase Open

Steps 1 and 2 - Wrap forward (Figure 20-9a-c). This action encourages the shoulder blades to move forward and amplifies lengthening techniques.

Step 3 - Wrap backward (Figure 20-9d-e).

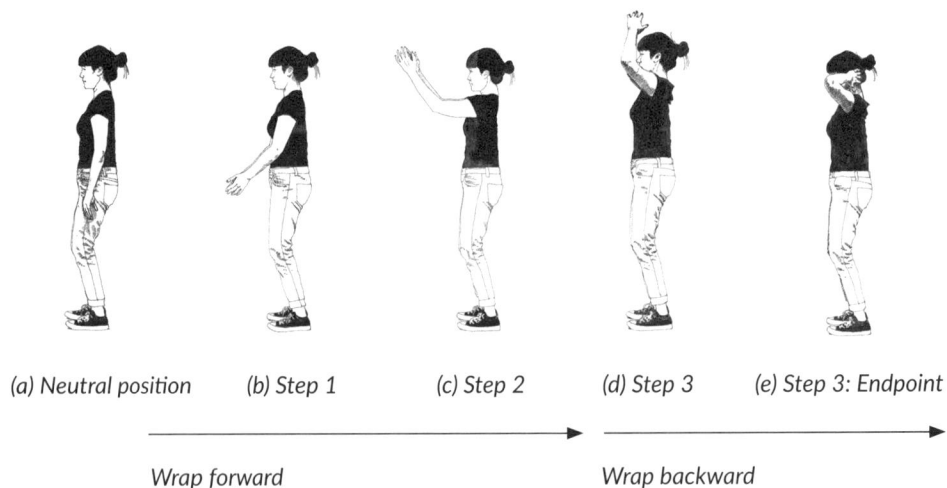

(a) Neutral position   (b) Step 1   (c) Step 2   (d) Step 3   (e) Step 3: Endpoint

Wrap forward   Wrap backward

Figure 20-9:
First-Phase Open—Wrap Forward and Backward

Second-Phase Close

Steps 4-7 - Wrap forward (Figure 20-10).

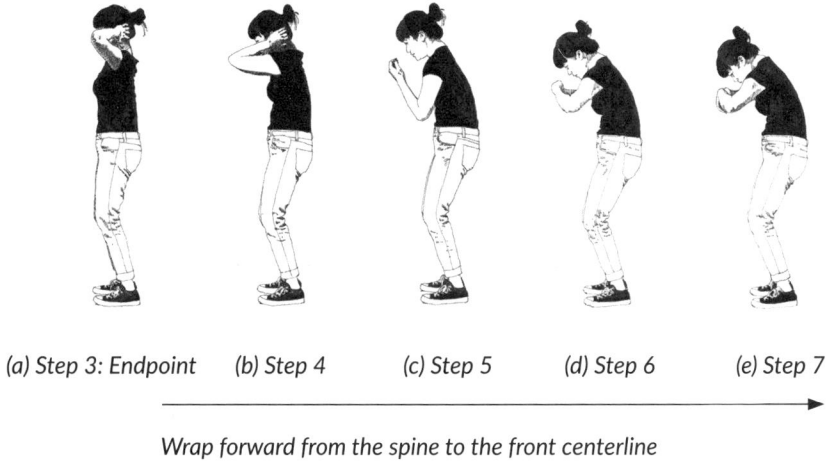

(a) Step 3: Endpoint   *(b) Step 4*   *(c) Step 5*   *(d) Step 6*   *(e) Step 7*

Wrap forward from the spine to the front centerline

Figure 20-10: Second-Phase Close—Wrap Forward

Third-Phase Open

Step 8 - Allow the torso tissues to return to neutral as your shoulder blades sink downward (Figure 20-11).

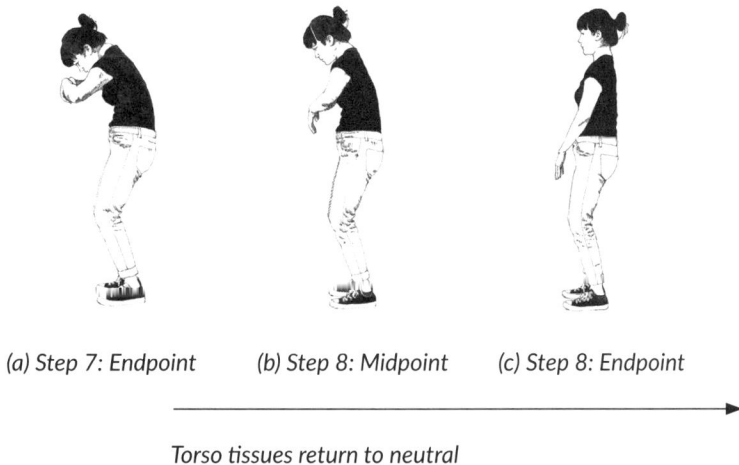

(a) Step 7: Endpoint   *(b) Step 8: Midpoint*   *(c) Step 8: Endpoint*

Torso tissues return to neutral

Figure 20-11: Third-Phase Open—Tissues Return to Neutral

MICROCOSMIC ORBIT

Fourth-Phase Close

Steps 9-11 - Emphasize wrapping backward (Figure 20-12).

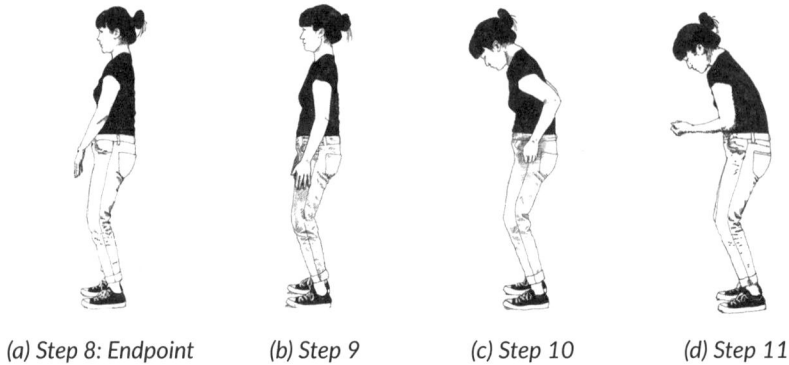

(a) Step 8: Endpoint   *(b) Step 9*   *(c) Step 10*   *(d) Step 11*

Wrap the tissues back toward the spine

Figure 20-12: Fourth-Phase Close—Wrap Backward

Fifth-Phase Open

Steps 12-13 - Emphasize wrapping forward (Figure 20-13).

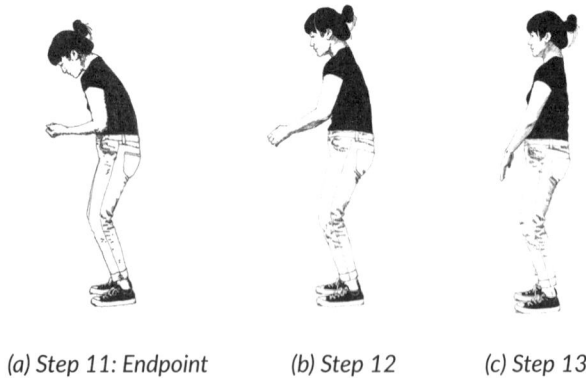

(a) Step 11: Endpoint   *(b) Step 12*   *(c) Step 13*

Wrap the tissues forward to the front centerline

Figure 20-13: Fifth-Phase Open—Wrap Forward

NEUTRAL

Sixth-Phase Release

Step 14 - Release into the neutral position by completely letting go and allowing your tissues to relax and regain slack (Figure 20-14).

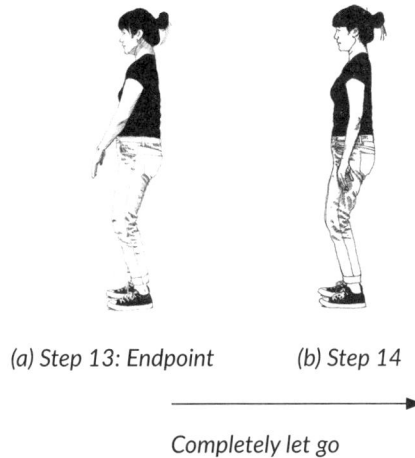

(a) Step 13: Endpoint   (b) Step 14

Completely let go

Figure 20-14:
Sixth-Phase Release

Heaven and Earth both begins and finishes with wrapping forward. Therefore, you must let go of your torso tissues and nerves on the sixth-phase release in order to allow the space required to wrap forward once again on the next repetition.

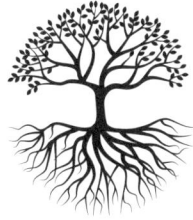

CHAPTER 21:

CLEANSING THE BRAIN

This particular qi technique removes excess blood and stagnant qi from the brain, which is invaluable in this age of big data, stress and visualizations. Modern living involves use of technology and endless mental projections, processing that draws blood and qi up to the head, where they can easily become stuck—especially when coupled with a sedentary lifestyle. The brain literally heats up from constant rising yang energy, which prevents blood and energy from being re-circulated back into the body. If left unattended for prolonged periods, brain-body imbalances become exacerbated and can lead to serious health issues.

The brain comes first in the body's hierarchy for receiving nutrients and resources. During normal functioning, the brain requires approximately 20 percent of the blood and qi in circulation, which is significantly more than its relative mass. This is why the Chinese say the brain can "eat" the body when the body is constantly depleted as a result of hyperactivity in the brain.

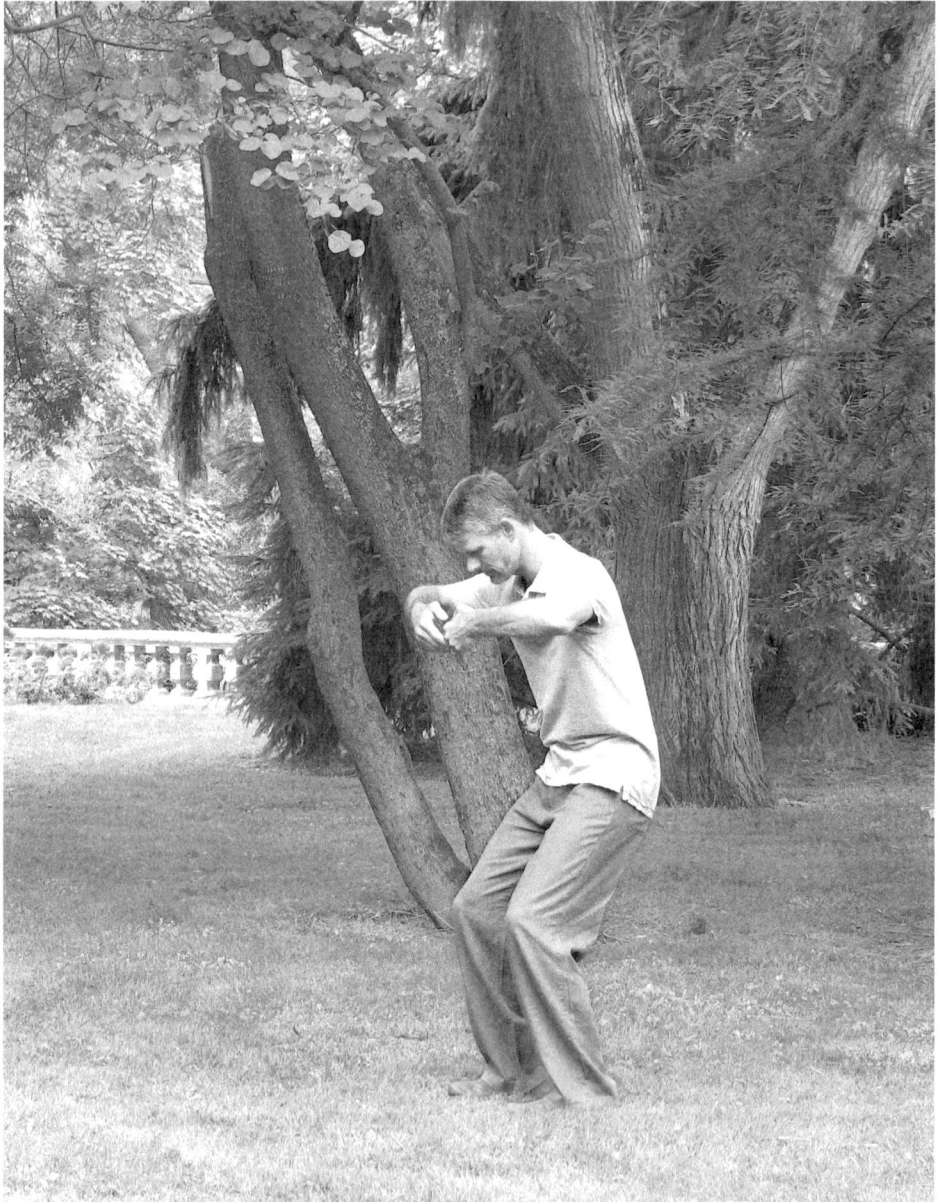

Paul Cavel, Senior Student of Master Frantzis, transitions from the end of the first close to the second open in the Heaven and Earth form, where the energy of the brain is dropped back into the body

PHOTO BY H.L. CAVEL

HOW TO CLEANSE THE BRAIN

The brain cleansing technique is activated in the macrocosmic orbit and:

- Starts from the moment the first-phase open is complete (Figure 21-1a)
- Continues through the second-phase close (Figure 21-1b-e)
- Finishes at the beginning of the third-phase open (Figure 21-1f).

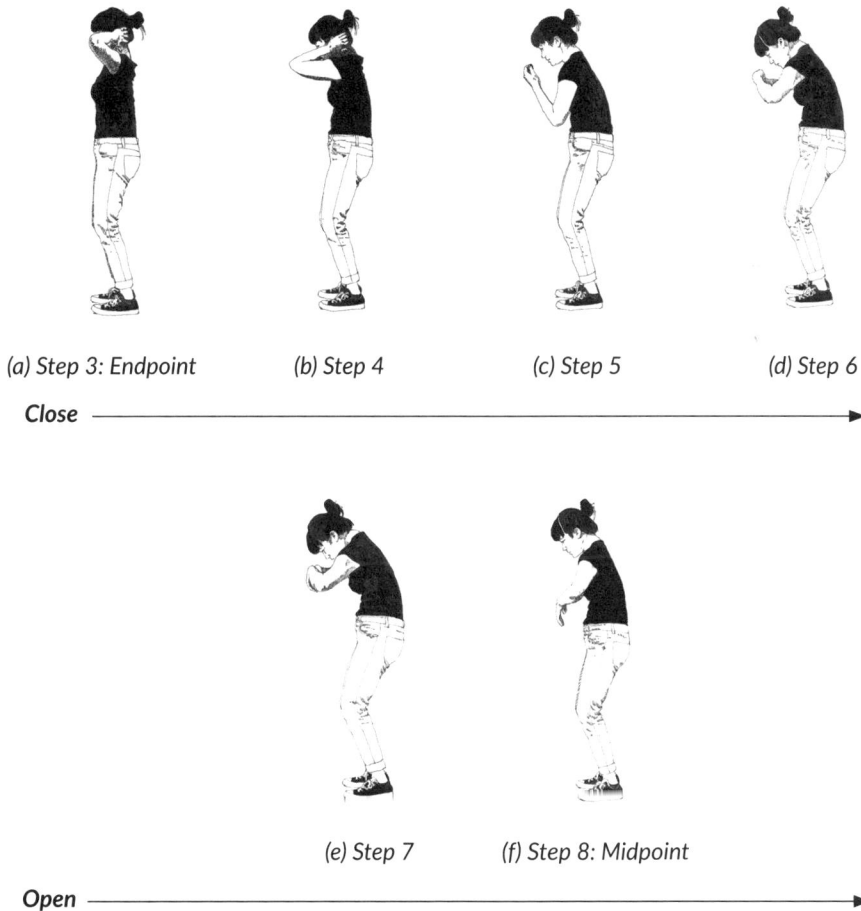

| (a) Step 3: Endpoint | (b) Step 4 | (c) Step 5 | (d) Step 6 |

Close ⟶

| (e) Step 7 | (f) Step 8: Midpoint |

Open ⟶

Figure 21-1:
Cleaning the Brain in Heaven and Earth Qigong

MACROCOSMIC ORBIT

End of the First-Phase Open

Step 3 - The brain cleansing technique starts at the moment the fingers touch the occiput at the end of the first open.

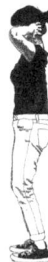

Second-Phase Close

Step 4 - As your elbows drive forward and toward each other, the etheric field of the inside of your forearms projects qi into:

- The left and right hemispheres of your brain
- If you can, the corpus callosum in the center of your brain.

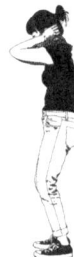

Step 5 - As your hands come over your head and in front of your face:

- Use the closing of your joints in your hands to pull qi from the back of your brain
- Then over the top of and to the front of your brain.

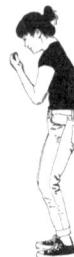

Step 6 - As your elbows widen and rise up, continue to use the closing of your hands to influence the qi of your brain. Pull qi from the center to the outside of your brain.

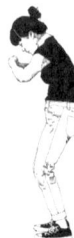

Step 7 - As you rotate your palms and drop your fingers, drop the qi from the crown of your head into your brain, then out of the bottom of your brain. This will also drop the blood out of the brain, allowing it to return to the heart, where it can be recirculated and, thereby, re-oxygenated.

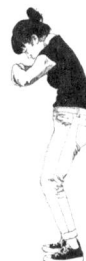

Third-Phase Open

Step 8 - Sink qi and let it continue to move the blood and qi out of the bottom of your brain and back down into your body.

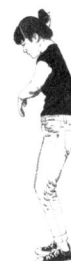

These qi techniques enable you to:

- Release stagnant qi from your brain.
- Open up the blood vessels within your brain.
- Improve circulation within your brain over time, so that blood and qi do not stagnate.

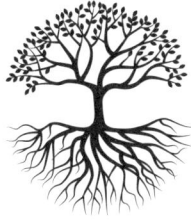

CHAPTER 22:

THE MACROCOSMIC AND MICROCOSMIC ORBITS OF ENERGY

At one level the two parts of the Heaven and Earth movement are very similar, except in external form. They both contain the same neigong—bending-and-stretching, leading from the kwa, the spinal bow, breathing, twisting, opening-and-closing, lengthening, wrapping and more—but the purpose of each part differs considerably.

- The first part, which involves the macrocosmic orbit, directly circulates qi throughout all the energy channels and associated tissues of the entire body.
- The second part, which primarily involves the microcosmic orbit, is localized in the torso, neck and head. All the body's energy channels become indirectly activated as points along the microcosmic pathway are activated during the movement.

The differences do not stop there.

The actual quality of how qi moves varies too: the macrocosmic orbit employs a yang methodology while the microcosmic orbit uses a yin one; together the two strike yet another balance between two extremes to create harmony in body, mind and qi.

This is played out in the form: during the macrocosmic half of the motion, energy is projected through the channels in a yang manner, like blowing through a straw into a glass of water and making bubbles; whereas, in the microcosmic half of the motion, energy is pulled into and through the appropriate channels in a yin manner, like drawing water through a straw to take a drink. The macrocosm and microcosm form a matched and interactive pair, which guides the practitioner to develop both opposites separately, then balance them and integrate the two.

In order to embody the deeper aspects of the macrocosmic and microcosmic orbits of energy, first practice with a focus on each quality independently, then recombine them again and again to accurately separate out the two distinct qualities. Only then will you be able to apply them in the correct sections of the form for optimal results. This ability to weave neigong into distinctly different qualities is the underlying reason why tai chi, bagua and hsing-i can all be constructed from the same neigong building blocks yet produce completely different forms, styles and qualities of motion.

MACROCOSMIC ORBIT:
THE PHYSICAL AND THE SPIRITUAL

Taoism's Fire and Water traditions both use the macrocosmic orbit to obtain a connection to the universe or all that is outside of oneself. At the most basic physical level, the macrocosmic orbit is about how energy moves from the soles of the feet up to the crown of the head and fingertips, and back down again. The Taoist concept of the macrocosmic orbit is that for a human being to be fully integrated within the universe, they must merge their energy with both the planet on which they live, the Earth, and the rest of the universe, the heavens—that which is below and above them.

Human beings naturally connect to the Earth through their feet and the heavens or universe through the crown of their head. But what most people do not realize, due to lack of sensitivity, is that they are constantly being influenced by the energy of the Earth rising up from its core beneath them, and the energy of Heaven raining down from above them. These energies enter into and commingle within us on a daily basis. We are in effect a marriage or union of these energies—a byproduct, if you like, of the joining of these yang and yin energies.

While practicing the Marriage of Heaven and Earth form, the aim is to allow in and absorb these natural energies, then join them within your lower tantien. This unification is generally done after each round as you release to neutral and more completely at the end of a practice session (as will be covered in Chapter 24). This not only allows you to circulate and increase your qi, but also to balance and integrate yang and yin opposites within yourself.

The traditional metaphors for this process are the marriage, union, joining, confluence or coming together of Heaven and Earth. All of these names are in effect describing a basic opening-and-closing of yang and yin energies. These are metaphors for two opposites continually coming together at a point and dividing again. They separate to circulate and join in storage. This is a sophisticated energetic play that emulates the natural activity and rest cycles of all beings on the planet, performed in such a way as to activate and develop each and every aspect of the human body, mind and qi.

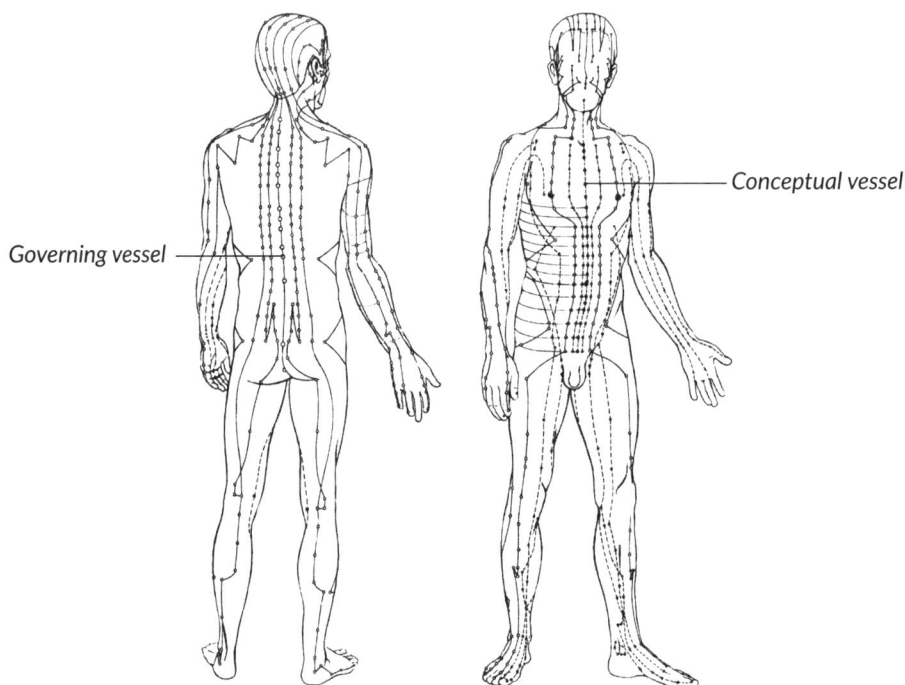

Figure 22-1
The Governing and Conceptual Vessels

MICROCOSMIC ORBIT: THE PHYSICAL AND THE SPIRITUAL

The standard pathway works two of the extraordinary meridians in acupuncture: the governing and conceptual vessels, which run up the length of the spine, from the perineum to the crown of the head, and back down the front centerline to the perineum again (Figure 22-1). Along these pathways there are many energetic points that connect to various parts of the internal anatomy, such as muscles, tendons, ligaments, blood vessels, organs and glands, as well as the 12 acupuncture meridians.

The main concept behind the health benefits gained by unblocking and cir-culating qi through the microcosmic orbit is that, when qi flows strongly, it will—via numerous subsidiary channels—seep into all the connected anat-omy and generate vitality. If qi flow is strong enough in the microcosmic orbit, all the attached anatomy will function reasonably well. Therefore, the microcosmic orbit offers a very simple yet effective method for opening up your channels and flooding your body with life-sustaining qi.

FIRE VERSUS WATER TRADITION PERSPECTIVES

From a spiritual perspective, many of the practice methodologies of the Fire and Water traditions vary greatly. The focus in the Fire tradition is on circu-lating a ball of light, which is basically achieved by condensing energy into the lower tantien to create immense heat until eventually—literally not met-aphorically—the heat transforms into a viscerally experienced ball of light. Once the ball of light has been generated, it is then circulated around the microcosmic orbit to clear energetic blockages. Depending on the skill of the practitioner, it is possible to neutralize emotional and mental blockages, unleash the entirety of an individual's psychic abilities and, at the highest levels, release and transform karma. However, the vast majority of people never get past the visualization stage and therefore do not reach the point of actualizing the ball of light and all the benefits that come with it.

In the Water tradition, the microcosmic orbit is worked at a more superficial level in order to develop qi and the parts of the physical body to which that qi connects. This process continues until the practitioner is at or near the (Seventh) Body of Individuality, that is personal rather than universal enlightenment. The reasons for practice to reach this level are discussed in depth in Master Frantzis' meditation books (see the Bibliography). The focus in this text is on the principle of unifying the body and qi within Heaven and Earth Qigong, rather than its more profound spiritual aspects.

Qi is the power upon which your body runs and therefore that energy must interface with the physicality of your body. Just having qi and not connecting it to something will do nothing for you, just as a printer has to be connected to a computer to both receive and print an image. Again, visualizing the flow is only a beginning stage. Eventually you must connect to your qi with your intent (via specific neigong techniques), pull that qi into the relevant channels and draw it through your body.

FEEL INTO YOUR BODY

Generally all qigong practice aims to get you out of your head and instead feel inside your body. Intellectually understanding a concept is not the same as directly experiencing and embodying it. Just moving your hands in space and visualizing will not necessarily get your qi to move. It is important to feel and *listen*.

> In Chinese medicine and healing arts, *listening* is the ability for the mind to become quiet and focused enough to directly perceive in the flesh the effects of qi techniques—whether in your own or someone else's body. Listening makes use of all the senses.

This principle is also true for the macrocosmic movements of qi: the flow through the whole is the goal. It is both progressive—from the feet to the fingertips—and continuous, that is through the whole stream when the practitioner arrives at the designated point in the form.

Once the flow is activated, qi must connect to the hardware—the physicality—enabling the software to upgrade the system, i.e., increase health through improved functionality of the internal anatomy. The form of Heaven and Earth is an excellent container and its unique neigong weave is incredibly sophisticated, but it is all about the qi. Qi is what gives life to the body and tells it how to grow, repair and replicate cells to manifest an ever-more efficient system. Flowing, unrestricted qi is responsible for longevity and rejuvenation.

BALANCING TWO OPPOSITES

The pathways of the macrocosmic and microcosmic orbits have already been discussed to some extent in the sections on lengthening, wrapping and brain cleansing (covered in Chapters 19, 20 and 21, respectively). However, there are a number of refinements and specific neigong threads that dominate at specific points of the form in order to produce the desired flavor of motion and qi. Practice becomes complex at this level of training, so do your best not to juggle between neigong techniques. Instead, emphasize what is being used to influence the quality of the qi you are developing within each phase of the Heaven and Earth form.

First become familiar with the two circuits of energy within the form. Then refine neigong in order to manifest the correct quality of qi and bodily motion. Do your best not only to visualize, which creates a conceptual map of the journey of qi through your flesh instead of enabling you to take steps on the journey itself. Feel your body and experience the motion directly via your kinesthetic sense.

ACTIVATING THE MACROCOSMIC AND MICROCOSMIC ORBITS

Begin in the neutral standing posture with the insides of your hands resting on the outside of your thighs, and sink your torso down through your legs into your feet while keeping your spine erect—without leaning forward, backward or to either side. This movement is small and not a close, more of a sinking to the bottom of neutral in order to give you more space to open and lengthen at the beginning of the form.

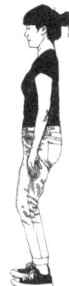

MACROCOSMIC ORBIT

First-Phase Open

Step 1 - Begin to open and shift forward as you bring your arms parallel. Link your hands to the soles of your feet, especially the bubbling-well points, in order to assist the qi rising up the body.

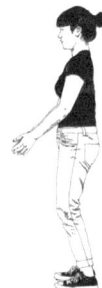

Step 2 - Emphasize opening, lengthening and raising your arms:

- Project your qi from the soles of your feet to the outside of your feet and ankles.
- Project your qi up the outside of your calves and thighs, through your hips and buttocks to your back, up your back to between your shoulder blades.
- Finally the qi flow splits and travels up the outside of both of your arms and your neck, ideally to your fingertips and the crown of your head.

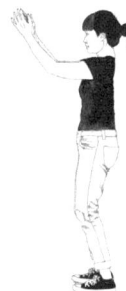

Step 3 - Wrap your torso tissues backward to join and deliver more qi to the flow rising up your yang tissues. Keep projecting your qi to your upper extremities until your fingers come to touch your occiput.

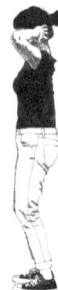

Second-Phase Close

Throughout the entire second-phase close, there is a continual movement of qi as a result of wrapping and lengthening techniques, where you simultaneously:

- Dropping qi from the crown of your head, down your face to your chest.
- Drawing qi from your fingers, down the inside of your arms to your chest.
- Wrapping qi from your spine to the front of your torso via flooding the collateral meridians.

Additionally, there is a sequential movement of qi as detailed in steps 4-7 that follow.

Step 4 - Drive the qi in the etheric field between your forearms into your brain.

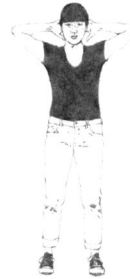

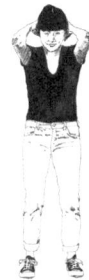

Step 5 - Draw the qi from the back of your brain to the front of your brain.

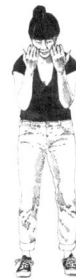

Step 6 - Pull the qi from the center of your brain to the periphery of your brain.

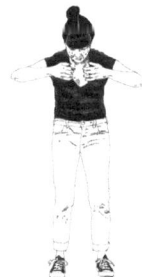

Step 7 - Drop the qi from the crown of your head down to and out of the bottom of your brain.

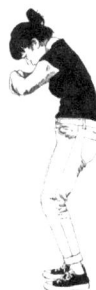

Third-Phase Open

Step 8 - Pick up the accumulated qi collected on the front of your torso and the qi dropping out of the bottom of your brain, and project it downward via opening and lengthening down your body:

- From the front of your torso to the inside of your legs
- To the inside of your ankles
- To the soles of your feet and bubbling-well points
- Then, along the centerlines of the soles of your feet to the back of your heels.

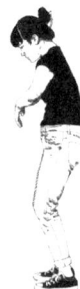

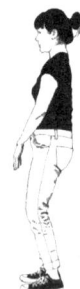

MICROCOSMIC ORBIT

Fourth-Phase Close

Step 9 - As you relax to neutral and allow your palms to come to the outside of your thighs, link your palms to your perineum in order to assist in drawing qi up your body.

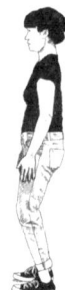

Step 10 - As your spine begins to bow and your elbows bend to pull your hands backward and upward to initiate the circle, pull qi from your perineum to your tailbone. As your hands rise, lengthen up your back, drawing qi up your spine.

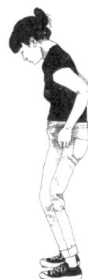

Step 11 - Continue using closing, lengthening and twisting in to draw qi all the way up your spine to the crown of your head.

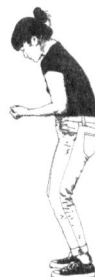

Fifth-Phase Open

Step 12 - As you release the stored energies from the closing action, twisting inward, the spinal bow and the release of air in the lungs produces the out-breath, allow qi to release and start dripping down from your crown along the centerline of your body.

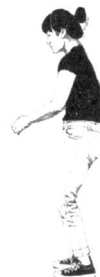

Step 13 - Continue to let go and, with a yin intent, open and lengthen downward in order to allow qi to sink of its own accord to your perineum.

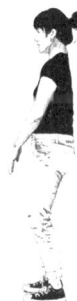

NEUTRAL

Sixth-Phase Release

Step 14 - Deepen the sense of letting go, sink into the arches of your feet and allow the natural capillary action generated by all your joints and tissues releasing to neutral to draw your qi toward and into your lower tantien, where the energies of Heaven and Earth merge.

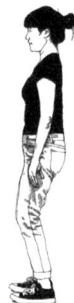

THE SLOW ROAD LEADS TO EMBODIMENT

Even though there are obvious threads of neigong that are more prominent at specific times during the practice, all of Heaven and Earth's neigong techniques should be present, balanced and simultaneously integrated into the form. That being said, it is impossible for any individual to expect that they can learn all of the neigong threads at the same time. The Taoist Principle of Separate and Combine misleadingly appears to be the longer route. However, if you try to throw too many neigong components into the mix too early on, it does not yield embodiment of any one thread. Your mind simply juggles through components and overall practice results are greatly diminished.

Generally it could take as much as a year or two of daily practice to cycle through all the material presented in this book, but that certainly does not mean you have concluded your Heaven and Earth training. The first pass allows you to become familiar with the material at play and, from there, decide if you wish to dedicate considerably more time to fully embodying it. If so, over the years and decades of your life you will cycle through the material and, with each rotation, increase your vitality and wellbeing, rejuvenating your body, mind and qi. Your life is not a singular event, but rather an ever-evolving process as you age. This is one reason why deep, Taoist neigong practice is regarded as a life path. *Tao* translates as "the path" or "the way"—the journey, not the destination.

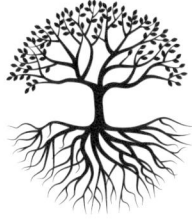

CHAPTER 23:

I CHU DZUO VERSUS *CHI CHU DZUO*

I chu dzuo, or indirect movement of qi, and *chi chu dzuo*, or direct movement of qi, are the two primary methods for developing energy in qigong. The first method involves moving qi via some form of influence, such as body motion, visualization or imagination. The second method involves directly moving qi with the mind while contacting, physically feeling and guiding the internal movement within the body. Nobody can jump entirely into directly moving qi without first developing the power of their intent and subsequently fusing that intent with their qi.

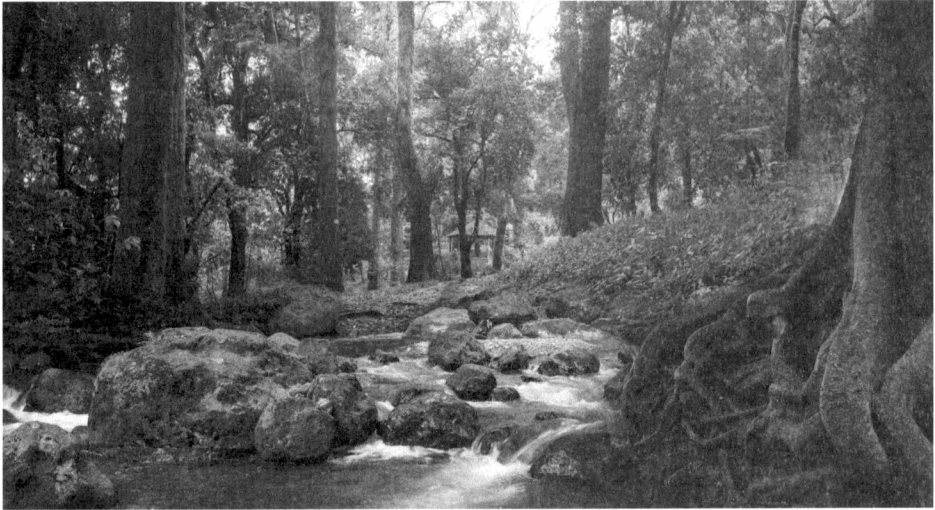

© IROCHKA/ADOBESTOCK

I CHU DZUO: INDIRECTLY MOVING QI

Most qi methods developed in China, especially the popular ones, are indirect and start with visualizations. While visualizing qi movement during qigong practice is an acceptable stepping stone to feeling the body and serves to wake up the nerves so you can feel, the Taoist Water tradition's primary method focuses on *feeling* rather than visualizing.

With this in mind, indirectly moving qi has two primary stages:

- Visualizing, imagining or some use of the mental capacities to jump-start the system.
- Consciously moving the flesh and/or the fluids of the body to influence qi movement.

The latter method is preferred in the Water tradition. At the most fundamental level, the purpose of practice is to become present to the here and now, so you can be aware of what is actually happening and, equally, that which is not. Any time spent in visual paradise, however fantastic, may not develop your ability to accept or change the set of circumstances in which you actually find yourself.

That said, we live in a hyper-visual era, where the majority of people are considered visual learners. This is in stark contrast to when Heaven and Earth was developed. So if initially visualizing helps you step into the world of feeling, it can be used in the very early stages of training.

Eventually though, your mind must attach to your body and fuse with your qi in order for you to get into the qigong driver's seat and unlock deeper qi techniques and health benefits. Up to this point, all of the material presented is based upon the fact that if you breathe, bend and stretch, twist, lengthen and wrap the various soft tissues and open and close the joints of your body, you will move and develop your qi to some extent. As you do so on a sustained basis, your energy grows and so too does your ability to feel more deeply, which can open the door to directly perceiving your qi. All of the practices in this text are within the realms of i chu dzuo, indirectly sensing, moving and cultivating your qi. When developed over long periods, the results can be profound.

MAKING CONTACT WITH THE ETHERIC FIELD

One important method of i chu dzuo not covered so far is making contact between the palms of your hands and your etheric field. This is one of the reasons for keeping your hands one to two fist(s) width away from your body during certain parts of the exercise. When you do so, your hands run along the edge of your etheric sheath and you can generate an indirect connection between the qi of your palms/hands and the qi of your torso, head and thighs.

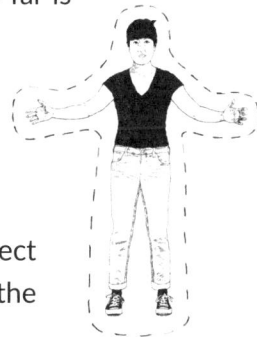

As your hands come over your head in the second-phase close and down the front of your body in the third-phase open, their movement causes the qi on the surface of your body to also move. Depending on the skill of the practitioner, the contact and movement of qi could also be deeper. Once a practitioner has tuned into this aspect of the Heaven and

Earth form, the movement of their hands can make a link throughout the rest of their form, and influence qi flows in the entirety of the macrocosmic and microcosmic orbits.

When this level of control is integrated with all other active threads of nei-gong in Heaven and Earth, an incredibly strong flow of qi begins to build in the body. Do not be in a rush to pass up this fundamental aspect of training for some perceived benefit from learning the more advanced chi chu dzuo practices. I chu dzuo training is precisely what enables a practitioner to enter into and experience chi chu dzuo.

CHI CHU DZUO: DIRECTLY MOVING QI

Neigong practices, as with classic Hatha yoga and Tibetan Buddhism, follow the same hierarchical training protocols for bridging i chu dzuo and chi chu dzuo methods of moving qi. For example, Tibetan Buddhists make use of images and deities to evoke visualizations, which are representative of the ways in which qi moves inside the practitioner. The image is just a mental construct that has the practical effect of beginning to train the mind and nervous system to stay aware of specific locations in their body. So when the practitioner conjures up the mental picture and focuses the motion of their mind, they can activate their nerves throughout their body. Eventually they can simultaneously move qi inside their body in tandem with the visual-ization—at least that is the goal. In Taoist neigong, visualizations are used to wake up the nerves in order to feel the body, which is a preparatory stage; however, most Westerners do not penetrate beyond this level.

The instructions in this text, if you practice them well, provide the founda-tion for moving into deeper studies, specifically the second phase of Taoist arts training to do with directly moving qi through your body (chi chu dzuo). So even though the techniques presented herein are all in the realm of indi-rectly moving qi (i chu dzuo)—since it is actually your intent moving through your body and not necessarily qi itself—you are forging the connections that make it possible for you to directly connect to and move your qi in later stages of practice. That is to say, Heaven and Earth serves as an i chu dzuo method through which you can progressively work through and open up all the energy lines of your body. Then, via consistent Taoist neigong training supported by transmissions from a genuine master, the barrier can be breached where you not only move your flesh, but directly merge with and move your qi through all the various channels of your body.

THE INTENT MOVES QI, QI MOVES THE BODY

One of the disadvantages of too much mental processing, that is visualizing or mind mapping the qi flows of the body, is the mind's movement of qi does not necessarily fuse with the physical body. When the intent moves qi, the aim is to merge that qi with the body and, thereby, move the body via the mobilized qi. When your body is open, free from tension, internally flexible and alive from i chu dzuo-powered neigong, you will have set the ideal conditions for your mind to meld with your qi—chi chu dzuo, where the mind and qi become one.

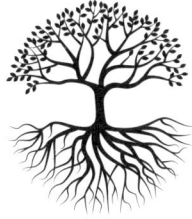

CHAPTER 24:

CLOSING THE PRACTICE SESSION AND BANKING QI

At the end of any internal arts practice session, the closing procedure culminates in banking the qi you have generated to maximize potential benefits. You must bank your qi in order to make use of it later.

CLOSING PROCEDURE FOR HEAVEN AND EARTH QIGONG

1. At the end of the fifth-phase open, slowly begin to *let go of:*

    (a) All the effort you put into stretching, twisting, opening, lengthening and wrapping

    (b) Your soft tissues and nerves

    (c) Your mind and your qi.

(a) Step 13: Open   *(b) Step 14: Release to neutral*

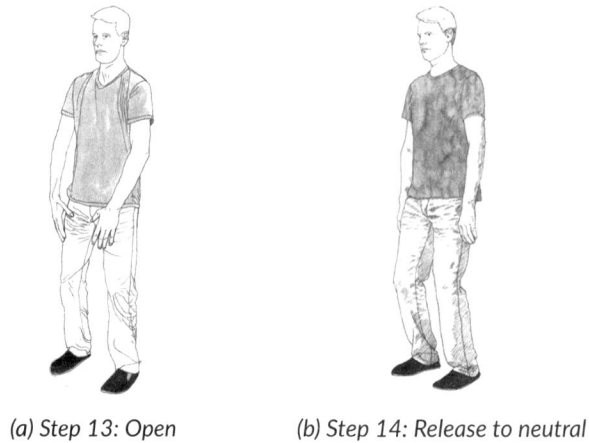

Figure 24-1:
Closing Procedure

2. Drop your mind into the area where your lower tantien is located, just below your naval in the middle of your body, and allow your qi to move from every part of your body and gather around your lower tantien. Continue to rest your mind in your lower tantien and gently condense your qi—without the use of tension—into a ball of qi no bigger than a golf ball. A little smaller is better, if possible for you.

3. Once all the qi that you can influence has gathered around your lower tantien, use the very outer edges of the ball of qi to form an energetic containment field or barrier for the rest of your qi.

4. Relax your body and mind yet deeper to allow the qi inside the ball to become smooth and quiet.

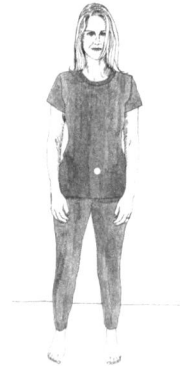

5. When your qi has become quiet and still, drop your mind yet deeper into your lower tantien at the center of the ball of qi.

6. Gently open your lower tantien and begin to absorb the qi without igniting any sense of force, strain or excess effort. Just allow your qi to naturally sink into your lower tantien.

7. Once you have absorbed as much qi as you can, close your lower tantien.

8. Release the containment field and allow whatever qi is left in the ball to spread throughout the entirety of your body and out to your five extremities—head, fingertips and tips of your toes.

The qi you bank is for future use, whenever your system needs it. For instance, if you become ill or when you have a lot of work to do. The qi you spread around your system is for the here and now—the rest of your day.

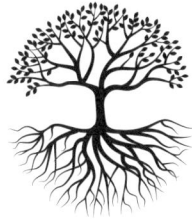

AFTERWORD

In this text you were introduced to many different techniques individually and, where relevant, in combination with others in order to practice the Marriage of Heaven and Earth Qigong and gain potential benefits from doing so. Eventually all of the neigong shown here—*plus a whole lot more*—seamlessly integrate into one fluid continuum (see Appendix A for the 16 neigong).

QI IS NOT BOUND TO SPACE AND TIME

Some neigong components influence qi in different ways to others, which often creates a bit of conflict for the Western mind. One example is opening-and-closing versus lengthening techniques. If you followed the methods presented in the pulsing section, you moved qi out of your spine to your fingers and toes on the open, and toward and into your spine on the close. This generates a center-to-periphery, periphery-to-center qi flow. Then, when lengthening, you learned to direct your qi up and down your body, from bottom to top and top to bottom. These two qi flows are the two primary methods of moving qi in the human body and both must be embodied, first independently of each other and then in combination with one another. If you cannot achieve each flow separately, they cannot become integrated as one. Once combined they are both active at the same time yet they do not interfere with each other. There is not any conflict as qi is non-physical and therefore does not require physical space in which to move. Qi can move in both directions in the same channels at the same moment in time without diminishing either. In fact, each qi flow completes and supercharges the flow of the other.

INTENT VERSUS AWARENESS

In the beginning phases of training, you have the intent to initiate one stream or flow of qi and to maintain that flow. As you progress in your training—both in a single practice session and over time as you cycle through the various aspects of practice—eventually the seemingly opposite or different flows will come alive together. At this stage, your intent passes the baton to your awareness and your awareness observes that which is in the flow. The intent can only focus on a few specifics at any one point in time, whereas the most profound aspects of awareness, called the Heart-Mind by Taoists, has the potential to observe the whole gamut of neigong—simultaneously. So your awareness observes and when something is lacking or missing, your intent takes over to fix the problem. When the specific technique or component is up and running, your awareness regains the reins and observes the whole once again. This interplay between your intent and your awareness is how you manage and practice a growing load of neigong components. In this way, you are aiming toward the sixteenth thread, that is, integrating the entire neigong system in body, mind and qi, which can only be achieved by fully developing your Heart-Mind. This is the basis of all Taoist qi practices.

SYSTEMATIC AND PROGRESSIVE TRAINING

At the beginning levels, Heaven and Earth Qigong is practiced to engage and upgrade your body's physical, internal and energetic systems; at more advanced levels, it is practiced to develop deeper spiritual balance and integration in your body, mind and qi, which is of great importance within Taoism.

In the Water tradition, qigong training is systematic and progressive, always beginning with the body:

1. First you open and balance your body—arms, legs and torso. For example, you would not want most of your effort to be in the upper body when you move with little happening in the lower body, or too much or too little in the limbs or spine. The five bows of your body (arms, legs and torso) want to be in balance with one another.

2. Next you open and balance all the layers of soft tissue techniques. Too much bending and stretching or twisting, for example, will diminish other techniques, such as wrapping or lengthening the yang and yin surfaces of the body.

3. You also balance fluid pressures in all the joints, cavities (not covered in this text) and soft tissues of the body.

4. The same balancing act is applied to all the layers of qi, from the etheric field to the left, right and central channels of energy (also beyond the scope of this text).

5. Finally you balance all active layers of neigong within your body and integrate them into one seamless whole.

WEAVING NEIGONG IN HEAVEN AND EARTH QIGONG

In Heaven and Earth Qigong, each layer of whichever neigong thread you focus on must be engaged, activated and honed before adding the next. You will need a certain degree of embodiment at each layer before progressing, or you will simply revert to juggling layers rather than integrating them. There is a reason the joker or court jester is often depicted juggling!

In each Heaven and Earth practice session, you repeat each individual layer several or more times in order to bring alive any given aspect of neigong and stabilize it within the other layers you have already assimilated. Then, when focusing on the next layer, you once again have the possibility of integrating that thread in your form. If any layer is intermittent or just outside of your ability to stabilize it, spend time at that stage, adhere to the methods for embodying tai chi and qigong principles, and cultivate your practice without allowing yourself to become too enticed by the next carrot. For example, according to the Taoist Principle of Separate and Combine, if you want to develop your skill with pulsing, you must start with sitting and standing while focusing on and engaging the pulse with as few distractions as possible. In time and with practice, you eventually want to transfer your ability to open and close to all Taoist arts, not just Heaven and Earth, but other qigong sets, tai chi, hsing-i, bagua, qigong tui na, Taoist yoga and Taoist meditation.

ACHIEVING THE INTEGRATION YOU DESIRE

The most common issue is that students move through the material much too quickly and end up building a glass ceiling. Unless you are a prodigy, you must be patient and allow your path to unfold with time and sustained effort. Visualizations alone are not enough. The tried-and-true method of focusing on and feeling individual threads, then slowly weaving them in over time allows practitioners to achieve integration and master higher-level neigong training.

Any imbalance within your system diminishes the overall effect and prevents full integration from occurring. True integration requires balance across the board, as well as smooth operation of the body, mind and qi within your comfortable range and ability. This protocol will allow you to achieve the balance and integration you desire.

Practice well,
Master Bruce Frantzis
and Paul Cavel

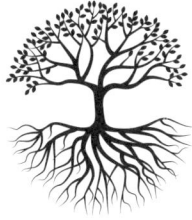

APPENDIX A:

THE 16 NEIGONG

The 16 components that make up the Taoist neigong system are:

1. Breathing methods, from simple to complex, taking many years to fully engage.

2. Developing the ability to feel, move, transform and transmute internal energies along the descending, ascending and connecting energy channels of the body.

3. Adhering to and maintaining ever-more precise body alignments—both externally and internally—to prevent the flow of energy from being blocked or dissipated; practicing these principles yields exceptional and refined biomechanical alignments, as well as better qi flow within the internal organs and the brain.

4. Dissolving blockages in the physical, energetic, emotional and mental bodies to strengthen and develop the body, energy and mind.

5. Moving energy through the main and secondary meridian channels of the body, including all the energy gates.

6. Bending and stretching the body's soft tissues (including the muscles, tendons, ligaments and fascia) from the inside out and the outside in, as well as along the direction of the yin and yang acupuncture meridian lines.

7. Opening and closing all parts of the physical body (joints, muscles, soft tissues, internal organs, glands, blood vessels, cerebrospinal system and brain), as well as all aspects of the body's subtle energy anatomy.

8. Manipulating the energy of the external aura outside the body.

9. Making circles and spirals of energy inside the body, controlling the spiraling energy currents of the body, and moving energy to any part of the body at will, especially to the glands, brain and internal organs.

10. Absorbing energy into and projecting energy away from any part of the body.

11. Controlling all the energies of the spine.

12. Gaining control of the left and right energy channels of the body.

13. Gaining control of the central energy channel of the body.

14. Learning to develop the capabilities and all the uses of the body's lower tantien.

15. Learning to develop the capabilities and all the uses of the body's upper and middle tantiens.

16. Connecting every part of the physical and other energetic bodies into one unified energy.

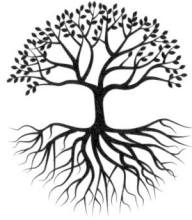

APPENDIX B:

TAOISM—A LIVING TRADITION

Many traditions that are based on ancient philosophies and religions have vibrantly continued into modern times. Because they manifest in our lives today, they are called living traditions. These include Christianity, Islam, Judaism, Buddhism, Yoga and Taoism. The latter three actively involve physical exercises and energy practices.

Taoism is the least known of the living traditions. Although its main literary works—the *I Ching*, the writings of Chuang Tzu and the *Tao Te Ching* by Lao Tzu—are well known and available in many translations, the practical methods and techniques of implementing Taoist philosophy in daily life are hardly documented in the West. One branch of living Taoist philosophy is about developing and using one's personal qi or life-force energy to strengthen, heal and benefit oneself and others.

This branch encompasses two broad traditions: Water and Fire. The Water tradition, based on the philosophies of Lao Tzu, emphasizes effort without force, relaxation and letting go, as a flow of water slowly erodes rock.

The Taoist lineages that Bruce Frantzis holds are in both the Fire and Water traditions, the latter of which has received little exposure in the West. Part of his lineage empowers and directs him to bring practices based on the Water tradition to Westerners.

While Master Frantzis studied with his main teacher, Grandmaster Liu Hung Chieh, texts were presented as: "This is what they say; this is what they mean; this is how to do them." Frantzis offers an unprecedented bridge to this pragmatic approach to spirituality; in fact, the authors are not aware of any other English or European language source for this style of teaching. It means that spirituality is not just an aspiration for which people strive in the dark—"in a mirror, darkly,"—to quote St. Paul, but it can become a genuine, accomplishable reality.

THE ENERGY ARTS SYSTEM

CORE PRACTICES

The Energy Arts® System includes six primary qigong courses that, together with the Taoist Longevity Breathing® program, progressively and safely incorporate all the aspects of neigong—the original qi cultivation (qigong) system in China that originated from the Taoists. Although the qigong techniques are very old, Master Frantzis' system of teaching them is unique. It is specifically tailored to Westerners and the needs of modern life.

The core practices consist of:

- Taoist Longevity Breathing
- Dragon and Tiger Medical Qigong
- Opening the Energy Gates of Your Body™ Qigong
- The Marriage of Heaven and Earth™ Qigong
- Bend the Bow Spinal™ Qigong
- Spiraling Energy Body™ Qigong
- Gods Playing in the Clouds™ Qigong

The core qigong programs were deliberately chosen because they are among the oldest, most effective and most treasured of Taoist energy practices. They are ideal for progressively incorporating the major components of neigong in a manner that is comprehensible and understandable to Westerners. They provide students with the foundation necessary for clearly and systematically learning and advancing their practice in Taoist qi arts.

SUPPORTING PROGRAMS

The Energy Arts® System also includes the following supporting programs:

- Taoist Longevity Yoga
- Qigong Tui Na Energy Healing
- Shengong
- Taoist Meditation
- Tai Chi and Bagua as Health and Meditation Arts
- Tai Chi, Bagua and Hsing-i as Internal Martial Arts

BIBLIOGRAPHY

Cavel, Paul, *The Tai Chi Space: How to Move in Tai Chi and Qi Gong*. Aeon Books, 2017.

Chuang Tzu, *The Book of Chuang Tzu*, translated by Martin Palmer. Penguin Books, 1996, 2006.

Chuang Tzu, *The Way of Chuang Tzu*, translated by Thomas Merton. Shambhala Publications, 2004.

Frantzis, Bruce, *Dragon and Tiger Medical Qigong: Health and Energy in Seven Simple Movements*. North Atlantic Books, 2008, 2010.

Frantzis, Bruce, *Opening the Energy Gates of Your Body: Chi Gung for Lifelong Health*. North Atlantic Books, 1996, 2006.

Frantzis, Bruce, *Relaxing into Your Being: Breathing, Chi and Dissolving the Ego*. North Atlantic Books, 1998, 2001.

Frantzis, Bruce, *The Great Stillness: Body Awareness, Moving Meditation and Sexual Chi Gung*. North Atlantic Books, 1999, 2001.

Jarmey, Chris, *The Concise Book of Muscles*. Lotus Publishing and North Atlantic Books, 2003.

Lao Tzu (also Laozi), *Tao Te Ching (also Daodejing)*, various English translations available.

Musashi, Miyamoto, *A Book of Five Rings*, translated by Victor Harris. The Overlook Press, 1974.

Myers, Thomas W., *Anatomy Trains: Myofascial Meridians for Manual and Movement Therapies*. Churchill Livingstone, 2001.

Netter, Frank H., *Atlas of Human Anatomy: Fourth Edition*. Saunders, 2006.

Olson, Stuart Alve, *Steal My Art: The Life and Times of T'ai Chi Master T.T. Liang*. North Atlantic Books, 2002.

Pankrnier, David W., *Astrology and Cosmology in Early China: Confirming Earth to Heaven*. University Printing House, 2013.

Scranton, Laird, *China's Cosmological Prehistory*. Inner Traditions, 2014.

The Original I Ching Oracle, translated by Rudolf Ritsema and Shantena Augusto Sabbadini. Watkins Publishing, 2005.

Tucker, Louise, *An Introduction to Anatomy and Physiology*. EMS Publishing, 2000.

Walker, Brad, *The Anatomy of Stretching: Your Illustrated Guide to Flexibility and Injury Rehabilitation*. Lotus Publishing and North Atlantic Books, 2007.

Wayne, Peter M., *The Harvard Medical School Guide to Tai Chi: 12 Weeks to a Healthy Body, Strong Heart and Sharp Mind*. Shambhala Boulder, 2013.

OTHER BOOKS AND MULTI MEDIA COURSES
BY MASTER BRUCE FRANTZIS

Tai Chi Mastery Program Online Course

Bagua Mastery Program Online Course

Hsing-i Mastery Program Online Course

Opening the Energy Gates of Your Body: Qigong for Lifelong Health

Dragon and Tiger Medical Qigong:
Health and Energy in Seven Simple Movements

Relaxing into Your Being (Taoist Meditation, Vol. 1)

The Great Stillness (Taoist Meditation, Vol. 2)

Tao of Letting Go: Meditation for Modern Living

Chi Revolution: Harness the Healing Power of Your Life Force

Taoist Sexual Meditation

The Power of Internal Martial Arts and Chi:
Combat and Energy Secrets of Bagua, Tai Chi and Hsing-I

Bagua and Tai Chi:
Exploring the Potential of Chi, Martial Arts, Meditation and the I Ching

BY PAUL CAVEL

The Five Keys to Taoist Energy Arts Online Course

The Tai Chi Space: How to Move in Tai Chi and Qi Gong

CONTACT INFORMATION

MASTER BRUCE FRANTZIS

Teaching Center: The Tao Space
1602 9th Avenue
Longmont, CO 80501
USA

Phone: (415) 454-5243
Email: support@energyarts.com

www.EnergyArts.com

PAUL CAVEL

P.O. Box 179
Launceston
Cornwall
PL15 0BW
United Kingdom

Phone: +44 (0)7411 418 018
Email: qi@paulcavel.com

www.PaulCavel.com